3 9087 02374908 0

DATE DUE

ANTIBODIES

VOLUME 1: PRODUCTION AND PURIFICATION

ANTIBODIES
VOLUME 1: PRODUCTION AND PURIFICATION

Edited by

G. Subramanian
Littlebourne, Kent, United Kingdom

Kluwer Academic / Plenum Publishers
New York, Boston, Dordrecht, London, Moscow

Library of Congress Cataloging-in-Publication Data

Antibodies / edited by G. Subramanian.
   p. ; cm.
   Includes bibliographical references and index.
   Contents: v. 1. Production and purification -- v. 2. Novel technologies and therapeutic use.
   ISBN 0-306-48245-2 (v. 1) -- ISBN 0-306-48315-7 (v. 2) -- ISBN 0-306-48334-3 (divisible set)
   1. Monoclonal antibodies--Synthesis. 2. Monoclonal antibodies--Therapeutic use. 3. Monoclonal antibodies--Biotechnology. I. Subramanian, G., 1935-
   [DNLM: 1. Antibodies, Monoclonal--isolation & purification. 2. Antibodies, Monoclonal--therapeutic use. 3. Biotechnology--methods. 4. Chromatography--methods. QW 575.5.A6 A6283 2004]
   TP248.65.M65A55 2004
   615'.37--dc22

2003069160

ISBN: 0-306-48245-2 (volume 1)
ISBN: 0-306-48315-7 (volume 2)
ISBN: 0-306-48334-3 (divisible set)

©2004 Kluwer Academic / Plenum Publishers, New York
233 Spring Street, New York, N.Y. 10013

http://www.wkap.nl/

10 9 8 7 6 5 4 3 2 1

A C.I.P. record for this book is available from the Library of Congress

All rights reserved

No part of this book may be reproduced, stored in a retrieval system, or transmitted in any form or by any means, electronic, mechanical, photocopying, microfilming, recording, or otherwise, without written permission from the Publisher, with the exception of any material supplied specifically for the purpose of being entered and executed on a computer system, for exclusive use by the purchaser of the work..

Permissions for books published in Europe: *permissions@wkap.nl*
Permissions for books published in the United States of America: *permissions@wkap.com*

Printed in the United States of America

Preface

In the last century since the technology was developed for producing monoclonal antibodies, numerous methods have been applied to their purification. Prominent examples include ion exchange chromatography, hydrophobic interaction chromatography, protein A affinity chromatography, hydroxyapatite chromatography and others. Even among this small subset, virtually none of the methods have been exploited to their full potential and some have been overlooked almost entirely, all to the detriment of the industry. Also, all methods have weaknesses, some very serious and many critical limitations have been overlooked, likewise to the detriment of the industry. Meanwhile product applications have become steadily more sophisticated and demanding, regulatory agencies have become more knowledgeable and assertive and the place of market development continues to exert ever greater pressure for rapid time to market.

If the antibody industry is to achieve its full potential in the next decade, the individual technical potentials must be exploited, the limitations must be addressed, and lessons learned must be applied both to current purification methods and to the new technologies that continue to emerge.

This book presents an overview of the current advances applied in the manufacture of monoclonal antibody.

I am indebted to the international group of contributors who have come forward to share their practical knowledge and experience. Each chapter represents an overview of its chosen topics. Chapter one presents the concepts in development of manufacturing strategies for monoclonal antibodies. Importance of antibody fragments and the methods of production have been presented in chapter two. Application of chromatography method development in production and purification is discussed in the subsequent three chapters. Chapter six discusses the quality control aspect of antibodies.

The effect of expression on the antibody properties is presented in chapter seven. Removal of virus and its safety in antibody production is discussed in chapter eight. The next two chapters cover the aspects of contract manufacturing and the pharmacokinetics and pharmacodynamic consideration for monoclonal antibodies. The regulatory aspect in the manufacture of therapeutic antibody is documented in the last chapter.

My thanks to all the contributors for their enthusiasm and patience during the production of the book.

It is to be hoped that this book will be of great value to all of those who are actively working in the field of antibodies and that it will stimulate further progress and advancement in this field to meet the ever increasing demands in the product. I should be most grateful for any suggestion, which could serve to improve future editions of the book.

My deep appreciation to Jo Lawrence of Kluwer Academic/Plenum publishers for her continuous help throughout this project.

G. Subramanian

Contributors

Dominique Bourel
Department of Research and Development
LFB Biotechnologies
3, Avenue des Tropiques
B.P.305, Les Ulis
F- 91958 Courtaboeuf cedex
France

Malcolm K. Brattle
Q–One Biotech Ltd.
Todd Campus
West of Scotland Science Park
Glasgow, G20 0XA
UK

John Bray
Q–One Biotech Ltd.
Todd Campus
West of Scotland Science Park
Glasgow, G20 0XA
UK

Christophe de Romeuf
Department of Research and Development
LFB Biotechnologies
3, Avenue des Tropique
B.P 305, Les Ulis
F- 91958 Courtaboeuf cedex
France

Brendan Fish
Downstream Processing Department
Cambridge Antibody Technology
Milstein Building
Granta Park
Cambridge, CB1 6GH
UK

Matthias Frech
Merck KgaA
Life Science Products
Frankfurter Strasse 250
64293 Darmstadt
Germany

Ruth Freitag
Chair for Bioprocess Technology
University of Bayreuth
D-95440 Bayreuth
Germany

Christine Gaucher
Department of Research and Development
LFB Biotechnologies
3, Avenue des Tropiques
B.P.305 Les Ulis
F-91958 Courtaboeuf cedex
France

Arnaud Glacet
Department of Research and Development
LFB Biotechnologies
3, Avenue des Tropiques
B.P. 305 Les Ulis
F- 91958 Courtaboeuf cedex
France

David J. Glover
GlaxoSmithKline
South Eden Park Road
Beckenham
Kent, BR3 3BS
UK

Contributors

David B. Haughey
Prevalere Life Sciences Inc.
1 Halsey Road
Whitesboro
N.Y.13492
USA

Andreas Hermann
Cardion AG
Erkrath
Germany

David P. Humphreys
Celltech R&D Ltd
208 Bath Road
Slough
Berkshire, SL1 3WE
UK

Lothar R. Jacob
Merck KgaA
Life Science Products
Frankfurter Strasse 250
64293 Darmstadt
Germany

Paula M. Jardieu
Prevalere Life Sciences Inc.
1 Halsey Road
Whitesboro
N.Y.13492
USA

Sylvie Jorieux
Department of Research and Development
LFB Biotechnologies
3 Avenue des Tropiques
B.P.305 Les Ulis
F-91958 Courtaboeuf cedex
France

Mark Jostameling
Newlab Bioquality AG
Max-Planck-Strasse 15A

D-40699 Erkrath
Germany

Glenwyn Kemp
Millipore (UK) Ltd
No 1. Industrial Estate
Medomsley Road
Consett
County Durham
DH8 6SZ
UK

Philippe Klein
Department of Research and Development
LFB Biotechnologies
3, Avenue des Tropiques
B.P.305 Les Ulis
F- 91958 Courtaboeuf cedex
France

Kerstin Muller
Newlab Bioquality AG
Max-Planck-Strasse 15A
D-40699 Erkrath
Germany

Paul O'Neil
Euroflow (UK) Ltd.
8 Elton Avenue
Stratham
NH 03885
USA

Martin Pitshke
Evotec Technologies GmbH
Erkrath
Germany

Andreas Richter
Newlab Bioquality AG
Max-Planck-Strasse 15A
D-40699 Erkrath
Germany

Lincoln Tsang
Of Counsel
Arnold & Porter
Tower 42
25 Old Broad Street
London, EC2N 1HQ
UK

Leo A. van Der Pol
DSM Biologics Company BV
Zuiderweg 72/2
P.O.Box 454
9700 AL Groningen
The Netherlands

Caroline Vandevyver
Laboratory of Chemical Biotechnology
Faculty of Basic Science
Swiss Federal Institute of Technology
Lausanne
Switzerland

Douwe F. Westra
DSM Biologics Company BV
Zuiderweg 72/2
P.O.Box 454
9700 AL Groningen
The Netherlands

Contents

1. Concepts in Development of Manufacturing Strategies for
   Monoclonal Antibodies   1
   Brendan Fish

2. Antibody Fragments: Production, Purification and Formatting
   for Therapeutic Applications   25
   David J. Glover and David P. Humphreys

3. Large Scale Production of Therapeutic Antibodies: Considerations
   for Optimizing Product Capture and Purification   75
   Glen Kemp and Paul O'Neil

4. Scale-Up of Antibody Purification. From Laboratory
   Scale to Production   101
   Lothar R. Jacob and Matthias Frech

5. Purification of Antibody by Chromatographic Methods   133
   Caroline Vandevyver and Ruth Freitag

6. Quality Control of Antibodies for Human Use   169
   *Andreas Richter, Mark Jostameling, Kerstin Müller,
   Andreas Herrmann and Martin Pitschke*

7. Expression of Human Anti Rh(D) Monoclonal Antibodies into
   Different Cell lines: Influence on their Functional Properties   189
   *Christophe de Romeuf; Christine Gaucher; Arnaud Glacet;
   Silvie Jorieux; Philippe Klein and Dominique Bourel*

8. Monoclonal Antibody Production: Minimising Virus Safety Issues 199
   John Bray and Malcolm K. Brattle

9. Contract Manufacturing of Biopharmaceutical Grade Antibodies 227
   Leo A. Van Der Pol and Douwe F. Westra

10. The Pharmacokinetics and Pharmacodynamics of Monoclonal Antibodies 249
    David B. Haughey and Paula M. Jardieu

11. Regulatory and Legal Requirements for the Manufacture of Antibodies 275
    Lincoln Tsang

Index 289

Chapter 1

CONCEPTS IN DEVELOPMENT OF MANUFACTURING STRATEGIES FOR MONOCLONAL ANTIBODIES

Brendan Fish
Downstream Processing Department, Cambridge Antibody Technology, Milstein Building, Granta Park, Cambridge CB1 6GH, UK

1. INTRODUCTION

In the mid 1970's researchers at the Laboratory for Molecular Biology in Cambridge, U.K., successfully fused a myeloma cancer cell with an immune cell creating an immortal antibody producing cell, a hybridoma (Kohler and Milstein, 1975). Since the first mouse monoclonal antibodies were produced, the idea of using them as therapeutics or "magic bullets" has been viewed as major exploitation of this technology. This is, in part, due to the fact that they are both natural in action, mimicking a natural process in the body, and because they lack the inherent toxicity often associated with "unnatural" small molecule chemical drugs – making them ideal therapeutic candidates. Additionally the problems associated with the early use of murine monoclonal antibodies as therapeutic agents (they cause the development of human anti-mouse antibodies as they are recognised as being foreign) have largely been overcome. Developments over the past decade include the production of chimaeric, complementary-determining region grafted ("humanised") monoclonal antibodies or fully human monoclonal antibodies (Adair and Bright, 1995 and Winter et al, 1994, Fig 1.1) all of which are significantly superior to murine antibodies.

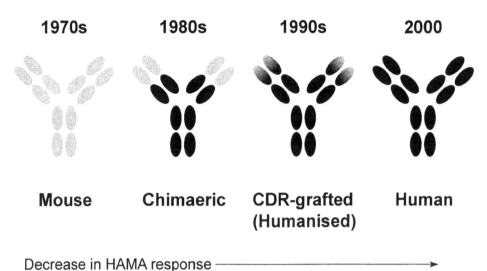

Figure 1.1. The evolution of monoclonal antibody therapeutics

Consequently monoclonal antibodies have become the most rapidly growing class of biopharmaceutical with sales in 2001 of $2.9 billion (Robinson, 2002). The biopharmaceutical industry's large antibody pipelines reveal the allure of antibodies as therapeutics. More than 250 antibody based therapeutics were in development in 2002 (Fig 1.2).

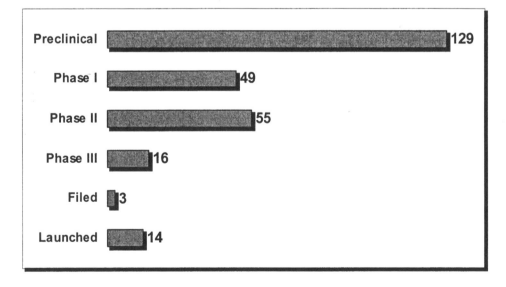

Figure 1.2. Monoclonal antibody therapeutics in development (Source CAT internal database, October 2002)

This staggeringly large number of antibody products in development may imply, to the novice, that the process of moving from concept, through the clinic and to approval is straightforward. In actual fact there is good news and bad news. The good news is that to date 14 antibody products have been launched, which in itself demonstrates that the process is achievable in a profitable manner. The bad news is that this is not necessarily an easy or quick process and that billions of dollars are spent in striving for the ultimate goal of in-market supply. In addition the considerable competition for resources and financing for such programmes means that mistakes are costly and potentially catastrophic to some of the smaller companies undertaking this challenge.

Regardless of this attractiveness, the development of a human or humanised antibody is just the start of the process. Clearly, an effective large scale manufacturing process must be selected and industrialised in order to fulfil the primary reason for developing antibodies in the first place – to supply a patient population with a protein with therapeutic potential and thus contribute to health.

It is the supply question that causes many of the issues with selection of an appropriate process. Monoclonal antibodies are typically administered in large doses and thus require large manufacturing capacity and highly efficient production processes. In recent years this requirement for large manufacturing capacity has raised concerns, as some analysts predict that worldwide manufacturing capacity will have to increase significantly to meet the demands of antibody products in development (Sinclair, 2001). Although, given unlimited resources, production capacity can be built, there is extreme pressure to drive up expression levels and improve production efficiency whilst maintaining ever increasing regulatory requirements for increasing purity and level of characterisation.

Manufacturing antibody therapeutics (like all biopharmaceuticals) is complicated, although the concept is elegantly straightforward. It is "nature" that does all the hard work, the biotechnologist simply exploits cells to do what they do naturally – synthesise proteins.

The task of the biotechnologist is to control the cellular growth and biochemistry to produce the desired protein, to recover that protein as a highly purified entity and to formulate it as a stable medicine in a way that can be safely delivered to the patient. The aim being manufacture at a scale and quality that can meet the demands of in-market supply and the strict regulation placed on such medicines.

The aim of this chapter is to provide a summary of some of the current manufacturing strategies available that take into account the factors mentioned above and to highlight the main concepts in bioprocess design. The process development of monoclonal antibodies is primarily driven by drug safety, efficacy, product quality and the economics of the process itself. The importance of these drivers is reflected in the sections covered below and although this is not intended to be an exhaustive discussion of all the individual methods it should give an overview of the current strategies employed to meet these criteria.

2. UPSTREAM PROCESSING - THE SOURCE MATERIAL

In industrial biotechnology the actual generation of the therapeutic product in a live organism is often referred to as upstream processing. Typically this involves some form of cell culture that utilises many, inexpensive, raw materials (making up the growth media) and few unit operations. Upstream processing however involves large investments in capital equipment and facilities and thus the systems available all need careful consideration when deciding upon a manufacturing strategy. Some of the key attributes of the main methods for antibody production currently applicable to large-scale manufacture are outlined below. For more a more comprehensive review of the available technologies see Andersen (2002).

2.1 Industrial mammalian cell systems

Animal cell culture is the most important source of therapeutic monoclonal antibodies. All of the current marketed monoclonal antibody products are derived from this source. Over the past decade there has been extensive development of mammalian protein expression systems facilitating very high levels of recombinant protein expression. Despite slow growth rates and relatively low productivity (compared to bacterial, yeast or transgenic systems) the ability of animal cells to generate fully processed products and functional proteins is seldom matched by other systems. This ability to correctly process proteins is allied to the functional activity of monoclonal antibodies, as this often depends upon complex and correct posttranslational processing such as disulphide bond formation and glycosylation (Werner et al, 1998). In order maintain these functionally important attributes the expression of glycoproteins in mammalian cells is often required.

Stable recombinant cell lines are produced by inserting the genes coding for the desired antibody heavy and light chains into the genome of an immortalised cell line from primary cell lines such as Chinese hamster ovary (CHO-DHFR, CHO-NEOSPLA, CHO-GS), mouse myelomas (GS-NS0) or baby hamster kidney (BHK) cells. The choice of vector, site of integration into the chromosome, copy number and promoter all influence the final expression levels obtained. Usually the heavy and light chains are combined into a single vector for transfection as this often gives more balanced expression of both chains. Once this has been completed extensive cell line selection is carried out to find stable cell lines that produce high levels of the desired antibody. Techniques to speed up and improve the effectiveness of this cell line development have been examined in order to maximise the return on development effort (Trill et al, 1995 and Bilila and Robinson, 1995).

For antibody production the systems producing the highest titres are either CHO based or NS0 based and to date these have become the methods of choice for large-scale mammalian cell antibody expression. Refinements of vector construction, use of selectable markers and high throughput screening methods have allowed routine construction of recombinant cell lines with specific productivities as high as 50pg/cell/day

The CHO-DHFR system utilises a vector containing various promoters driving the production of the genes for the antibody and dihydrofolate reductase (the selectable marker). The selective agent for this enzyme is methotrexate, which is applied to the cultures in order to amplify the expression. Using this strategy cell lines have been produced that express in excess of 1g/L of monoclonal antibody in 11 days (Werner et al, 1998).

The main alternative to CHO cell production of monoclonal antibodies is the mouse myeloma cell line GS-NS0. In this system the vector plasmid used to integrate the genes into the chromosome contains the glutamine synthetase gene as the selectable marker and methionine sulphoximine (MSX) is used as selection pressure for this GS gene. Fed batch suspension culture in serum free media using GS-NS0 cells have been able to produce 1g/L of monoclonal antibody from stable cell lines without the use of MSX selection (CAT internal data). The lack of requirement for glutamine also gives the advantage that cytotoxic ammonia accumulation is eliminated from these cell cultures.

The absolute requirement of NS0 cells for cholesterol and the difficulties in delivering this fatty acid to the cells in protein free media (bovine serum albumin is often included in cell culture media to facilitate the transport of cholesterol) has led to the development of a cholesterol independent mutant of NS0 (Keen 1995). Such cell lines may have significant advantages for future development of monoclonal antibodies as increasing regulatory pressure for the use of protein free media reduces the acceptability of bovine serum albumin as a culture medium component.

2.2 Microbial Expression Systems

The primary host for microbial expression of recombinant antibodies or antibody fragments is *E. coli.* and reviews of the use of this system for production of recombinant proteins have recently been published (Swartz, 2001 and Baneyxm, 1999). This expression system is well established with many highly characterised expression vectors for introduction of the antibody genes into the host. Additionally the cells are inexpensive, easily grown and quickly produce small amounts of target protein for evaluation. Unfortunately a big disadvantage with this system is the inability of *E. coli* to perform post-translational modifications such as glycosylation that can be a requirement for antibody function. Also, expressed proteins often accumulate in inclusion bodies in the cells as insoluble aggregates. Although active protein can frequently be recovered the process of solubilisation and refolding can be lengthy and time consuming and add to the total cost of goods for the product.

Although it is possible to express both full length antibody heavy and light chains intracellularly in *E. coli* and then recover and refold full IgG, yields are low and the products are not glycosylated (King, 1998). This has led to the almost exclusive use of *E. coli* for the production of antibody fragments. For example scFv, which are made up of the antibody heavy and light chain variable regions held together and stabilised by a flexible linker, can be expressed in *E. coli* either into the periplasmic space or secreted into the media (Kipriyanov et al, 1995 and Sinacola and Robinson 2002). Similarly the expression of Fab fragments in *E. coli* is now well established (Humphreys, 2001).

Expression of such antibody fragments can be highly efficient and relatively inexpensive compared to mammalian cell culture. Thus, if there is no requirement for effector function in the therapeutic antibody and if a simple and cost effective means of increasing the circulatory half life can be developed (e.g. PEGylation of the Fab) this expression system may have appeal as an alternative to mammalian cell expression.

2.3 Other sources of monoclonal antibody

Recombinant monoclonal antibodies are proving to be one of the great successes in the biotechnology industry although paradoxically this success is proving to generate concerns in the industry regarding a looming deficit in biomanufacturing capacity. It has been predicted that twenty new monoclonal antibodies may be commercialised between now and 2012 which would require a 200% increase in worldwide manufacturing capacity (Dove, 2002).

Table 1.1. Summary of the expression systems currently available for monoclonal antibody production

Expression System	Advantages	Disadvantages
Mammalian cell culture	Usually correctly fold and process the proteins (post translational modifications correct). Can secrete protein. Regulatory track record. Suitable for large and complicated proteins.	Slow growth and expensive complex media. May require animal derived proteins in media (ie, BSA). Potential for adventitious agents dictates extensive characterisation (mycoplasma and virus testing). Complex purification and often high cost of goods.
Bacteria	Well understood genetics. Established regulatory safety record. Cheap media and easy and quick to grow. High expression levels. Simple characterisation and few adventitious agents.	No posttranslational modifications. Proteins not secreted and cell disruptions can damage protein. Contain endotoxins. Microheterogenous.
Yeasts	Considered "safe" from a regulatory perspective. Long history of use. Proteins secreted. Fast growth in inexpensive media. Correct folding of proteins and some posttranslational modifications. No endotoxins or viruses.	Can cause problems with inappropriate glycosylation of protein. Can contain immunogenic host cell proteins. Protein folding not always correct.
Insect Cells	Correct protein folding and posttranslational modification. Product secreted at high expression levels. Baculovirus harmless to humans.	Little regulatory experience and history. Slow growth in expensive media. Can contain immunogenic host cell proteins. May be infected with mammalian viruses.
Transgenic animals	Can process complex and large proteins. Correctly folded. High expression levels and easy scale up. Low cost of goods.	Unproven regulatory experience. Variable expression levels. Safety issues with viruses and prions. Continuous production and thus definition of a batch or lot is complex. Questions relating to purification and cGMP compliance on farms. Public perception problems.
Transgenic Plants	Very low cost of goods. Simple and rapid scale up. No safety issues as plant infectious agents cannot harm man.	Limits on glycosylation. Potential problems with proteolysis. Containment issues.

In order to address this predicted "capacity crunch" several new technologies are being developed that utilise transgenic mammals, chickens or plants (for reviews see Sensoli and Bonernmann Chapters in Volume II of this book). Additionally many other researchers have produced antibodies or antibody fragments in yeast and insect cell based systems (reviewed in King 1998 and Daly et al 2001) although potentially having many commercial benefits none of these systems are currently in a position to be routinely adopted for large-scale therapeutic manufacture of antibodies.

A number of different systems have been developed for the production of monoclonal antibodies for large scale therapeutic use – the key attributes of each of these systems is outlined in Table 1.1.

Currently CHO and NS0 mammalian cell fermentation systems predominate the industry, and this trend is will continue unless the "capacity crunch" or economic pressures in biomanufacturing force the industry momentum to overcome the many regulatory, environmental and public perception issues associated with transgenic production.

3. DOWNSTREAM PROCESSING – PRINCIPLES AND PRACTICES

The series of operations that begins with the output from upstream processing, ie, the fermenter output containing the desired antibody, and ends with a stable purified protein product is referred to as downstream processing. Large-scale purification of antibodies as drug products is a highly complex process that often utilises numerous unit operations. These unit operations must be sequenced and integrated using a rational approach that maintains the requirements of purity, yield and throughput. Frequently a pragmatic approach is taken in the design of the process as the only way to determine the behaviour of a particular protein during a particular unit operation is by experiment. However, in taking this pragmatic approach there are some general guidelines that should be applied:

- Remove the most abundant impurities early in the process – this is usually water, although not strictly an impurity the main effort of most early unit operations is to remove water and concentrate the antibody product.
- Run the easiest separations early in the process – when there are large volumes of dilute culture, simple and inexpensive process steps are required to rapidly recover the bulk of the product.
- Run the difficult and/or expensive separations at the end of the process – the product is most valuable at the end of the process and is usually in a partially purified form. Thus, the difficult separations are easier to

Concepts in manufacturing strategies for monoclonal antibodies 9

achieve and cheaper when smaller volumes of purer product are being used as the starting material.
- Select separation steps that exploit differences in the properties of the antibody and contaminating impurities – affinity methods are particularly valuable for antibodies due to their extremely high specificity.
- Order the unit operations in an orthogonal manner to exploit different separation mechanisms – typically a monoclonal antibody purification process would utilise three chromatography steps each with a different mechanism of action ie, affinity, ion-exchange and gel filtration.

At Cambridge Antibody Technology (CAT) we generally follow these rules of thumb in combination with three key principles that we work to in design of large-scale processes for novel monoclonal antibodies. These are design in scalability early in the development process, tailor generic purification schemes and keep it simple.

3.1 Manufacturing processes are different from research processes

The design of a large scale manufacturing process for a biopharmaceutical is not the same as the creation of processes in the laboratory in early stage research and development. Although appearing obvious this is an important concept that is often neglected when taking a process from the bench to clinical production and beyond. Aspects that are clearly different include the quantities required (scale), regulatory requirements, raw materials, equipment, process costs (economics) and formulation and stability of the final product (Table 1.2).

Table 1.2. Differences in process requirement when moving from bench to large scale manufacture

Process attribute	Bench or laboratory scale	Large scale manufacturing process
Scale	Usually small scale – limited amounts required for characterisation	Multi kilogram amounts required
Purity	Purity desirable but not essential – many analytical methods can cope with 10 – 20% impurities (ie, sequencing)	Purity absolute – as far as it can be measured
Regulatory	No regulatory constraints	Significant regulatory compliance required with the process ie, validation, robustness, control
Raw materials	Any available laboratory reagent or method can be used	Raw material quality, costs and availability in sufficient quantity have an impact

Process attribute	Bench or laboratory scale	Large scale manufacturing process
Equipment	Designed for flexibility to perform many different experiments quickly with many variations. Not usually validated and often designed for small volumes or quantities of protein.	Designed for robustness and reproducibility – repeat the same operation reliably over and over again. Validated and deal with large volumes or quantities of protein.
Costs	Very rarely an issue at this stage.	Excessive costs are very undesirable. Cost models often used to identify areas of the process that can be focussed on.
Formulation and stability	Long-term stability not often required. Formulation in exotic buffers acceptable for many analytical methods	Long-term stability of the product is critical; hence final formulation and administration to patient requires careful consideration.

Consideration of these differences in how the target monoclonal antibody is purified leads to a better understanding of how the process should look when being used at scale. It also leads to a series of questions that must be answered when taking processes forward.

Firstly in the design of a manufacturing process you need to ask "How much product do you need?" This clearly depends upon the potency of the antibody, the proposed clinical indication (patient population) and the route of administration. Often this information is not available when designing the manufacturing process as pharmacology, toxicology and early clinical data are required to set dosing regimes. However, it is important to understand the scale required in putting together a strategy. For example, gel filtration chromatography is limited compared to other modes of chromatography in its throughput and capacity. Thus, if the process uses this step, alternatives may have to be found before production at very large scale can be economically justified.

The equipment and methods used at scale clearly have to be very different from those used within a laboratory environment and need to be considered at the outset. An obvious example is the method of clarification. Filtration is often used in laboratories and is scaleable to a degree, but commercialised biotechnology processes create new challenges in filtration technology. Centrifugation may produce efficient economies of scale and may be the unit operation of choice for large-scale processes. It is important therefore, to understand the scale-up and validation issues associated with centrifuges early in the development of a manufacturing process.

Another substantive difference between processes used in therapeutic production and those used in research is the requirement of the manufacturer to follow a framework of regulatory requirements for the production and

quality control of monoclonal antibodies. These legal requirements define the steps in the development process that take an antibody into large scale production. The major activities directly related to the manufacturing process include:
- Establishment of a cell banking system that includes a Master Cell Bank, a Manufacturers Working Cell Bank and a Post Production Cell Bank.
- Creation of the manufacturing process including scale-up, purification and formulation of the monoclonal antibody.
- Generation of a reference batch of antibody.
- Validation of the production process including any in-process controls, process limits studies and chromatography matrix lifetime studies.
- Validation of the ability of the purification process to clear or inactivate process impurities or adventitious agents.
- Demonstration of consistency of the manufacturing process at the intended scale of operation.

Thus, for a process to receive regulatory approval there is an obligation that these activities are covered successfully. Consequently process design must refer to these requirements continually during the development phase so as to ensure that the process being created is capable of meeting them. This is often neglected in the research environment and is a clear distinction between laboratory and manufacturing.

3.2 Purity, potency and identity matter

Monoclonal antibodies destined for the clinic must meet very high standards of proof of identity, purity, potency, safety and stability. Often these standards may be higher that those applied to conventional biologics due to the availability of large quantities of very pure protein. Ultimately therefore, the process chosen will be required to meet these standards at the same time as being economically sound. Increasing the number of purification steps in a process will improve purity at the expense of cost and thus for large scale commercial production quality control testing during the development stages is an important consideration. Extremely sensitive chromatographic, immunological and spectroscopic methods combined with the ever-increasing sophistication and sensitivity in analytical instrumentation has led to the requirement for an in depth analysis of purified products. Quality control testing of biotechnology products has been extensively reviewed (Federici 1994), however, for process development scientists the key considerations are raw materials and in-process testing. Are raw materials available at the desired purity and in the desired quantities? Do the manufacturers of process chemicals, chromatography matrices and filter membranes have regulatory compliant validated production facilities and processes? Are there any environmental issues with disposing of large quantities of buffers containing exotic chemicals? Do analytical methods exist for the potential process impurities derived from any of the raw materials or product contact materials intended at large scale?

Another facet of monoclonal development which is again often neglected until late stage development, is final formulation and drug delivery. Usually monoclonal antibody products are solutions that are delivered by either subcutaneous or intravenous injection. Stability and concentration of the monoclonal, the final formulation buffer and the requirement of excipients all influence the process chosen, as they affect the final unit operations. These final operations are under most scrutiny as they are at the point where the product is closest to the patient and where it is most valuable; that is, alterations to the process at this point are very costly.

3.3 Process economics matter

Downstream processing costs are a very important factor in the development of monoclonal antibody therapeutics as they can account for up to 80% of the overall cost of production (Sadana and Beelaram 1994). The desired level of purity is not the only factor to consider when evaluating the overall cost of manufacture. In terms of downstream processing it is important to consider the final scale of equipment, the batch size, the level of automation and the amount of labour required to run the process, all of which interact in complex ways to determine the final cost of goods. Affinity chromatography is often expensive, centrifugation requires costly equipment and levels of labour have a significant impact on the overall process economics. High process costs may be offset by increased yields or purity although the complex interactions of the whole process, rather than the individual unit operations, need to be looked at and optimised in a holistic way.

The complexity and increasing industry wide focus on economics, in what is a very competitive market, has meant that process cost models have become an important tool for the downstream process developer. Cost modelling of a process assists in development of the manufacturing strategy, allows assessment of commercial feasibility to be made and will also give confidence when evaluating new products as potential therapeutics. At CAT we employ a detailed computer model that encompasses process parameters, equipment, facility and materials costs to build up a model of final cost of goods for any particular process. The key elements of any process cost model and how they are used to calculate the process economics are depicted schematically in Fig 1.3.

Concepts in manufacturing strategies for monoclonal antibodies 13

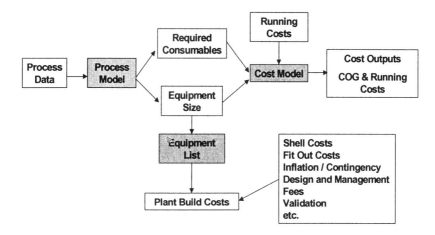

Figure 1.3. Elements employed in a process cost model. Grey boxes indicate key elements for a computational model

All cost models should be designed to be transparent such that assumptions made are easily seen and so that sensitivity analysis is easily undertaken. This is complementary to process development and allows for attention to be focussed on the most expensive areas of the process.

3.4 Generic processes for monoclonal antibodies

The similarities between monoclonal antibodies make the use of a generic purification process the obvious choice when starting development of a process for a novel antibody. A typical large scale purification process is often built around the use of immobilised Protein A as the primary capture and purification step in combination with ion exchange and/or gel filtration (Fig 1.4).

Protein A is a cell wall component from *Staphylococcus aureas* that has four binding sites, two of which are capable of binding with pronounced specificity for the constant domains on a broad range of antibodies. (Huse et al 2002).

Thus, when this molecule is immobilised (covalently bonded) to a solid phase a highly effective stationary phase is produced that, in theory, will only bind to antibody molecules. Fractionation of the antibody target from host cell and other contaminants is achieved by lowering the neutral or mild alkali binding pH to mild acidic conditions (pH < 4 for human IgG). Protein A has become well established as a large scale unit operation in antibody manufacture due to this high specificity, high yields (typically >85% recovery), and high purity (typically >95%) from unmodified culture

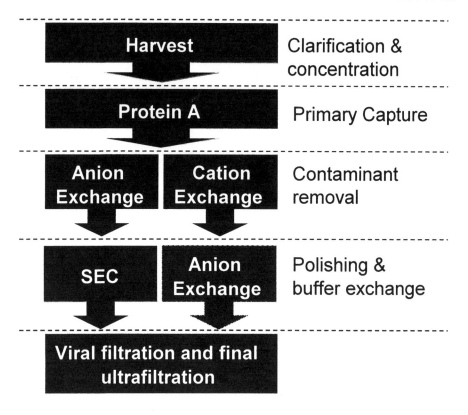

Figure 1.4. Typical generic monoclonal antibody purification processes

supernatants. Additionally there exist a variety of commercially available matrices all with high antibody capacity (typically 15 – 20g IgG /L of matrix).

Disadvantages with this approach include the high cost of this affinity matrix, the potential for Protein A to leach from the matrix and remain with the product and the low resistance of immobilised proteins to traditional sanitisation regimes. However, these disadvantages are often offset by the very high levels of purity obtained which have yet to be achieved by any other method in a single step.

The remaining steps in the process represent conventional purification methods for large scale biopharmaceutical manufacture combined in a rational way usually based on the rules of thumb outlined above. The main purpose of these steps is to clear major process impurities and polish the product to the final purity and formulation desired. Detailed discussion of the theoretical and practical aspects of downstream processing and secondary purification are outside the scope of this assessment of general approaches to monoclonal antibody manufacture but have been extensively reviewed by other authors (Kaul and Mattiasson 1992, Jungbauer 1993, Labrou and Clonis 1994, Gagnon 1996, Huse 2002 and Lydiatt 2002).

4. APPLYING THE CONCEPTS

4.1 Generic in principle, specific in practice

It must be remembered that the rules of thumb and the generic process outlined above are just guidelines and cannot always be followed explicitly, as all proteins are different. This is a good thing, as otherwise it would be impossible to separate them (ie, in order to remove protein contaminants from the target therapeutic we must exploit some biophysical difference in the molecules). However, as well as allowing us to exploit these differences for purification purposes this also means that the purification process will be different for each different biopharmaceutical. This is also the case for monoclonal antibodies, as although, as a class of molecule they are similar in many respects, they are sufficiently different that there is no such thing as a standard monoclonal antibody purification process.

Antibodies derived at CAT from Phage Display libraries can be constructed in very similar ways, resulting in molecules that can potentially be identical in terms of the constant domains and framework regions, differing only in the amino acids that make up the complementarity determining regions of the variable domains on the heavy and light chains. Although these may seem relatively minor changes they not only give the antibodies exquisite specificity they also have a profound effect on the physical and chemical characteristics of the antibody. Monoclonal antibodies vary in their solubility, isoelectric point and resistance to extremes of pH. This can have significant effect when applying them to a generic purification scheme.

Even affinity steps, of which Protein A could be considered to be the most generic for antibodies, need modification on a case-by-case basis. We have demonstrated this during the application of a generic Protein A affinity capture step to the purification of a novel therapeutic human antibody (Bannister and Fish 2001). In this study purification of the antibody on Protein A, following an existing generic process (pH 3.75 elution) resulted in purified material, but with a significantly tailing peak with an approximate volume of 6.9 column volumes (Fig 1.5).

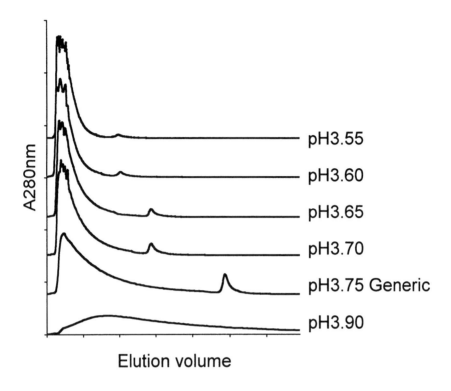

Figure 1.5. Effect of elution pH on antibody eluate peak volume on Protein A Sepharose

Increasing the pH of Protein A elution buffer resulted in an increased volume and an increased loss of IgG to the strip fraction (Fig 1.5). At pH 3.55, and below, precipitation of IgG in the eluate was observed. This was not seen with elution at pH 3.65 and above. Thus, in tailoring this generic step for large scale chromatography multiple factors had to be considered, the recovery of antibody, the volume of elution and the effect of low pH on the stability of the molecule. A compromise must be found between efficient elution conditions that generate smaller volumes that are easier to handle at scale and detrimental effects on the antibody molecule itself.

In the generic processes shown above anion exchange is typically used in a negative mode. In this mode conditions are selected in which the antibody being purified does not bind to the matrix but impurities do. This step is often used for DNA removal, as being an acidic molecule it will bind tightly to the negatively charged matrix under conditions in which most antibodies fail to interact with the matrix. This method is applicable to many antibodies although again like Protein A, generic approaches will require modification. We have observed at CAT significant differences in performance of this step when using generic conditions with different antibodies. In some instances the generic conditions do not promote flow through of the novel antibody and significant tailing and losses can be seen. This however can be relatively easily solved by taking an empirical approach to adjustment of running pH and salt concentration (Fig 1.6).

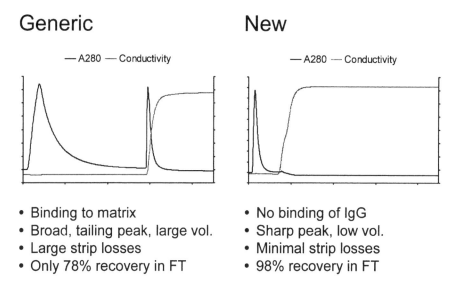

Figure 1.6. Purification of a monoclonal antibody using generic and modified conditions on anion exchange chromatography run in negative 'flow through' mode

Another aspect of generic processes that needs evaluation is whether it is suitable for the scale intended. For example, gel filtration chromatography is often included in generic purification schemes to remove both aggregates and fragments commonly encountered in monoclonal antibody purification processes. At very large scales gel filtration is not economically or practically viable for many products and thus alternatives for aggregate removal may have to be developed. A relatively simple solution to this problem has been achieved with the use of cation exchange chromatography in a bind and elute mode. The antibody and any associated multimeric protein are bound to the column under mildly acidic conditions followed by step elution of the monomeric antibody with sodium chloride leaving the multimers bound (CAT unpublished data). This method has been shown to produce 99% monomeric antibody with high recoveries combined with significantly increased processing efficiency compared to gel filtration.

4.2 Keeping it simple

Economic pressures on processes driving speed, efficiency and yield have not surprisingly had a big influence on process design in recent years. Current trends are to use fewer steps and to maximise the benefit of each of these steps (Ultee, 1999 and Francis, 2002). This reduction in complexity brings about improvements to yields, increases process robustness (as there are less things to go wrong in manufacturing!) and reduces the overall processing time. The use of affinity chromatography is advocated as a means of reducing the number of process steps as it can be used early in processes to very efficiently recover highly purified protein from very crude starting materials (Roy and Gupta 2002). This clearly relates to the attractiveness and widespread adoption of Protein A affinity chromatography for monoclonal antibody purification.

Expanded bed adsorption (EBA) has the potential to simplify processes as it combines the harvest, initial capture, purification and concentration steps into a single unit operation. Although having much promise EBA matrices have had little uptake in monoclonal antibody processes. This may be due to the significant decreases in dynamic capacity and limited number of cycles seen with Protein A EBA matrices and the reduced efficiencies seen with anion exchange EBA matrices when used for antibody purification (Blank et al 2001).

Process intensification can be achieved with rationalisation and reduction of unnecessary steps such as ultrafiltration for conditioning of chromatography loads or unnecessary concentration steps. Reordering of process steps can often result in feed streams that are suitable for the next chromatography step without further modification.

At CAT we have redesigned existing generic strategies to replace gel filtration with cation exchange and rationalise the process to allow for removal of unnecessary concentration and diafiltration steps, reduce buffer volumes, increase column capacities and flow rates and utilise a common buffer system for all steps (Fig 1.7). These relatively simple changes had a dramatic effect on costs and recovery, reducing costs per gram by over 40% with no effect on product quality (Fish 2001).

4.3 Bringing it all together – a holistic approach to process design

During the development of antibody purification strategies researchers will have to grapple with all of the issues discussed above. Increasing the quantities of antibody from the tiny amounts required for research protocols (such as the nanograms required for the estimation of molecular weight by

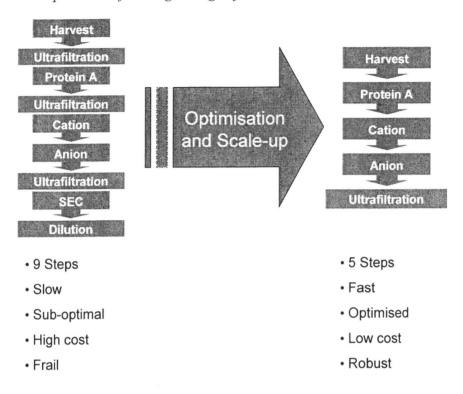

Figure 1.7. Monoclonal antibody process simplification

mass spectrometry) to the requisite amounts for a chronically administered pharmaceutical may range over many orders of magnitude. Such a massive amplification means that process design considerations will be radically different. Generic processes are valuable approach though there is considerable scope to rationalise these on a case-by-case basis. Ultimately there is no truly generic process. All monoclonals are slightly different and generic simply represents a starting point that will require modification for effective scale up. Overall the process development scientist needs to take a view of the bigger picture and have a holistic approach that balances all of the facets of what can be a very complex process. This approach to scale up balances the needs of robustness, purity, yield and economics the aim being to generate scaleable processes that work from day one. Planning for scale early in development is an essential part of this approach. Ultimately the ideal would be to work with processes that from their very early use in small-scale research translate to large-scale production without the need for reconstruction. Getting it right first time may not always be achievable but striving towards this goal will dramatically shortcut the process of moving from the laboratory to the clinic with corresponding reductions in cost, time and effort.

5. THE FUTURE OF PROCESS DESIGN

Since 1982, when Genentech received approval from the Food and Drug Administration to market genetically engineered human insulin, the technologies associated with the biotechnology industry have developed enormously. The worldwide trend for rapid progression and change, seeking improvement to existing manufacturing strategies continues and it may not be possible to accurately predict the future. However, trends in purification development can be discerned in what has been a discipline relatively slow to adopt radical or novel protein purification methodologies.

Large scale chromatography remains the method of choice for purification of all biopharmaceuticals and thus it is unlikely that these methods will be phased out completely. Clearly more automation and greater resolution will be applied to such methods and the involvement of engineers and engineering solutions to large scale production issues will increase as the demand for large scale equipment increases. Examples of this are the introduction of large scale pack-in-place chromatography columns and chromatography media designed to tolerate crude and viscous feed stocks (Williams et al 2002). Another engineering derived development is the use of radial flow chromatography columns (Wallworth 2000). This type of chromatography provides an alternative to traditional axial columns with the advantages of simple packing techniques, lower pressure drops and smaller footprints.

Additionally much improvement is continuing to be made in the development of novel chromatography matrices with alternative modes of action, together with the introduction of several high density, high performance matrices enhancing the selectivity for monoclonal antibodies (Table 1.3 and Lyddiatt 2002).

Table 1.3. Developments in chromatographic methods applicable to purification of monoclonal antibodies

Mechanism	Remarks	Reference
High charge density ion exchange media	CM-HyperD™, a cation exchanger composed of an inorganic macroporous support filled with a viscoelastic gel with a high charge density for use in capture of antibodies direct from cell culture supernatants	Necina (1998)
Protein A mimetic used in EBA chromatography	FastMabs A™ - an agarose matrix derivatised with a low molecular weight Protein A mimetic stable to 1M sodium hydroxide. Can be used in expanded bed adsorption mode at high ionic strength	Lihme (1997)

Hydrophobic charge induction	Dual mode ionisable ligands that support hydrophobic binding of antibodies but also become charge sufficiently under elution conditions to overcome this interaction and facilitate desorption	Schwartz (2001)

Some of the problems associated with the use of packed bed chromatography at scale may potentially be overcome by the use of synthetic macroporous and microporous membranes as chromatographic media. If this technology can overcome the current issues of low binding capacity, membrane pore size distribution and uneven membrane thickness their future in large scale manufacturing will be promising (Ghosh 2002).

For a more comprehensive review of the current trends in purification and novel technologies the reader is directed to the remaining articles in this volume and the companion volume "Biopharmaceutical antibodies: Novel Technologies"

ACKNOWLEDGEMENTS

I am grateful to Karen Bannister, Richard Turner, Jin Langstone, Anne Laver, Carl Spicer and Pascale Diesel at Cambridge Antibody Technology who generated much of the data in this chapter.

REFERENCES

Adair, J.R. and Bright, S.M. (1995) Progress with humanised antibodies – and update. *Expert Opinion on Investigational Drugs* **4**, 863-870

Andersen, D.C. and Krummen, L. (2002) Recombinant protein expression for therapeutic applications. *Curr. Opin. Biotech.* **13**, 117-123

Baneyxm F. (1999) Recombinant protein expression in *Escherichia coli. Curr. Opin. Biotechnol.* **10**, 411-421

Bannister, K. and Fish, B. (2001) Tailored optimisation of a generic process as applied to CAT-213 an anti-eotaxin antibody. Poster presentation at IBC 8th International Antibody Production and Downstream Processing Conference, San Diego USA.

Bilila, T.A. and Robinson, D.K. ((1995) In pursuit of the optimal fed-batch process for monoclonal antibody production. *Biotechnology Progress* **11**, 1-13

Blank, G.S., Zapata, G., Fahrner, R., Milton, M., Yedinak, H., Knudsen, H. and Schmelzer, C. (2001) Expanded bed adsorption in the purification of monoclonal antibodies: a comparison of process alternatives. *Bioseparation* **10**, 65-71

Daly, S.J., Dillon, P.P., Brennan, J., Dunne, L., Fitzpatrick, J. and O'Kennedy, R. (2001) Production and analytical applications of scFv antibody fragments. *Anal. Lett.* **34**(11), 1799-1827

Dove, A. (2002) Uncorking the manufacturing bottleneck. *Nature Biotech.* **20**, 777- 779

Federici, M.M. (1994) The quality control of biotechnology products. *Biologicals* **22**, 151-159

Fish, B. (2001) Taking a monoclonal antibody from mg to kg scale production: strategies, issues and successes. Presentation at IBC's 3rd International Conference Scaling-up from Bench to Clinic and Beyond. San Diego, USA

Francis, R (2002) Commercialisation of manufacturing processes for therapeutic antibody products Presentation at IBC Accessing Production Capacity, Partnerships and IP Issues Seminar. London UK

Gagnon, P (1996) *Purification tools for monoclonal antibodies.* Validated Biosystems Inc., Tuscan, AZ, USA.

Ghosh, R. (2002) Protein separation using membrane chromatography: opportunities and challenges. *J. Chrom. A* **952**, 13-27

Humphreys, D.P. and Glover, D.J. (2001) Therapeutic antibody production technologies: molecules, applications, expression and purification. *Curr. Opin. Drug. Disc. Dev.* **4**, 172-185

Huse, K., Böhme, H-J. and Scholz, G.H. (2002) Purification of antibodies by affinity chromatography. *J. Biochem. Biophys. Methods* **51**, 217-231

Jungbauer, A (1993) Preparative chromatography of biomolecules. J. Chrom. **639**, 3-16

Kaul, R. and Mattiasson, B. (1992) Secondary purification. *Bioseparation.* **3**, 1-26

Keen, M.J. and Hale, C. (1995) The use of serum-free medium for the production of functionally active humanized monoclonal antibody from NS0 mouse myeloma cells engineered using glutamine synthetase as a selectable marker. *Cytotechnology* **18**, 207-217

King, D.J. (1998) *Production of monoclonal antibodies. Applications and Engineering of Monoclonal Antibodies*, pp.161-185, Taylor and Francis Ltd, London.

Kipriyanov, S. M. Moldenhauer, G. Little, M. (1997) High level production of soluble single chain antibodies in small-scale *Escherichia coli* cultures *J. Immunol. Meth.* **200**(1/2), 69-77

Kohler, G. and Milstein, C. (1975) Continuous cultures of fused cells secreting antibody of pre-defined specificity. *Nature* **256**, 495-497

Labrou, N. and Clonis, Y.D. (1994) The affinity technology in downstream processing. *J. Biotech.* **36**, 95-119

Lihme, A and Hansen, M.B. (1997) Protein A mimetic for large-scale monoclonal antibody purification. *American Biotech. Lab.***15**, 30-32

Lyddiatt, A. (2002) Process chromatography: current constraints and future options for the absorptive recovery of bioproducts. *Curr. Opin. Biotech.* **13**, 95-103

Necina, R., Amatschek, K and Jungbauer, A. (1998) Capture of human monoclonal antibodies from cell culture supernatant by ion exchange media exhibiting high charge density. *Biotech. Bioengin.* **60**, 689-698

Reference from Ray/Diane on cholesterol free mutant of NS0

Robinson, K. (2002) An industry comes of age. *BioPharm International* **15** (11) 20-24

Roy, I. and Gupta, M. (2002) Downstream processing of enzymes/proteins. *Proc. Indian Natn. Sci. Acad. (PINSA)* **2**, 175-204

Sadana, A. and Beelaram, A. (1994) Efficiency and economics of bioseparation: some case studies. *Bioseparation* **4**, 221-235

Sinacola, J.R. and Robinson, A.S. (2002) Rapid refolding and polishing of single-chain antibodies from *Escherichia coli* inclusion bodies. *Protein Expres. Purif.* **26**, 301-308

Sinclair, A. (2001) Biomanufacturing capacity: Current and future requirements. *Journal of Commercial Biotechnology* **8**(1), 43-50

Swartz, J.R. (2001) Advances in *Escherichia coli* production of therapeutic proteins. *Curr. Opin. Biotechnol.* **12**, 195-201

Schwartz, W., Judd, D., Wysocki, M., Guerrier, L., Birck-Wilson, E. and Boschetti, E. (2001) *J. Chrom. A* **908**, 251-253

Trill, J.J., Shatzman, A. and Ganguly, S. (1995) Production of monoclonal antibodies in COS and CHO cells. *Current Opinion in Biotechnology* **6**, 553-560

Wallworth, D.M. (2000) Practical aspects and applications of radial flow chromatography. From: *Methods in Biotechnology, Vol 9: Downstream processing of proteins: Methods and protocols.* Ed M.A.Desai, Humana Press Inc., Totowa, NJ. USA

Werner, R.G., Noe, W., Kopp, K. and Schlüter, M. (1998) Appropriate mammalian expression systems for biopharmaceuticals. Arzneimittel Forschung $\underline{48}$(8), 870-880

Williams, A., Taylor, K., Dambuleff, K., Persson, O. and Kennedy, R.M. (2002) *J. Chrom. A* **944**, 69-75

Winter, G., Griffiths, A.D., Hawkins, R.E. and Hoogenboom, H.R. (1994) Making antibodies by phage display technology. *Annu. Rev. Immunol.* **12**, 433-455

Ultee, M.E. (1999) The design of antibody purification for manufacturing. Presentation at the 5th Annual IBC Conference on Antibody Production and Downstream Processing, San Diego.

Chapter 2

ANTIBODY FRAGMENTS
Production, purification and formatting for therapeutic applications

David J. Glover[1] and David P. Humphreys
Celltech R&D Ltd., 208 Bath Road, Slough, Berkshire SL1 3WE, UK
[1]*Current address: GlaxoSmithKline, South Eden Park Road, Beckenham, Kent BR3 3BS, UK*

1. INTRODUCTION

Monoclonal antibodies have become widely accepted as safe and effective therapeutics in indications as diverse as oncology, inflammation, and cardiovascular and infectious diseases. This is largely due to the development of technologies that enable the generation of antibodies of high specificity and low immunogenicity with relative ease (Maynard and Georgiou, 2000). The specificity of all antibodies is determined by the nature of their binding to antigen but the mode of action, *i.e.* the way an antibody-based drug uses antigen binding to mediate a therapeutic effect, varies considerably. Whilst full-length immunoglogulin (Ig) G (Fig. 2.1) has been used widely it is not the optimal antibody format for all therapeutic applications. In addition production of correctly folded and glycosylated IgG using mammalian cell culture is expensive and limited in scale, which may be prohibitive for certain clinical indications. Consequently a variety of antibody fragments and conjugates have been developed that address specific applications and facilitate their production using low cost, microbial expression systems. This chapter will review key considerations in the formatting of antibody fragments for specific therapeutic applications, how they are modified to confer effector function or improved pharmacokinetics, and methods used for their expression and purification. Particular attention will be given to expression in *Escherichia coli*, which has become the preferred production method for most antibody fragments. Furthermore, the relative merits of antibody fragments and their conjugates will be compared to full-length antibodies by reference to IgG function where possible.

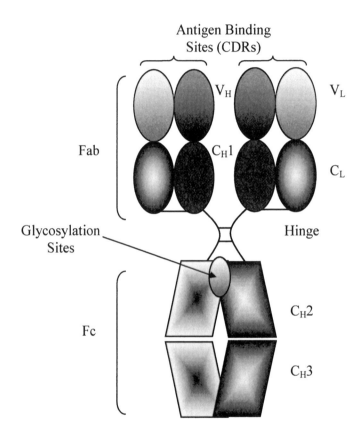

Figure 2.1. Schematic representation of full-length IgG (human gamma 1 isotype). Native IgG consists of two heavy chain and two light chain polypeptides. Each heavy chain has four domains: one variable (V_H) and three constant (C_H1-hinge-C_H2-C_H3). Each light chain has two domains: one variable (V_L) and one constant (C_L). The two heavy chains are covalently linked by disulphide bonds and each light chain is attached to a heavy chain by a disulphide bond. In native human IgG carbohydrate is attached to each heavy chain at Asn297 in the C_H2 domains.

2. FORMAT, FUNCTION AND THERAPEUTIC APPLICATIONS

2.1 Antibody format

Various antibody-based structures have been designed to meet the requirements of specific applications (*e.g.* valency, multiple specificity, tumour penetration, pharmacokinetics) as well as the need for measures that improve stability (*in vitro* and *in vivo*) and production yield. Table 2.1 shows the structures, nomenclature and relative merits of antibody fragments in common use. The structures fall into two groups: those that have been the subject of major protein engineering modifications and those that resemble native fragments of IgG. The former have issues associated with potential immunogenicity where amino acid alterations from native human sequences or the introduction of protein linkers make these fragments unlikely to be suitable for repeat dosing therapies.

Antibody constructs must remain stable under physiological conditions and upon prolonged storage. The smallest antibody domain that retains an acceptable affinity is the V_H domain but these are usually very unstable and prone to aggregation. Exceptions include the V_H domains of camelids (camels and llamas), which occur naturally without light chain pairing and yet are stable whilst possessing high affinities (Hamers-Casterman *et al.*, 1993). Sequences from camelid V_H domains have been used to 'camelise' human V_H domains that then demonstrate improved stability (Riechmann and Muyldermans, 1999). In general, however, both V_H and V_L domains are required for stability and antigen binding. Fv fragments consist of V_H and V_L domains held together by weak, non-covalent interactions and are thus prone to dissociation and aggregation. Stabilisation of Fv fragments can be achieved using protein engineering methods to introduce an inter-domain disulphide bond (Glockshuber *et al.*, 1990) or a peptide linker between the C-terminus of one domain and the N-terminus of the other such that the Fv can be produced as a single chain polypeptide *i.e.* scFv (Bird *et al.*, 1988; Huston *et al.*, 1988). The linker most frequently used to span the 35-40 Å distance between the two termini is the 15 amino acid sequence $(Gly_4Ser)_3$. Many scFvs are susceptible to aggregation with dimers and larger species being formed (Raag and Whitlow, 1995). This is because V_H and V_L domains tend to dissociate under some conditions and reassociate with the variable domains of a second dissociated scFv, an event known as domain swapping. Factors influencing scFv stability include the nature of the V_H/V_L interface, protein concentration, linker length, solvent system, temperature and presence of antigen. In recent years much attention has been directed towards improving the stability of scFvs (Wörn and Plückthun, 2001). Strategies for improved stability include deliberate protein engineering approaches such as grafting antigen binding residues onto stable frameworks and specific amino acid mutations that increase intrinsic domain and / or inter-domain stability. Alternatively evolutionary approaches have been used where phage or ribosome display technologies are used to select scFvs on the basis of stability and affinity. All of these methods, however, result in scFvs that contain amino acid sequences significantly different from natural human antibodies and thus carry immunogenicity concerns. By contrast, Fab fragments are highly stable due to non-covalent interactions that occur over a large interface between heavy and light chain polypeptides and the presence of a stabilising disulphide bond between the C_H1 and C_L domains. Fab' fragments consist of an Fab component with a heavy chain C-terminal hinge region which is often used for dimerisation to make $F(ab')_2$ or for conjugation to additional functional groups.

For many applications the increased avidity conferred by multi-valent antigen binding fragments is important. Consequently various strategies have been developed for linking antibody fragments whereby increased avidity or multiple specificity (Section 2.2.2.1) is achieved. Peptide linkers have been used for the production of dimeric scFv (Mallender and Voss, 1994) and $F(ab')_2$ (Zapata et al., 1995) but this approach can result in reduced antigen binding for one or both binding sites. An alternative approach has been the fusion of Fv fragments with leucine zippers, proteins that naturally form dimeric structures (Pack and Plückthun, 1992; Horn et al., 1996). Leucine zippers are peptides of approximately 30 amino acids that naturally form amphipathic helices with leucine residues lining up on the hydrophobic face of the helix. The hydrophobic faces of two zipper peptides associate through hydrophobic interactions and are typically stabilised further by engineering a disulphide bond between the dimerisation domains. C_H3 domains, which help drive dimerisation of IgG heavy chains through non-covalent interactions, have also been used to drive the formation of $scFvC_H3$ dimers, sometimes referred to as minibodies (Hu et al., 1996). Dimers are then stabilised by inclusion of a hinge region containing cysteine residues to allow disulphide bond formation (see Table 2.1).

Natural or engineered hinge regions can be used for the direct expression of divalent $F(ab')_2$ (Carter et al., 1992; Humphreys et al., 1997). Hinge regions containing a single cysteine residue result in little $F(ab')_2$ formation but increasing hinge cysteines to two and three has resulted in 10-30 % and 70% $F(ab')_2$ formation respectively (King et al. 1992; Better et al. 1993;

Rodrigues *et al.* 1993). F(ab')$_2$ assembly did not improve and in some cases was abolished when 5 or 6 hinge cysteines were used, presumably because these lengthy hinge regions fold to form intra hinge disulphides (Humphreys *et al.*, 1997). Alternatively, recombinant Fab' can be recovered and re-oxidised *in vitro* to form F(ab')$_2$ (Humphreys *et al.*, 1998).

Multivalent antibody fragments can also be formed by chemical cross-linking. Usually a single cysteine is engineered into the hinge region of Fab' or scFv' for site-specific attachment of linker. Following activation of the hinge thiol cross-linking occurs *via* two or more thiol reactive groups, usually maleimides (Glennie *et al.*, 1987). Trimeric and tetrameric antigen binding proteins have been made successfully using tri- and tetra-maleimide reagents (Schott *et al.*, 1993; King *et al.*, 1994) or, alternatively, using polyoxime chemistry (Werlen *et al.*, 1996). Longer linkers may also improve avidity by ensuring enough mobility for separate antigen binding domains to reach between potentially distant surface epitopes.

2.2 Function and therapeutic applications

Therapeutic antibodies function as antagonists, by blocking the interactions of two macromolecules; as agonists by, for example, binding to a cell surface receptor and activating a downstream event; or by targeting an active function to a particular cell type. Central to each of these modalities is the binding of antigen *via* complementarity determining regions (CDRs) that reside within the Fv regions of antibodies. The Fc domains of an antibody confer prolonged *in vivo* circulation times through binding to the neonatal Fc gamma receptor (FcRn) and their contribution to overall mass, which prevents clearance by renal filtration. Various functions are also mediated *via* the Fc domain *e.g.* recruitment of effector cells or complement for cell killing.

When designing an antibody-based drug for a therapeutic application the mode of action required should be considered. For those modalities where Fc functions are not required or may be undesirable (*e.g.* antigen blockade) then the only antibody domains required are those containing antigen-binding properties (Fv, Fab). In some circumstances avidity may be important for activity and divalent species may be required *e.g.* diabody, di-Fab, scFv zipper. Conjugation technologies have enabled antibodies to be used for delivery of cytotoxic drugs, radionuclides and enzymes for additional functionality. Some of these functions are dependent upon the internalisation of antigen bound antibody conjugates into specific cells. Antibody fragments may also offer some pharmacokinetic advantages over full-length antibodies such as improved tumour penetration or rapid clearance from circulating serum where desirable. It is this versatility that has made antibody fragments

Table 2.1 Antibody fragments produced in *E. coli*. (Adapted from Humphreys (2003) and printed with the kind permission of Thomson Current Drugs, London, U.K)

Name	Structure	Strengths	Weaknesses	References
scFv		High yield. Small size / good tumour penetration.	*In vitro* aggregation (storage and affinity measurement issues). Potential immunogenicity of linkers, peptide junctions, exposed surfaces. Purification with affinity tags (immunogenicity). Low thermal stability. Intellectual property burden.	Bird *et al.*, 1988; Huston *et al.* 1988; Nieba *et al.*, 1997
Diabody		Small size and avidity beneficial for tumour penetration. Potential for bispecificity. High yields demonstrated.	Purification issues as for scFv. Purification problems increased if bispecific protein is required.	Holliger *et al.*, 1997; Zhu *et al.*, 1996; 1997
Triabody		Small size and avidity beneficial for tumour penetration. Potential for multispecificity.	High yields not demonstrated. Purification issues as for scFv with increased problems if multi-specific protein is required.	Atwell *et al.*, 1999; Reviewed by Todorovska *et al.*, 2001.

scFv-zipper.		High yields possible. Small size and avidity beneficial for tumour penetration.	Potential immunogenicity of linkers, peptide junctions, exposed surfaces and coil. Purification with affinity tags (immunogenicity).	Pack and Plückthun, 1992; Rodrigues et al., 1992
Minibody (scFv linked to C_H3).		Intermediate size and avidity confer good balance between serum half life and avidity for tumour penetration.	Potential immunogenicity of linkers, peptide junctions, exposed surfaces.	Hu et al., 1992
ScAb (scFv linked to C_L).		More stable than scFv.	Potential immunogenicity of linkers, peptide junctions, exposed surfaces. Purification with affinity tags. Low thermal stability.	Grant et al., 1995; Dooley et al., 1998

Linear F(ab')$_2$		Production of an avid F(ab')$_2$ in a single polypeptide / process.	Low yield. Purification of full length F(ab')$_2$ difficult. Steric obstruction of second antigen binding site.	Zapata et al., 1995
Bispecific miniantibodies. (scFv linked to both C$_L$ and C$_H$1).		Potential for producing an avid or bispecific F(ab')$_2$ in a single polypeptide / process.	Potential immunogenicity of linkers, peptide junctions, exposed surfaces. Purification with affinity tags (immunogenicity). Potential for C$_L$ driven homodimers. Low yield.	Müller et al., 1998
Fab'		High yielding. Readily purified. Demonstrated in vitro modifications through hinge cysteine. Basis for dimeric and bispecific F(ab')$_2$.	Monomeric binding. Short serum half life of unmodified Fab'.	Carter et al., 1992; Forsberg et al., 1997 Humphreys et al., 1998; Chapman et al., 1999 Glennie et al., 1987

Antibody Fragments

Fab-scFv		Bispecificity and potential for trispecificity.	Potential immunogenicity of linkers, peptide junctions and exposed surfaces. Purification with affinity tags (immunogenicity). Low yield. Steric problems for 2nd antigen binding demonstrated.	Lu et al., 2002

Key for Table 1:
Disulphide bond —
Peptide linker ╱
Antigen A ◯
Antigen B ◇

the focus of much attention for diagnostic and therapeutic purposes over many years.

2.2.1 Tissue targeting and penetration

Some antibody-based therapies deliver cell-killing agents such as radionuclides and toxins (see Section 2.2.2) by targeting cell specific antigens, particularly those expressed on tumours. Selection of the antigen target is of prime importance since some tumour associated antigens are normal proteins that are simply over expressed in some cancerous tissues. Other antigens are shed into the circulation as well as being attached to the tumour. Consequently, a proportion of an injected dose of antibody may simply bind to non-tumour associated antigen, potentially increasing the toxic dose received by normal tissue. Blood tumours are readily accessible to antibody-mediated therapies but this is not usually the case for solid tumours, which may be poorly vascularised. In these circumstances an antibody format with good tumour penetrating properties is required. Antigen and bound antibody need to be internalised when using toxins to inhibit protein synthesis or microtubule formation or degrade DNA, but this is not essential for radionuclides which are able to deliver a toxic ionising dose from the cell surface.

The ideal antibody conjugate for tumour therapy should localise at the tumour in large amounts whilst clearing rapidly from the circulation and rest of the body thus minimising non-specific toxicity. In this respect, antibody fragments offer many advantages over IgG. Smaller antibody constructs are thought to show greater mobility than IgG following extravasation to reach parts of the tumour remote from the vasculature. Their reduced size and lack of Fc domains also results in rapid clearance from the circulation (see Section 3). For example, ^{131}I-F(ab')$_2$ showed superior tumour penetration and less toxicity when compared to IgG against the same antigen (Buchegger *et al.*, 1990; Pedley *et al.*, 1993). In practice the optimal antibody construct must not be cleared so rapidly that there is not sufficient accumulation at the tumour site yet must not persist in the circulation too long to risk non-specific toxicity. Size of antibody construct must therefore reflect a balance between these two factors.

Avidity is also an important consideration for tumour targeting. Multimeric antibody fragments have slower off-rates (rates of dissociation) than their corresponding monomers, as each binding site must simultaneously disengage from the antigen for antibody-antigen dissociation. Reduced off-rates result in prolonged retention of the antibody construct at the tumour site thereby allowing more time for their internalisation. Trivalent Fab's have been prepared by chemical cross-linking with tris-maleimide (TFM) (King *et al.* 1994). When compared to their IgG counterpart TFM conjugates show prolonged retention at the tumour site, increased rates of internalisation, rapid clearance from the circulation and reduced rates of toxicity (King *et al.*, 1994, 1995; Antoniw *et al.*, 1996; Weir *et al.*, 2002).

An alternative means of improving retention of the therapeutic entity at the tumour site is to use antibodies of high affinity, which usually have slow off-rates. However, antibodies with very high affinities (*e.g.* <10^{-10} M) may be less effective because they tightly bind to antigen bearing cells close to the capillaries forming an impeding line against penetration into the bulk of the tumour (Saga *et al.*, 1995; Adams *et al.*, 1999, 2001). Low affinity (10^{-7} M) antibody fragments do not show significant tumour retention (Adams *et al.*, 1998) so it would appear there is an optimal window of antibody affinity for solid tumour therapy.

2.2.2 Engineering effector function

Natural antibody effector functions include antibody dependent cellular cytotoxicity (ADCC), phagocytosis, complement dependent cytotoxicity (CDC) and half-life / clearance rate (see Section 3 for a discussion of half-life / clearance rates). ADCC and phagocytosis are mediated through interaction of cell bound antibodies with Fc gamma receptors (FcγR) on the surface of effector cells such as natural killer (NK) cells, neutrophils, macrophages and B cells. FcγR are comprised of three distinct classes: FcγRI, FcγRII and FcγRIII. The molecular diversity found amongst these receptors is demonstrated by their classification into further sub-divisions and the existence of polymorphisms. FcγR interact with the Fc portion of antibodies which triggers the effector cell to destroy the target cell. The mechanism of destruction is dependent on the specific effector cell type but can include induced apoptosis, phagocytosis, release of cytoplasmic granules containing perforin and granzymes, or release of toxic substances such as superoxide and hydrogen peroxide. CDC is mediated by interaction of cell bound antibody with proteins of the complement system which cascade to form a complex that kills cells. Proteins of the complement system also bind to the Fc portion of cell bound antibodies. Natural effector functions may be desirable for certain therapeutic modalities but equally, one or more function may be undesirable in certain contexts (see Section 2.2.3). Interactions between Fc and FcγR or complement are influenced by degree and type of glycosylation of the Fc (Jefferis *et al.*, 1998). This is an important consideration when selecting a means of production if natural effector functions are important for therapy since differences in glycosylation pattern are observed amongst expression systems.

Antibody fragments lacking Fc domains are unable to elicit cell killing *via* natural effector functions in the conventional manner (*i.e.* Fc interactions). However, bispecific constructs can be made that recruit natural effector functions through traditional antibody / antigen interactions. Alternatively, novel functions can be introduced such as targeting radionuclides, toxins or drugs to kill unwanted cells. Each of these options is discussed further below.

2.2.2.1 Bispecific antibodies

Bispecific antibodies contain two distinct binding specificities for different epitopes, usually on two separate antigens. They can be used for the juxtaposition of any two molecules in any application but are of particular interest for their capacity to redirect effector cells against tumour, virally infected and other unwanted cells. Typically one binding specificity will be directed against a specific cell surface antigen of the target cell and the other against a 'triggering' molecule on the surface of the effector cell *e.g.* one of the FcγR or the CD3 / T cell receptor complex. In doing so the bispecific antibody overrides the specificity of an effector cell for its natural target and redirects it to kill a target that it would otherwise ignore. Different cytotoxic cells express different triggering molecules (receptors). Thus, by varying the specificities of target and effector binding domains a variety of effector responses can be directed against most types of target cells. Alternatively, the full range of effector functions (*i.e.* ADCC, phagocytosis, complement activation and extended serum half-life) can be conferred by targeting one binding specificity to serum immunoglobulin (Holliger *et al.*, 1997). Bispecific antibodies have been evaluated in several cancer clinical trials (van Spriel *et al.*, 2000). Others have been used to target viruses, virally infected cells and bacterial pathogens as well as to deliver thrombolytic agents to blood clots thus demonstrating the diversity of potential applications for bispecific antibodies (Cao and Suresh, 1998; Koelemij *et al.*, 1999; Segal *et al.*, 1999).

Various antibody formats have been used to convey multiple specificities (see Table 2.1). Bispecific IgG have been expensive and difficult to produce using conventional hybridoma technology as expression of light and heavy chain genes coding two different specificities results in up to nine unwanted chain pairings in addition to the desired combination (Carter, 2001). Although heavy chain engineering for heterodimerisation to reduce the number of unwanted pairings and use of a light chain common to each specificity are possible solutions (Carter, 2001), the problems are readily circumvented by production of simpler antibody fragments in *E. coli*. Diabodies can be formed in *E. coli* by fusion of the V_L of one antibody with the V_H of another with a short linker and coexpression of the V_L of the second antibody fused to the V_H of the first. The two polypeptide chains associate though natural V_L/V_H interfacing and can be stabilised by further protein engineering strategies (Zhu *et al.*, 1997). Yields in excess of 500 mg/l have been reported for functional heterodimer produced during high cell density fermentation (Zhu et al., 1996). Chemical linkers, leucine zippers and engineered hinge regions containing multiple disulphides (as discussed in Section 2.1; also see Table 1) can all be used for the production of bispecific scFv and Fab (Cao and Suresh, 1998; Todorovska et al., 2001). Similarly, these strategies can be used to form constructs with multiple specificities (triabodies, tetrabodies) where desired (Todorovska et al., 2001).

2.2.2.2 Attachment of radionuclides

Radionuclides are attached to antibodies and antibody fragments for therapeutic (radioimmunotherapy), imaging and experimental purposes. The attachment is generally by use of a cyclic ion specific chelating agent, such as DOTA or DTPA, for the metallic radionuclides, directly to thiols (^{99}mTc) or using traditional random attachment chemistries such as via tertiary amine groups (Bolton and Hunter, 1973; Goldenberg, 2002).

There are a number of radionuclides that may be considered for use in radioimmunotherapy (Table 2.2). The therapeutic aim is to deliver a killer dose of ionising radiation to a localised piece of tissue, such as a tumour. Hence high energy α and β particles are often used to inflict maximum cellular damage. The path length (or maximum particle range) and energy of the emitted particle are of prime consideration. A very short path length (say 1-3mm) may restrict tissue damage to very close to the point of rest of the antibody, whereas longer path lengths (10-50 mm) may inflict unnecessary damage on healthy tissue. For blood tumours where individual cells are targeted the former may indeed be preferential. A longer path length can be attractive for the treatment of larger, solid tumours. If the tumour is poorly vascularised, or the tumour specific antigen is not internalised, or the antigen is very prevalent on the outer surface of the tumour the radiolabelled antibody may not gain access to all areas of the tumour. Here longer path lengths may be desirable, where cells that do not have antibody attached to them may be killed simply due to their proximity to other tumour cells (sometimes referred to as the bystander effect). Indeed even if a radiolabelled antibody is internalised and degraded by a cell, the radionuclide will remain locally and cause cell damage until its decay is complete or it is cleared from the locale.

Radioimmunotherapy presents a series of practical challenges associated with the generation of the radionuclides, shipment around the world, hospital storage and dosing of patients without harming healthcare workers. Generally the usable α-emitters have a short half-life (minutes to hours) and so have to be generated locally and used promptly. ^{90}Y and ^{131}I have longer half-lives and so can be generated in bulk and shipped around the world. Radioactivity can damage the protein of the antibody itself so it is preferable to attach the radionuclide to the antibody just prior to patient dosing.

Table 2.2 Potentially useful radionuclides for radioimmunotherapy

Radionuclide	Emission	Half-life (h)	Maximum particle range (mm)	Maximum energy (MeV)
^{131}I	β	193	2.0	0.61
^{90}Y	β	64	12.0	2.28
^{67}Cu	β	62	1.8	0.58
^{77}Lu	β	161	1.5	0.50
^{186}Re	β	91	5.0	1.08
^{188}Re	β	17	11.0	2.12
^{212}Bi	α	1	0.09	8.78
^{213}Bi	α	0.77	<0.1	>6.00
^{211}At	α	7.2	0.08	7.45

Thus some formulations have been developed where the antibody is shipped with a chelating agent pre-conjugated to the protein. The radionuclide can then simply be mixed with the antibody in the hospital and unbound radionuclide removed using an easy to use and disposable desalting column.

Practical issues associated with dosing radiolabelled antibodies may be overcome with a two-step targeting approach. Naked antibody (*i.e.* without radiolabel) can be dosed allowing sufficient time to achieve maximum 'tumour to blood' ratio. This is followed by a second treatment with a highly radioactive component that associates rapidly with the pre-targeted antibody. One approach makes use of the high affinity of the interaction of biotin and streptavidin for each other (Goodwin *et al.* 1988; Sharkey *et al.* 1997). An antibody with streptavidin attached is used as the pre-targeting molecule, and is chased some time later with radiolabelled biotin. A second approach uses some form of bispecific antibody that has dual antigen specificities: one for the tumour associated antigen and another that binds the radionuclide or its relevant chelating agent (Bardiés *et al.* 1996; Barbet *et al.* 1999). In both examples, the small molecular size of the 'chase' molecule delivering the radionuclide facilitates its rapid clearance from the circulation if not associated with the antibody. Renal filtration causes rapid loss (~30 minutes) of any molecule much smaller than 60 to 70 kDa unless it associates with other cellular or blood proteins. With these two-step approaches damage to normal tissue may be reduced in which case an increased amount of radioactivity can be given to the patient. However, the former at least has been found in practice to be of restricted use due to the immunogenicity of streptavidin.

The most successful application of radiolabelled antibodies in the clinic so far has been for tumours of the blood, which are more readily accessible than the solid tumours. For example, Zevalin (^{90}Y-ibritumomab tiuxetan; IDEC Pharmaceuticals / Schering AG) and Bexxar (^{131}I-tositumomab; Corixa Corp./ GlaxoSmithKline) are radiolabelled anti-CD20 antibodies approved for the treatment of non-Hodgkin's lymphoma.

Radiolabelled antibodies may also be used for imaging of diseased tissue and have some of the same considerations as those used for delivery of a therapeutic dose of radioactivity. In the simplest form of imaging, patients due for surgical removal of tumour are pre-dosed with a radiolabelled antibody specific for their tumour type. Surgery can then be performed as normal but with surgeons using small hand held detectors to enable identification of small metastases or non-obvious tumours. Dosing and surgery must be separated in time sufficient to allow clearance of unattached antibody to reduce the dose of radioactivity received by the surgeon. More sophisticated approaches using external imaging machines remove the risk to the surgeon and require the use of isotopes with γ or positron emissions that reach outside of the body. In its most elaborate forms (using the bi-directional decay of positrons) imaging can generate a 3-dimensional image of the tumour relative to the rest of the organs hence increasing the chances of finding the tumour during subsequent surgery or enable targeting of traditional beam radiotherapy.

A high tumour to normal tissue ratio with respect to radiolabelled antibody is required for tumour imaging. In practice this is achieved by selecting the antibody format optimal for circulating half-life and avidity (Sections 2.1 and 2.2.1). The major obstacle encountered is that normal clearance from the body of non-tumour associated antibody molecules is through the kidney or liver. The signal received from these organs is often so strong that it masks any signal from tumours located in those parts of the body. This is especially troublesome since these organs are often the site of the very small metastatic tumours that any prospective tumour imaging technique would aim to capture.

2.2.2.3 Attachment of toxins

Cell killing properties are also conferred to antibodies and their fragments by conjugation with toxic agents. Such agents may be protein toxins (Ng and Khoo, 2002) or small-molecule toxins (Garnett, 2001). Protein toxins evaluated in cancer therapy include the plant toxins ricin, abrin, gelonin, saporin and the pokeweed anti-viral protein (PAP) and bacterial toxins, such as diphtheria toxin and *Pseudomonas* exotoxin. All of these are potent inhibitors of protein synthesis. Protein toxins however, are highly immunogenic which limits the number of doses that can be administered to the patient. Alternatives include extremely potent small-molecule toxins from drug classes called the enediynes, which function by site-specific cleavage of DNA, and the maytansinoids that work by inhibiting microtubule formation.

Toxins offer advantages over radionuclides for specific cell killing. For example, the issues associated with distribution, storage and safety of radionuclides do not apply to most toxins in use. However, antibody-toxin conjugates are generally limited to antigens that are efficiently internalised since most toxins need to be inside the cell to exert their effect. Toxins and cytotoxic drugs potentially have less bystander effect than radionuclides which makes them less attractive for treatment of certain tumours but does mean that they may be considered as antibody conjugates for treatment of non-life threatening diseases. Radionuclides would not be considered for this purpose because of the general health risks posed by ionising radiation.

Various linkage chemistries have been used for the attachment of toxin usually through lysine, cysteine or the carbohydrate residues of antibodies (Garnet, 2001). These linkages must remain stable in circulation yet be readily cleaved to allow release of the toxic agent from the antibody once internalised. One approach is to use an acid labile linker such as hydrazone, which remains stable at the neutral pH encountered during circulation but is hydrolysed at low pH values found in lysosomes (Hamann *et al.*, 2002a, 2002b). Indeed this is the mechanism used by an anti-CD33 antibody-calicheamicin conjugate called Mylotarg (gentuzumab ozogamicin; Celltech Group / Wyeth-Ayerst Research), which is approved for the treatment of acute myeloid leukaemia. If a protein toxin is used then conjugation can be achieved by translational fusion of toxin and antibody (Benhar and Pastan, 1995). Conjugation of enough toxin to the antibody to confer sufficient potency can be challenging. Multiple toxin molecules can be randomly attached to antibody lysines but risks some loss of antigen binding (Firestone *et al.*, 1996). Site-specific attachment to cysteines (Willner *et al.*, 1993) and carbohydrate moieties (Rodwell *et al.*, 1986; O'Shannessy *et al.*, 1987; Stan *et al.*, 1999) avoids the risk of disrupting antigen binding but limits the number of toxic molecules per antibody. The use of more potent toxins such as those from the enediynes (*e.g.* calicheamicin) and maytansinoids reduces the number of toxin molecules that need to be attached to the antibody.

An alternative approach is to use a pre-targeting antibody to direct an enzymatic function to the target cell, which is used to convert a non-toxic pro-drug into a toxic drug (Melton and Sherwood, 1996; Jung, 2001; Xu and McLeod, 2001). This is known as ADEPT (antibody directed enzymatic pro-drug therapy) and has the dual benefits of reducing the non-specific toxicity of a systemically dosed toxin whilst retaining some bystander effect, since the toxic form of the drug may be liberated outside of the target cell. The activated drug may then be taken up by nearby tissue by non-specific

Antibody Fragments 41

pinocytosis. The enzymatic portion of ADEPT can be an enzyme conjugated or genetically fused to the targeting antibody. Alternatively, bispecific antibodies can be made with binding specificity for tumour associated antigen as well as catalytic activity (Wentworth *et al.*, 1996). Such catalytic antibodies have been notoriously difficult to generate and often have catalytic efficiencies considerably lower than a naturally evolved enzyme. Since the catalytic activity resides inside an antibody they can be considerably less immunogenic than direct antibody-enzyme fusions. This has important benefits if repeat dosing of these therapeutic agents is required.

2.2.3 Considerations for blocking antibodies

Many therapeutic antibodies function by blocking the interaction of a particular protein with its ligand. The therapeutic applications utilising this modality are extremely varied but include many examples from inflammatory disorders such as rheumatoid arthritis, multiple sclerosis, inflammatory bowel disease (IBD), psoriasis, transplant rejection and allergy. Inflammatory processes involve a complex series of interactions including both soluble pro-inflammatory cytokines and the up-regulation of cell adhesion molecules involved in migration of leukocytes from the vasculature. Pro-inflammatory cytokines, such as IL-1 and TNF, from macrophages have been targeted for disease intervention. For example, Remicade (infliximab; Centocor) is an anti-TNFα antibody approved for the treatment of rheumatoid arthritis and Crohn's disease. In another application of blocking antibodies the target antigen may not be a soluble protein but rather a cell surface receptor. ReoPro (abciximab; Centocor) is a chimeric Fab fragment that binds to the gpIIb/IIIa receptor on platelets and prevents interactions that lead to platelet aggregation. It is approved for the prevention of complications following coronary angioplasty, a surgical treatment for clearing blocked blood vessels.

Many of the blocking antibodies used for clinical applications have been IgGs where a long serum half-life conferred by the Fc portion is usually desirable. However, IgG interactions with FcγR can cause undesirable effects. For example, antibodies against the T cell surface proteins CD3 (Carpenter *et al.*, 2000) and CD4 (Reddy *et al.*, 2000) have been tested as immunosuppressive therapies in inflammatory diseases such as transplant rejection, rheumatoid arthritis and asthma. The mechanisms by which immunosuppression is mediated in both therapies are complex but essentially the aim is to prevent T cell activation, a primary aggravator of inflammation. However, in the former example Fc mediated cross-linking of T cells and FcγR bearing cells can result in T cell activation and consequent cytokine induced toxicity in patients (Carpenter *et al.*, 2000). Alternatively interactions of anti-CD4 bound antibody with FcγR bearing cells resulted in ADCC mediated $CD4^+$ T cell depletion, which if persistent during chronic therapy may compromise the immune status of patients. Whilst use of inactive IgG isotypes (*e.g.* human IgGγ2, IgGγ4) or Fc engineering approaches (Presta, 2002) can be taken to avoid FcγR binding, inactivation is not always complete or easy to achieve. An alternative approach is to use antibody fragments devoid of Fc. F(ab')$_2$ directed against L3T4, which is homologous to human CD4, has been shown to block immune responses to co-administered antigen and prevent the development of spontaneous autoimmune conditions in genetically susceptible mice (Carteron *et al.*, 1989). Circulating half-life can be improved by chemical modification of antibody fragments where desirable (Section 3.2). In another example, ReoPro (see above) is used as a therapeutic Fab fragment because the presence of an Fc might cause unwanted cell binding through FcγR, which would be counter productive to preventing cellular aggregation.

3. PHARMACOKINETICS

For many therapeutic antibodies, a long circulating half-life is beneficial for efficacy, dosing and cost of goods considerations. Natural, human IgG molecules (isotypes gamma 1, 2 or 4) have a $t_{1/2}\alpha$ (distribution phase half-life) of 18-22 hours and $t_{1/2}\beta$ (terminal elimination phase half-life) of 21-23 days in humans (King, 1998). The primary route for clearance of small molecules from circulating serum is filtration through the glomerulus of the kidney. IgG molecules are approximately 150 kDa in size which is considerably larger than the 60 to 70 kDa molecular size limit for renal filtration. In addition, a receptor-mediated mechanism is involved in maintaining serum half-life for IgG molecules (Ghetie and Ward, 2000). The receptor responsible is the neonatal Fc gamma receptor (FcRn), which is expressed in most human adult tissues. It is thought that circulating IgG is internalised into cells (probably of the endothelium) by non-specific pinocytosis where the low pH of the endosome results in tight binding to FcRn. Bound IgG is protected from degradation and is returned to the cell surface where the higher extracellular pH allows re-release into the circulation. FcRn thus regulates the level of serum IgG. When IgG levels decrease more FcRn is available for binding so that an increased amount of IgG is salvaged. Conversely, if IgG levels rise FcRn becomes saturated and an increased proportion of pinocytosed IgG is degraded. The receptor binding site is located between the C_H2 and C_H3 Fc domains and overlaps with the binding site for Staphylococcal protein A, commonly used for purification of IgG.

Antibody Fragments 43

Clearly, antibody formats lacking an Fc (see Table 2.1) cannot be maintained in circulation by FcRn mediated salvage. Thus, the serum half-life of such fragments will be determined primarily by their size. Strategies to bulk-up the size of antibody fragments have been used to improve serum half-life. Examples include conjugation of antibody fragments to low molecular weight dextrans (Fagnani *et al.*, 1995; Mikolajczyk *et al.*, 1996) or albumin (Smith *et al.*, 2001) and the use of bispecific diabodies with one specificity for target antigen and another for serum immunoglobulin (Holliger *et al.*, 1997). However the most common and favoured method for modulating the pharmacokinetics of therapeutic proteins is PEGylation, which will be the focus of further discussion below.

3.1 Pharmacokinetics of antibody fragments

Many studies have compared the pharmacokinetics of Fab and F(ab')$_2$ with IgG. In most cases the order of IgG > F(ab')$_2$ > Fab holds true with respect to serum half-life. The absolute residence times recorded are antibody dependent involving a mixture of factors which include, degree of immunogenicity, isoelectric point, affinity, location and tissue distribution of antigen. However, as a guide, a specific study in mice found residence times in the body of 8.5, 0.5 and 0.2 days for IgG, F(ab')$_2$ and Fab versions of the MOPC21 antibody respectively (Covell *et al.*, 1986). Similar patterns have been observed elsewhere using mouse, rat and cynomolgus monkey models (Brown *et al.*, 1987; Milenic *et al.*, 1991; King *et al.*, 1994; Chapman *et al.*, 1999). F(ab')$_2$ has also been shown to be cleared more rapidly than IgG in human studies. For example, a serum elimination half-life of 70 hours was observed for the chimeric MOv18 IgG compared to 20 hours for the F(ab')$_2$ version of the same antibody (Buist *et al.*, 1993).

Linkage format in the hinge region affects the pharmacokinetic properties of F(ab')$_2$ molecules. In particular, the number of disulphides in the hinge region appears to influence serum half-life. In a comparison of chimeric F(ab')$_2$ of human IgG isotypes, the γ2 version (four hinge disulphides) was retained in circulation longer than the γ1 and γ4 isotypes (two hinge disulphides each) (Buchegger *et al.*, 1992). It is possible that an increasing number of inter-chain disulphides results in a slower metabolism, either reductively or proteolytically, of F(ab')$_2$. As F(ab')$_2$ (~100 kDa) is above the molecular weight cut-off for renal filtration, degradation to smaller fragments probably plays a role in F(ab')$_2$ pharmacokinetics. Artificial F(ab')$_2$ fragments of the same isotype show an increasing half-life with number of disulphides (Rodrigues *et al.*, 1993; Humphreys *et al.*, 1998). Alternatively, Fab' fragments can be chemically cross-linked to form F(ab')$_2$. Such chemically cross-linked molecules have been shown to have longer serum circulation times than F(ab')$_2$ linked by a single hinge disulphide bond

(Rodrigues *et al.*, 1993; King *et al.*, 1994). Fv and scFv fragments are cleared from circulation just as rapidly as Fab in animal studies (Milenic *et al.*, 1991; King *et al.*, 1994; King, 1998). A useful property of smaller fragments can be their short biodistribution times ($t_{1/2}\alpha$ distribution half-life) which facilitates rapid access to extra-vascular antigens or tumour penetration as discussed in Section 2.2.1.

3.2 Modulation of serum half-life by PEGylation

The pharmacokinetics of antibody fragments are commonly modified by the attachment of poly(ethylene glycol) (PEG) moieties (Chapman, 2002). PEG can be conjugated to proteins by a variety of means (Zalipsky, 1995; Greenwald *et al.*, 2000), which include amine reactive (*e.g.* succinimidyl esters, *p*-nitro-phenol carbonates and tresylates), aldehyde reactive, thiol reactive (*e.g.* maleimide, vinyl sulphone and iodoacetamide) and alcohol reactive chemistries. Many types of PEG molecule derivatised with these functional chemistries are commercially available. Historically antibodies have been randomly PEGylated most commonly using amine reactive chemistry, such as *N*-hydroxysuccinimide ester functionality at the terminus of the PEG molecule. These react with lysine residues and potentially N-terminal residues in the target protein. However, random PEGylation frequently results in a significant reduction in antigen binding presumably due to attachment of PEG to lysine residues close to the antigen binding site. Antigen binding losses between 12 and 90% have been reported (see Chapman, 2002 for a literature comparison). More recently, methods have been developed for the site-specific attachment of PEG to a cysteine residue in an engineered hinge region of Fab' or F(ab')$_2$ molecules (Chapman *et al.*, 1999; Leong *et al.*, 2001). This approach ensures full retention of antigen binding and homogeneity of product. Specific activation of the hinge cysteine normally requires the use of a thiol based reducing agent such as β-mercaptoethylamine, dithiothreitol or cysteine that needs to be removed so that the subsequent oxidative reaction with activated PEG can occur.

Various studies have demonstrated the pharmacokinetic benefits of Fab' and F(ab')$_2$ PEGylation. In rats, non-PEGylated Fab' was found to have a half-life less than 4% of the intact IgG but the site-specific attachment of 25 kDa, 40 kDa and two 25 kDa PEG chains resulted in increases in half-life of seven-fold, 13.5-fold and 21-fold respectively (Chapman *et al.*, 1999). The same authors also report improved pharmacokinetics in a higher species, the cynomolgous monkey, where the half-life of 40 kDa PEG-Fab' conjugate was calculated to be 78% of whole IgG. PEGylation confers prolonged half-lives to antibody fragments primarily though size increments to prevent renal filtration. Attachment of one and two 40 kDa PEG moieties to humanised F(ab')$_2$ increased the serum half-life of F(ab')$_2$ in rabbits from 8.5 hours to 45 and 48 hours respectively (Koumenis *et al.*, 2000). The small difference observed between one and two 40 kDa PEG molecules suggests it may not be necessary to conjugate more than one large PEG molecule per antibody fragment or use longer chain PEGs to achieve optimised pharmacokinetics. Addition of PEG has a much larger effect on apparent molecular weight than the theoretical addition of the PEG alone. For example, a linear 40 kDa PEG-F(ab')$_2$ conjugate has a theoretical molecular weight of 135 kDa but its apparent molecular weight, as determined by size exclusion chromatography, is about 1600 kDa (Koumenis *et al.*, 2000) due to the large effect PEG has on hydrodynamic size. This 'hydration shell' effect of PEG is also thought to account for the reduced immunogenicity of PEGylated proteins in general and reduced proteolytic susceptibility thereby offering an additional mechanism for the enhancement of serum half-life.

4. PRODUCTION

There is a broad range of expression systems available for the production of biopharmaceuticals. These include mammalian cell culture (Racher *et al.*, 1999), transgenic animals (Rudolph, 1999; Dove, 2000), transgenic plants (Peeters *et al.*, 2001), yeasts and prokaryotic hosts such as *E. coli* (Humphreys, 2003). Each of these systems have their own relative merits with selection largely dependent upon complexity of expressed protein, need for post-translational modifications, production scale required, cost of goods (COG) and regulatory acceptance (see Humphreys and Glover, 2001 for a comparative review relating to antibody production). Historically mammalian cells have been preferred for production of IgG due to their capacity for folding and modification of complex proteins. However, simpler antibody fragments are amenable to expression using any of these systems. The emergence of transgenic expression systems offers the potential for very large scale production of antibodies at low COG. However, regulatory acceptance and the time taken to establish production herds and crops are significant barriers to overcome. High-level expression of antibody fragments in *E. coli* is a long established technology offering benefits in COG, production scale and development speed (discussed further in Section 4.1). Consequently *E. coli* remains the preferred method for the production of antibody fragments. This chapter will therefore focus on *E. coli* production methods whilst only briefly considering mammalian and transgenic expression systems, which are covered in more detail elsewhere in this book.

4.1 Use of *Escherichia coli* for the production of antibody fragments

4.1.1 General considerations

E. coli production methods offer a number of significant advantages when compared to conventional mammalian cell culture used for the production of antibodies. *E. coli* has a generation time in the order of minutes (10 minutes at the optimal growth temperature of 37 °C) compared with several hours for most mammalian cell types. Consequently, *E. coli* fermentation processes are complete within 1 to 3 days whereas mammalian cell culture typically takes 10 to 12 days to reach peak antibody titre (see Section 4.3). Presently mammalian cell culture technology is limited to the 20 000 litre scale of operation whereas fermentation technology for *E. coli* and yeasts is proven up to about 100 000 litres. The economies of scale associated with microbial fermentation strategies combined with rapid process time, use of simple media free from serum components and the lack of need for costly viral clearance steps all contribute to a greatly reduced cost of goods (COG). These factors combined make microbial production processes far more suited to addressing the COG and annual production requirements of large market indications. *E. coli* expression systems also facilitate rapid development times to the clinic and market. Uniformity of expression amongst *E. coli* clones is ensured because the genes of interest are expressed from an extra-chromasomally replicating plasmid. This negates the need for screening for high expressers. With mammalian cell transfection techniques the genes of interest are integrated into the chromosome and their expression is dependent upon the site and number of integrations. Although there are methods available for controlling these events invariably some gene amplification and screening for high expressing clones is required. The short generation time for *E. coli* enables cell lines and processes to be developed much more rapidly when compared to mammalian cell culture and transgenic expression systems.

Until recently *E. coli* has been limited to the production of aglycosylated fragments of antibodies due to the intrinsic limitations of its protein folding, disulphide bond forming and post-translational apparatus. However recently expression of full length IgG in *E. coli* has been achieved (Simmons *et al.*, 2002). Fine balancing of light chain and heavy chain expression, use of protease deficient strains and high cell density fermentation resulted in purified yields of full length IgG at up to 150 mg/l. The lack of effector functions on this aglycosylated IgG may actually be an advantage for clinical applications that simply require blocking / neutralisation. However, specific functions could be added back by conjugation of toxins or radionuclides as discussed in Section 2.2.2.

4.1.2 Periplasmic expression

Expression of proteins in the periplasm, the compartment between the inner and outer membranes of Gram-negative bacteria, favours disulphide bond formation. Natural antibody domains contain a single intramolecular disulphide bond. Hence, increasing the complexity of antibody fragments to contain multiple domains results in an increased requirement for disulphide bond formation. Furthermore, some fragments contain domains that are linked by intermolecular disulphides. For example, an Fab fragment contains four intramolecular disulphides (one in each domain) and a single intermolecular disulphide bond between the C_H1 and C_L domains. The formation of disulphide bonds involves cysteine oxidation. As the bacterial cytoplasm is usually a reducing environment antibody fragments are typically secreted to the oxidising environment of the periplasm. Following induction of expression, nascent polypeptides are targeted to the inner membrane by use of a well characterised leader peptide (*e.g.* OmpA, pelB, phoA) fused to the N-terminus of the antibody heavy and light chains. The leader peptide is cleaved by membrane peptidases upon translocation of the polypeptides. The *E. coli* inner membrane and periplasm contain an extremely adept machinery, consisting of oxidoreductases and isomerases, for the formation and rearrangement of disulphide bonds (Bardwell 1994; Missiakas and Raina, 1997; Åslund and Beckwith, 1999). Here the antibody fragment folds into its native state and can be recovered from the periplasm using a simple extraction procedure.

Periplasmic expression levels as high as 1-2 g/l have been reported for antibody fragments during high cell density fermentation (Carter *et al.,* 1992). However, the level of expression can vary considerably and is largely dependent upon the primary sequence of the protein: some antibody frameworks and CDRs express better than others. Those fragments that do not express well show a tendency to misfold or aggregate in the periplasm. Various protein engineering approaches have been taken in an attempt to overcome these problems. Yields of such fragments can be improved by specific amino acid substitutions that do not affect binding affinity but improve solubility. Up to 30-fold improvements in yield have been reported for specific amino acid substitutions in some poorly expressed scFvs but the yields and substitutions required vary on a case-by-case basis (Kipriyanov *et al.,* 1997; Wall and Plückthun, 1999). The approach is applicable to a range of antibody fragments including Fv, Fab and scFv (Knappik and Plückthun, 1995). Hydrophobic patches at the antibody variable / constant domain interface are inherently exposed during expression of Fv type fragments. Disruption of these patches at the V_H/C_H1 interface, in particular, has been shown to improve solubility of a poorly expressed scFv in the periplasm (Nieba *et al.*, 1997). Whilst such modified fragments certainly have many individual advantages, it is difficult to envisage that any protein with large numbers of amino acid alterations from native human sequences will be used as repeat dosage therapeutics to patients with anything other than the most immediate life threatening situations. Hence, these heavily engineered proteins may have limited therapeutic application. An alternative approach is to graft the CDRs belonging to the antibody of interest on to the framework of an antibody fragment known to express well in the periplasm of *E. coli*. Jung and Plückthun (1997) grafted the CDRs of a poorly expressed antifluorescein antibody on to the framework of the highly expressed, humanised 4D5 anti-HER2 antibody with big improvements in yield of the grafted scFv. Humanisation procedures designed to avoid problems of immunogenicity of non-human antibodies can therefore be combined with a strategy for improving soluble expression in the periplasm of *E. coli*. The use of phage libraries tends to generate fragments that express well in *E. coli* because phage selection has the potential to isolate both good binders and good expressers (Jung and Plückthun, 1997; Verma *et al.* 1998). Also, co-expression of periplasmic folding factors can improve the expression of antibody fragments in *E. coli*. The functional yield of various aggregation prone scFvs has been improved by co-expression of the periplasmic chaperones, Skp (Bothmann and Plückthun, 1998) and FkpA (Bothmann and Plückthun, 2000). FkpA possesses independent, but mechanistically related, isomerase and chaperone functions (Ramm and Plückthun, 2000; Ramm and Plückthun, 2002).

4.1.3 Cytoplasmic expression

The cytoplasm of *E. coli* is attractive as a site of expression due to the availability of native or heterologously expressed ATP driven chaperones that are not functional in the ATP free periplasm, lack of dependence upon the secretory apparatus and the productive potential offered by the greater volume of the cytoplasm compared to the periplasm. However, disulphide bonds do not form readily in the cytoplasm thus limiting production options to either protein refolding from inclusion bodies or soluble expression in highly engineered strains. A further consideration is the need for processing of N-terminal methionines inherently present in cytoplasmically expressed proteins.

The cytoplasm of *E. coli* is considered to be a reducing environment that disfavours the formation of disulphide bonds. Disulphide containing proteins are reduced in the cytoplasm *via* two independent systems, the thioredoxin and glutaredoxin pathways (Prinz *et al.*, 1997). The glutaredoxin system consists of the thiol-disulphide oxidoreductases glutaredoxin 1, 2 and 3, encoded by the *grxA*, *grxB*, and *grxC* genes respectively, and glutathione encoded by two genes, *gshA* and *gshB*. Glutathione plays a key role in maintaining glutaredoxins 1 to 3 in the reduced state and is in turn reduced by the *gor* gene product, glutathione reductase. Similarly, the thioredoxin system consists of the oxidoreductase thioredoxin (*trxA* gene product) which is maintained in the reduced state through the action of thioredoxin reductase (*trxB* gene product). Both pathways derive their reducing power from NADPH and function independently *i.e.* the glutathione and thioredoxin reductases are specific for their respective substrates. Consequently, a deliberate attempt to create an oxidising environment within the cytoplasm compatible with a high level complexity of disulphide formation requires disruption of both pathways. Indeed, strains mutant in *trxB* and *gor* have been identified that permit the formation of disulphide bonds in the cytoplasm.

The first isolates of the double *trxB gor* mutant had very poor growth properties unless DTT was added to cultures (Prinz *et al.*, 1997). However, a DTT-independent suppressor mutant of a *trxB gor* strain called FÅ113 has been isolated that exhibits normal growth properties (Bessette *et al.*, 1999). Using strain FÅ113, two Fab's have been expressed at 10-30 mg/l in shake flask cultures grown to 1.2-1.3 OD_{600} units (Venturi *et al.*, 2002). Co-expression of the chaperones / foldases GroESL, trigger factor, and cytoplasmic versions of DsbC and Skp, also improves expression of some Fab's and scFvs (Levy *et al.*, 2001; Jurado *et al.*, 2002). For scFvs, which have a low complexity of disulphide bonds, the *trxB* mutation alone may be sufficient for good yields (Proba *et al.*, 1995). From these studies some very good cytoplasmic yields of Fab' have been achieved in shake flask culture but, as with periplasmic expression, these seem to be protein sequence and plasmid system dependent.

Expression as inclusion bodies in the cytoplasm should not be overlooked due to the very high levels of protein expression, short fermentation time and the potential for a simple and highly enriching primary purification procedure. However, high yielding *in vitro* refolding of Fab' has yet to be reported. Concerns over the batch to batch quality for refolding of complex proteins along with the potential for the variable presence of N-terminal initiator methionines may mean that the inclusion body route may be limited both to the easier to refold monomeric scFv and to proteins destined for non-therapeutic applications (Hexham *et al.*, 2001; Lee *et al.*, 2002).

An alternative to using *trxB gor* mutant strains is to select scFv frameworks that can function without the intramolecular disulphides (Wörn and Plückthun, 2001). Such scFvs could be expressed in the natural reducing environment of the cytoplasm but have principally been developed to enable intrabody technology.

4.1.4 Plasmid biology

The major plasmid factors to be considered for optimal expression of antibody fragments are copy number, stability of the DNA structure and its maintenance, promoter / induction regime and resistance marker. Selection from these components will depend upon the type of antibody molecule to be expressed, its sub-cellular location and the likely achievable yields. Non-single chain antibodies, such as Fab and IgG, require expression of at least two genes, which code for the discrete light and heavy chain polypeptides. For these multi-chain proteins plasmid designs that optimise the ratio of light and heavy chain expression are also important for product yield (Carter *et al.*, 1992; Humphreys *et al.*, 2002; Simmons *et al.*, 2002).

Lactose, IPTG and phosphate starvation are commonly used as inducers of *lac, tac* or *phoA* promoters. The *tet*A (Skerra, 1994), arabinose promoter (Guzman *et al.*, 1995) and the T7/pLysS/BL21(DE3) system (Studier *et al.*, 1990) may be used where especially tight / low level expression prior to induction is required due to a need to express semi-toxic products. Where lack of chemical induction is the critical factor the *phoA* (Carter *et al.*, 1992) or *trp* promoters (Tacon *et al.*, 1983) may be useful.

The powerful T7 promoter system has been refined in a number of ways. In the usual system the gene to be expressed has a T7 promoter put in front of it. The gene for the T7 RNA polymerase is then typically placed under the control of the lacUV5 promoter placed on the chromosome of a recipient strain. Addition of IPTG induces the production of the T7 RNA polymerase and hence indirectly the gene of interest. In an adaptation, the T7 RNA polymerase is placed under the control of the *ara*BAD promoter (Chao *et al.*, 2002a). This benefits from the tight pre-induction control associated with the arabinose promoter (Guzman *et al.*, 1995) and the use of low levels of an inducer that is a safe metabolisable plant product. Additional control of expression is achieved by carbon source switching in fed-batch fermentation (see Section 4.1.5) using glucose (which represses the promoter) for the growth phase and glycerol during induction. Arabinose is added as the inducer.

Physical inducers, such as a temperature shift, are used for some plasmid systems. A temperature inducible R1 origin of replication has been used to express recombinant bovine somatotropin (Trepod and Mott, 2002). Notably this system uses a decrease in temperature from ~37°C to 28 °C to cause an increase in plasmid copy number and thus an increase in gene dosage and protein expression. This temperature regime is optimal for rapid pre-induction growth and controlled protein production. Others have used an upward temperature shift for induction, such as that used for the λP_L / λP_R tandem promoter (Chao *et al.*, 2002b). However, upward temperature shifts are particularly difficult to implement in large scale fermentations.

The stable inheritance of plasmids during large scale fermentation is essential for maintaining product yield, quality and process consistency. This is often achieved using antibiotic selection markers. Antibiotics added to fermentations are readily removed during product purification but validation of removal is necessary and may be expensive. Positive selection of plasmids in the absence of antibiotic selection can be achieved using plasmid borne complementation of a *pro*BA deletion in proline auxotrophic *E. coli* strains (Fiedler and Skerra, 2001). Cranenburgh *et al.,* (2001) have described a system known as repressor titration that can be used for antibiotic-free maintenance of plasmids. In this system, the *lac* operator is placed upstream of an essential gene on the chromosome and is also present on the plasmid. With the *lac* repressor expressed from the chromosome, the *lac* operator must titrate the repressor for the cell to grow. Improved control of copy number has been achieved by changing the nucleotide composition of the *col*E1 origin of replication, used in some plasmids (Grabherr *et al.,* 2002). Uncharged tRNA molecules, which are increased in number as a result of high rates of amino acid consumption during protein production, are thought to interact with and disrupt the proper function of the origin of replication. This prevents 'runaway' replication of plasmid.

4.1.5 Fermentation

Production of commercial scale quantities of recombinant protein is achieved by the application of fermentation strategies that increase specific productivity (protein produced per cell per unit time), and biomass concentration (Yee and Blanch, 1992; Lee, 1996). Usually a chemically defined medium is used to support growth to high cell densities because the concentration of individual nutrients is known and can be controlled during fermentation. A semi-defined medium may be used where a defined component is supplemented with amino acids or peptide based products for improved growth. Some nutrients become inhibitory above certain concentrations so high cell densities are usually attained using fed-batch batch processes where an initial batch culture phase is supplemented with additional nutrients during a fed-batch phase. Growth of the culture occurs at the maximum specific growth rate during the batch phase and is often limited by the rate of addition of a key nutrient during the fed-batch phase. Cell densities as high as 110 g dry cell weight (DCW)/l have been achieved at laboratory scale using conventional fed-batch fermentation (Riesenberg *et al.,* 1991) and up to 190 g DCW/l using dialysis fermentation (Fuchs *et al.,* 2002).

Fed-batch fermentation strategies can be used to address issues associated with high cell density culture at large scale. These cultures have high oxygen and cooling demands that may be difficult to satisfy at large scale. Both the heat generated and oxygen required are related to the total biomass and growth rate, the latter of which can be controlled by the rate of addition of a nutrient limiting feed. Usually the limiting nutrient is the carbon source, such as glucose or glycerol, and can be applied as a constant, exponential or increasing (gradual, stepwise or linear) feed. A constant feed is the simplest to apply but results in an ever-decreasing growth rate as the biomass concentration and volume of culture increase. Acetate production can be a problem in *E. coli* fermentations where glucose is in excess or during growth under anaerobic or oxygen limiting conditions. Growth rate, maximum biomass concentration and, in some cases, recombinant protein production can be compromised when acetate concentration exceeds 5 g/l at pH 7 (Lee, 1996). Acetate accumulation occurs because the carbon flux through the glycolytic pathway exceeds that through the tricarboxylic cycle. Thus, acetate production is avoided by controlling the supply of carbon with a limiting feed. Alternatively, glycerol has a slower uptake rate than glucose and does not result in acetate production by *E. coli* cultures (Holms, 1986). Other considerations for scale-up include the impact of reduced mixing efficiency on culture heterogeneity and CO_2 toxicity.

Recombinant protein expression is typically induced when high biomass levels have been attained during the fermentation. This allows cellular activities to be directed towards biomass generation during an initial growth phase and then towards recombinant protein production, often at the expense of biomass, in the induction phase. The demarcation of growth and induction phases may, but does not necessarily, coincide with transition between batch and fed-batch phases. Strong promoters and induction regimes are used for production of recombinant protein as inclusion bodies in relatively short fermentation times. The challenge is then to recover and refold product with high efficiencies. Accumulation of soluble product, however, is often best achieved by gradual but prolonged induction regimes that allow a slow rate of production compatible with improved protein folding (Fig. 2.2). Reducing fermentation temperature during induction is often beneficial for protein folding and soluble product accumulation (Lee, 1996). Also, at lower temperatures growth rate of *E. coli* is reduced and oxygen solubility increased, both of which help in satisfaction of oxygen demand. Control of growth rate during induction may also be important for control of product accumulation rate and solubility (Sandén *et al.* 2003). This can be achieved using carbon or nitrogen limiting feeds or phosphate depletion.

Recombinant proteins destined for therapeutic use are made according to good manufacturing practice (GMP) to ensure the product consistently meets its predetermined quality attributes. From a fermentation perspective key objectives include control of starting materials, asepsis during production and reproducible fermentation performance in terms of product yield, quality and host cell protein profile entering purification. Manufacture begins with the cell banks which must be prepared and characterised for purity and genetic stability. Consideration must also be given to the clearance or avoidance of fermentation additions such as antifoam or antibiotics used for plasmid selection and where possible animal derived components should be avoided or at least sourced from BSE free countries.

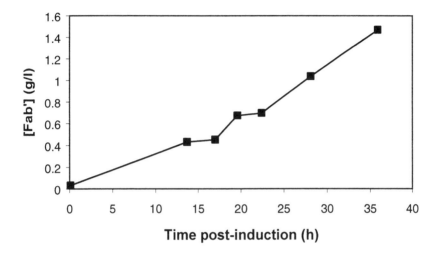

Figure 2.2. Expression of engineered Fab' in the periplasm of *E. coli* during a 10 litre high cell density, fed-batch fermentation. Gradual accumulation of Fab' over an extended induction phase is conducive to a high end of fermentation product titre.

4.2 Use of yeasts for the production of antibody fragments

The facts that yeasts possess eukaryotic secretion pathways and are amenable to high cell density fermentation may give them advantages over *E. coli* and mammalian cell culture methods for the production of recombinant antibodies. Despite the potential advantages far less work has been published on expression of antibody fragments in yeasts than in *E. coli*. Whole IgG and Fab have been expressed and secreted by *Saccharomyces cerevisiae* (Horwitz *et al.*, 1988) but yields have been low due to the limited secretory capacity of this yeast. Overexpression of the chaperone BiP and protein disulfide isomerase (PDI) has increased expression of five scFv fragments 2-8 fold, up to 20 mg/l in shake-flasks (Shusta *et al.* 1998). The methylotrophic yeast, *Pichia pastoris*, is capable of secreting up to 250 mg/l scFv in a shake-flask (Eldin *et al.*, 1997). More complex divalent scFv and scFvFc fusion antibody forms have also been produced by *P. pastoris* (Goel *et al.*, 2000). Powers *et al.*, (2001) reported the secretion of a scFvFc fusion into the medium of *P. pastoris* cultures. A prolonged serum half-life in mice and ADCC activity was demonstrated for the secreted protein. However, a high degree of glycosylation heterogeneity was also observed. Glycosylation of proteins at Asn-X-Ser/Thr motifs in yeasts differs considerably from that seen in higher eukaryotes (Gemmill and Trimble, 1999). Hence it is more likely that engineered aglycosylated antibodies will be produced for therapy using yeast systems.

4.3 Use of mammalian cell culture for the production of antibody fragments

Conventionally IgG therapeutics have been produced using mammalian cell culture. Common choices of mammalian cell line and expression system for the production of antibodies are the dihydrofolate reductase (DHFR) system in Chinese hamster ovary (CHO) cells (Wood *et al.*, 1990) and the glutamine synthetase (GS) system in murine myeloma cells, usually NS0 (Bebbington *et al.*, 1992). Transfection of the cell line with the expression vector results in random integration of the expression cassette into the host genome. Transfectants are selected for expression of a selectable marker (*e.g.* GS or antibiotic resistance), and thus antibody expression in appropriate selective media. Methotrexate blocks the action of the essential DHFR metabolic enzyme whilst glutamine synthetase is inhibited by methionine sulfoxamine. Increasing the concentration of these inhibitors in media selects for increases of integrated copy number and / or transcriptional activity (Peakman *et al.*, 1994; Racher *et al.*, 1999). Selection and amplification procedures increase production cell line development times although more rapid methods have been developed that enable site-specific recombination of the genes of interest into a transcriptionally active locus (Hollis and Mark, 1995; Karreman *et al.*, 1997).

Mammalian cell lines can be cultured at scale in stirred tank reactors and airlift fermenters using batch, fed-batch, continuous and perfusion production systems (Racher *et al.*, 1999). Yields of 1-2 g/l of IgG have been achieved in both CHO/DHFR and NS0/GS systems using such culture techniques. Use of serum in media is expensive and is subject to concerns over the presence of adventitious agents of animal origin. Adaptation of cell lines to serum-free media is possible but this further adds to the cell line generation time. Many mammalian cell lines are known also to harbour viruses. Therefore, validated viral clearance procedures need to be included in the production process. All these things combined together result in a relatively high cost of goods (COG) for mammalian cell culture derived therapeutic antibodies.

Antibody fragments have been expressed in mammalian cells using methods similar to those used for IgG expression. For example, chimeric and humanised Fab' fragments have been expressed in CHO and NS0 cells at yields up to 500 mg/l (King et al., 1994, 1995). Smaller fragments such as Fv and scFv have also been expressed in CHO and myeloma cells but yields were much lower (Riechman et al., 1988; King et al., 1993; Dorai et al., 1994). Mammalian cells may be more useful for the production of scFv fusion proteins, particularly if the fusion protein is complex or requires glycosylation e.g. scFv-IL2, scFv-B domain from Staphylococcal protein A (Dorai et al., 1994).

Before the advent of recombinant production technologies Fab and F(ab')$_2$ were produced by proteolytic digestion of IgG and is an established technique (King, 1998). ReoPro (abciximab; Centocor), a product used to prevent complications of coronary angioplasty, is a Fab produced by proteolysis of chimeric IgG expressed in mammalian cells. Proteolysis of IgG above the disulphide bonds in the hinge region with, for example, papain results in Fab fragments, which are monovalent for antigen binding. Alternatively, proteolysis below the disulphide bonds with enzymes such as pepsin results in the divalent F(ab')$_2$ fragment. Digestion with papain also results in the generation of an Fc fragment whereas this is substantially degraded if pepsin is used. Purification after proteolysis requires the separation of the desired Fab or F(ab')$_2$ from undigested IgG, other antibody fragments and the enzyme used for digestion.

4.4 Use of transgenic plants and animals for the production of antibody fragments

Antibodies and antibody fragments have been expressed in a variety of transgenic plant systems (Fischer and Emans, 2000; Peeters et al., 2001). The attractions of transgenic plants for production of therapeutic antibodies include the low cost of crop production in the field, the ease of huge scale production to meet commercial demand, the absence of animal or human pathogens, the existing methods for processing plant derived products and the possibility for stable storage of molecules in seeds and tubers. A variety of antibody formats including IgG, secretory IgA, IgM, Fab and scFv, have been expressed in plant systems (Fischer and Emans, 2000). The bacterium *Agrobacterium tumefaciens* can be used as a vehicle for transformation of plant cells with the Ti plasmid harbouring the recombinant antibody genes, which are inserted into the plant genome following transformation. Alternatively, recombinant viral vectors can be used for transient, but very high level, expression. Plant glycosylation patterns can be significantly different from those of human or CHO derived IgG (Faye et al., 1989; Cabanes-Macheteau et al., 1999) so many plant antibodies are made with null glycosylation sites to avoid potential immunogenicity. This is not an issue for most antibody fragments, which are not usually used for applications requiring glycosylated forms. The development and establishment of a transgenic crop producing significant quantity of therapeutic protein can be time consuming (about 20-24 months for transgenic maize). Regulatory acceptance, security of production (protection from climatic variations or plant disease), public attitudes towards growth of genetically modified crops and challenges in purification of antibodies from plant storage organs are also issues that may need to be addressed.

Transgenic animals also offer great potential for the production of therapeutic antibodies and antibody fragments, particularly with regard to scale-up, productivity (up to 14 g/l in goats milk), and enabling use of simple dairy-based product recovery from milk (Pollock et al., 1999). Recombinant proteins have been produced in the milk of various transgenic animals including sheep, goats, cows and pigs. Although production at scale is feasible using large herd sizes it can take 18 to 36 months before a large herd is established depending on the technologies and species involved. This is due to the inefficiencies of pro-nuclear microinjection methods used for introduction of recombinant protein genes (less than 5% of founders born are transgenic) and the need to allow the transgenic animal to mature and generate offspring to produce the herd (Rudolph, 1999; Dove, 2000). Cloning methods could reduce this time but technical difficulties and health concerns for herds mean that generation of large production herds by cloning is far from routine. Alternatively, production of antibodies in the eggs of transgenic chickens may be attractive due to the ability to grow large numbers of birds cheaply as well as their short generation time. Goat, cow and sheep IgG glycosylations show heterogeneity from human IgG but again, this is not an issue for applications involving aglycosylated antibody fragments. Concerns over the potential or perceived risk associated with human infective animal viruses and prions could, however, be an issue affecting public acceptance of transgenic animals as expression systems.

5. RECOVERY AND PURIFICATION

Biopharmaceutical protein formulations suitable for human administration must meet very high standards of purity. Common impurities that must be removed or inactivated can include host cell proteins, DNA, endotoxin and viral contaminants (dependent upon the expression system used for production). Furthermore, retention of biological activity and expected physicochemical characteristics of the active ingredient must be assured during any purification regimen. A variety of chromatographic techniques are used for the purification of antibody fragments, many of which are similar to those used for IgG purification. Typically these consist of various operating modes of solid phase matrices that are derivatised with

Antibody Fragments

specific chemistries to facilitate the selective adsorption and subsequent elution of product (see Lyddiatt, 2002 for a contemporary review of process chromatography). Antibody fragments used as therapeutics are often conjugated to molecules that modify their pharmacokinetics or confer effector function. Two phases of purification need to be considered for such conjugates: one that achieves purification of antibody fragment and another which purifies conjugated antibody fragments from non-conjugated fragments and free conjugation partner molecules. Some of the purification options available will be discussed here with key considerations for antibody fragments highlighted.

5.1 Primary recovery

True purification unit operations are frequently preceded by primary recovery procedures that perform one or more functions such as separation of cells or particulate matter from liquid broth, product concentration / dewatering, feedstock (process fluid) conditioning or primary capture. Feedstocks differ considerably dependent upon the production method used and thus different methods are required for primary recovery. Typically cells and particulate matter are separated from conventional fermentation broths by centrifugation or filtration. The fraction used for further processing depends on whether the product is cell associated or secreted. Cell associated material must be released by an extraction step which for intracellular product can be achieved using a homogeniser for cell disruption. However, this results in a complex mixture of proteins for subsequent purification steps. Release of antibody fragments from the periplasm of *E. coli* can be achieved by methods that disrupt the outer membrane without compromising inner membrane integrity *e.g.* osmotic shock, Tris and / or EDTA treatments. The *E. coli* periplasm contains significantly fewer proteins than the cytoplasm. The antibody fragment of interest is thus effectively concentrated making its purification less onerous. Initial purification can be enhanced further by the inclusion of a heat treatment step (Weir and Bailey, 1994). At elevated temperatures (>40 °C) correctly assembled IgG, Fab and Fab' are remarkably stable whilst many other proteins in the feedstock form precipitates and / or aggregates which can be easily removed during centrifugation, filtration or primary capture. The extracellular medium of both mammalian cell and *E. coli* cultures also contains relatively few proteins. However, secreted antibodies and antibody fragments typically reside in large volumes at dilute concentrations and may require concentration or use of expensive affinity matrices. Some proteins such as scFv have been demonstrated to be unable to withstand the high sheer forces generated by some microbial fermentation processes (Harrison *et al.*, 1998). Hence loss of product may occur if the scFv is secreted into the medium.

Some conditioning of the feedstock may also be required in preparation for the first purification step. For example, adjustments in pH or conductivity (ionic strength) may be required to favour binding of protein to the capture adsorbent. These may present challenges particularly where large volumes need to be conditioned possibly requiring large tanks for dilutions / adjustments, in-line dilution or diafiltration steps.

5.2 Adsorption chemistries

5.2.1 Affinity ligands

Antibody purification frequently involves the use of bacterial immunoglobulin binding proteins immobilised on a solid phase matrix. Protein A derived from *Staphylococcus aureus* or protein G from group C and G Streptococci bind with high affinity to the Fc region of antibodies at the C_H2/C_H3 domain interface. Some antibody fragments also bind *via* low affinity sites to protein A and G. Protein A binds to the V_H region of Fab's belonging to the human gene family sub-group 3 (V_H3) and specifically to sequences in the second CDR region and framework regions 1 and 3 (Potter *et al.*, 1996). Some Fab' fragments from mouse, rabbit and guinea pig have also been shown to bind to protein A (Young *et al.*, 1984; King, 1998). Consequently recombinant humanised Fab's expressed in both mammalian and *E. coli* systems have been successfully purified using immobilised protein A (Carter *et al.*, 1992; King *et al.*, 1995). Similarly, protein G has been used for purification of Fab's from either of these systems (Proudfoot *et al.*, 1992; Humphreys *et al.*, 1998). Structural studies have shown that protein G interacts with the C_H1 domain of Fabs (Derrick and Wigley, 1992). An alternative bacterial immunoglobulin binding protein that can be used for antibody purification is protein L derived from *Peptostreptococcus magnus*. Protein L binds specifically to light chain variable regions belonging to the human gene families κ1, λ2 and λ3 but not κ4 or λ1 (Åkerström *et al.*, 1994). For antibody fragments that bind relatively strongly to protein A, G or L the feedstock often requires little conditioning making these ligands ideally suited to purification from large volume solutions where product concentration is low. The product is then commonly eluted from the column by a reduction in pH.

Affinity purification using immobilised antigen is particularly useful for small fragments such as Fv or scFv which are not readily purified by other affinity methods (King *et al.*, 1993). The degree of purification achieved can be very high but disadvantages include the high cost of antigen, lack of availability of sufficient quantity of antigen and the possible requirement for

Antibody Fragments

harsh elution conditions such as extremes of pH or chaotropic agents which may be partially denaturing to the antibody fragment of interest.

An alternative approach for the purification of antibody fragments is the use of affinity peptide tags that are engineered into the protein, usually at the C-terminus, and removed later by chemical or proteolytic cleavage. The most commonly used peptide is the hexa-histidine tag which allows purification using immobilised metal-ion affinity chromatography (IMAC). Histidine residues bind to immobilised nickel, copper or zinc ions. The tagged protein is then eluted under gentle conditions using imidazole which competes for metal binding sites. Histidine tagged scFv has been purified using IMAC for clinical application (Casey *et al.*, 1995). Other systems used include strep-tag, a biotin mimetic peptide which binds to immobilised streptavidin (Schmidt and Skerra, 1994) and the FLAG tag which is captured using an immobilised antibody (Knappick and Plückthun, 1994). Peptide tags are often cleaved by proteases such as Factor X, Tev and thrombin for research preparations but these are undesirable in a therapeutic setting on cost grounds since production of the high grade proteases required is expensive. A number of chemical approaches have been used including cleavage by cyanogen bromide (Haught *et al.*, 1998), *o*-iodobenzoic acid (Hara and Yamakow, 1996) and site-specific cleavage by Cu^{2+} ions (Humphreys *et al.*, 2000). Use of self-cleavable inteins activated by thiol agents are certainly less harsh and may be very useful for production of thiol insensitive proteins (Chong *et al.*, 1998). Residual cleavage site amino acids can be an issue with all of these approaches, particularly with regard to immunogenicity.

Recent advances in affinity purification have focused on the identification of new synthetic ligands that are cheaper, more robust under stringent operating (adsorption, washing, desorption) and cleaning conditions, and compatible with resin reuse. Peptide ligands, which reversibly bind antibodies or mimic existing antibody-protein interactions (mimotopes), have been identified by screening phage-displayed, combinatorial peptide libraries with immobilised target protein (Zwick *et al.*, 1998; McConnel *et al.*, 1998). A synthetic version of the selected peptide is then immobilised on a suitable matrix (Murray *et al.*, 1997). Others have screened combinatorial chemistry libraries for antibody mimetic ligands that can also be immobilised on conventional matrices (Teng *et al.*, 2000; Sproule *et al.*, 2000). Affinity columns based on chemical ligands are likely to be cheaper and more robust than those based on synthetic peptides but the peptide display technologies offer greater ligand diversity to choose from.

5.2.2 Non-affinity ligands

Conventional chromatography resins are often used as alternatives to protein A and G for the purification of antibodies and their fragments.

Protein A and G are 10-20 fold more expensive than some of these resins and thus there is considerable commercial pressure to avoid affinity capture steps to reduce purification costs. Also some antibodies are unstable under the low pH conditions typically used for elution of antibodies from protein A and G and require other methods for purification.

Ion exchange chromatography uses differences in charge interactions for the selective adsorption of proteins from feedstocks. The isoelectric point of antibodies and their fragments varies widely, from about 4.5 to 9.0, and thus binding and elution conditions need to be determined for each antibody. However, most Fab' fragments are basic making cation exchange a good first step for purification although significant conditioning (pH, conductivity) of the feedstock may be required to ensure binding to the charged resin. Anion exchange chromatography is commonly used as a second step in purification after either cation exchange or affinity capture steps. DNA and endotoxin bind strongly to anion exchangers facilitating their removal whilst the basic antibody is collected in the flow-though. Endotoxin load and clearance is an important consideration where Gram negative bacteria such as *E. coli* are used for recombinant antibody production. A combination of cation and anion exchange can be used to give pure Fab' produced in either mammalian or *E. coli* systems in just two steps (King *et al.*, 1992; D. J. Glover *et al.*, unpublished results).

Hydrophobic interaction chromatography (HIC) separates proteins on the basis of hydrophobicity and is often used downstream of ion exchange chromatography to achieve highly pure preparations of antibody fragments. Adsorption takes place in high salt concentrations with desorption effected by lowering of salt concentration. Some antibodies are prone to precipitation and loss of antigen binding in the presence of high concentrations of salts, commonly used during adsorption, such as ammonium sulphate. Therefore, HIC may not be suitable for all antibody fragments and must be carefully optimised.

Gel filtration chromatography (although not an adsorptive process) is often used as a final 'polishing' step after other chromatography methods. It is particularly useful for removing aggregates which are a common problem in antibody preparations. However, gel filtration is time consuming and difficult to scale-up and is thus disfavoured at large scale.

5.3 Mode of operation and process integration

Selective adsorption ligands are immobilised on solid, (often) porous, beaded matrices which operate most commonly in fixed or expanded bed modes. Suitable materials used for the construction of beaded matrices include natural biopolymers such as dextran, agarose and cellulose (or their synthetic equivalents). These may be cross-linked by chemical treatment to

Antibody Fragments

confer additional strength and resistance to compression under hydrostatic pressure. Conventionally these adsorbents have been used in chromatography columns operated in a fixed, or packed, bed mode. However, a feedstock with high solids content is likely to cause blockage of a fixed bed column and must be clarified by centrifugation or filtration (Section 5.1). Expanded bed adsorption (EBA) offers an alternative mode of chromatography in which non-clarified feedstocks, such as whole fermentation broths or biological extracts, can be applied directly to the column (Anspach et al., 1999; Lihme et al., 2000). Upward application of the process stream causes expansion of the adsorbent allowing the free passage of solids through the column whilst product is selectively captured. Optimal design of adsorption bead size and density, column hardware and operating conditions ensure maintenance of bed expansion without loss of adsorbent in the column effluent. Product is then typically eluted in packed bed mode to minimise the volume of elution buffer required.

There has been a recent developmental trend towards process integration and intensification strategies that improve process efficiency and reduce COG. Advances in expression systems have resulted in the availability of relatively cheap production methods that have effectively increased the fraction of total manufacturing costs attributable to primary recovery and purification. Consequently, there has been an increased interest in downstream improvements. Labour and capital depreciation, major costs attributable to bioprocesses, are greatly reduced for faster, integrated processes. The application of EBA to a conventional fermentation process could replace centrifugation, filtration, concentration, and primary capture with a single column step. EBA has been used for the successful purification of both IgG from mammalian cell culture (Fahrner et al., 1999) and Fab' fragments from E. coli (Hansen et al., 1999). Processes may be further intensified by direct capture of product during fermentation of secreted products where broth is continually, or intermittently, circulated via an external loop containing adsorbent in an expanded, or fluidised[1], mode (Hamilton et al., 1999). Prompt removal from the fermentation broth reduces the risk of product degradation. The relatively high, or increasing, ionic strengths encountered during fermentation make affinity or mixed mode ligands most suitable for these applications (Hamilton et al., 2000).

---

[1] Expanded- and fluidized-bed adsorptions (EBA and FBA) differ in dispersion characteristics of adsorbent beads: in FBA adsorbent beads and feedstock are subject to uncontrolled, turbulent back mixing whereas the size and density distribution of adsorbent beads in EBA results in their restricted motion and plug flow of feedstock without back mixing.

6. CONCLUSIONS AND FUTURE PROSPECTS

This chapter has presented the various options and considerations for the expression and formatting of antibody fragments for different therapeutic applications. The use of antibody fragments and conjugates enables the optimal design of antibody-based drugs with respect to valency, pharmacokinetics and therapeutic function with far greater flexibility than can be achieved using standard IgG formats. Furthermore, these drugs can be manufactured using low cost microbial manufacturing technology at a scale compatible with supply for large market indications.

The choice of antibody format is broad and raises the question of which of the options discussed in this chapter are likely to prove to be the most useful in the clinic? Many antibody formats have been engineered to address issues such as stability, valency, expression yield, pharmacokinetics and tissue distribution. Highly engineered fragments containing peptide linkers and significant amino acid alterations from human sequences carry concerns over immunogenicity making them less desirable for repeat-dose therapy. The Fab' unit is made up of natural antibody domains and thus does not have these same concerns over immunogenicity (when using human / humanised antibody generation methods). Fab' can be expressed to high levels in *E. coli* (Carter *et al.*, 1992), can be chemically linked to other Fab's to confer multiple valency (King *et al.*, 1994), can be modified by site-specific PEGylation for optimised serum half-life (Chapman *et al.*, 1999) and is stable both *in vivo* and *in vitro*. These factors are likely to make Fab's the fragment of choice for many antibody based drugs. The most imminent application of Fab's will be as blocking antibodies. For example CDP870 (Celltech Group / Pfizer), an *E. coli* derived humanised Fab'-PEG conjugate that neutralises TNFα, has been evaluated in a phase II clinical trial and was shown to be well tolerated and effective in the treatment of rheumatoid arthritis (Choy *et al.*, 2002). This drug is now being evaluated in phase III clinical trials. Future applications are likely to include oncology where Fab's can be conjugated to highly potent toxins and the drug optimised for valency, pharmacokinetcs and tissue distribution.

There are a number of expression systems to choose from for manufacture of Fab' based drugs. Whilst transgenic plants and animals potentially offer low cost production on a huge scale there are a number of uncertainties regarding regulatory acceptance, security of production, public attitudes and potential or perceived risks associated with transgenic organisms. The relatively high cost and limited scale of operation are limiting factors for the use of mammalian cell culture. Consequently *E. coli* is likely to remain the preferred expression system for the production of low cost, high volume Fab' based drugs which will probably be purified using robust, low-cost, non-affinity capture methods. The next 5-10 years are likely to provide additional clinical and commercial evidence of which therapeutic molecules and expression strategies offer clear advantages for different applications.

REFERENCES

Adams, G.P., and Schier, R., 1999, Generating improved single-chain Fv molecules for tumor targeting. *J. Immunol. Methods* **231**: 249-260

Adams, G.P., Schier, R., Marshall, K., Wolf, E.J., McCall, A.M., Marks, J.D., and Weiner, L.M., 1998, Increased affinity leads to improved selective tumour delivery of single-chain Fv antibodies. *Cancer Res.* **58**: 485-490

Adams, G.P., Schier, R., McCall, A.M., Simmons, H.H., Horak, E.M., Alpaugh, K., Marks, J.D., and Weiner, L.M., 2001, High affinity restricts the localization and tumor penetration of single-chain Fv antibody molecules. *Cancer Res.* **61**: 4750-4755

Åkerström, B., Nilson, B.H.K., Hoogenboom, H.R., and Björk, L., 1994, On the interaction between single chain Fv antibodies and bacterial immunoglobulin-binding proteins. *J. Immunol. Methods* **177**: 151-163

Anspach, F.B., Curbelo, D., Hartmann, R., Garke, G., and Deckwer, W-D., 1999, Expanded-bed chromatography in primary protein purification. *J. Chromatography A* **865**: 129-144

Antoniw, P., Farnsworth, A.P.H., Turner, A., Haines, A.M.R., Mountain, A., Mackintosh, J., Shochat, D., Humm, J., Welt, S., Old, L.J., Yarranton, G.T., and King, D.J., 1996, Radioimmunotherapy of colorectal xenografts in nude mice with yttrium-90 A33 IgG and Tri-Fab (TFM). *Br. J. Cancer* **74**: 513-524

Åslund, F., and Beckwith, J., 1999, The thioredoxin superfamily: redundancy, specificity, and gray-area genomics. *J. Bacteriol.* **181**: 1375-1379

Atwell, J.L., Breheney, K.A., Lawrence, L.J., McCoy, A.J., Kortt, A.A., and Hudson, P.J., 1999, scFv multimers of the anti-neuraminidase antibody NC10: length of the linker between Vh and Vl domains dictates precisely the transition between diabodies and triabodies. *Prot. Eng.* **12**: 597-604

Barbet, J., Kraeber-Bodéré, F., Vuillez, J-P., Gautherot, E., Rouvier, E., and Chatal, J-F., 1999, Pretargeting with the affinity enhancement system for radioimmunotherapy. *Cancer Biotherapy & Radiopharmaceiticals* **14**: 153-166

Bardiès, M., Bardet, S., Faivre-Chauvet, A., Peltier, P., Douillard, J-Y., Mahé, M., Fiche, M., Lisbona, A., Giacalone, F., Meyer, P., Gautherot, E., Rouvier, E., Barbet, J., and Chatal, J-Y., 1996, Bispecific antibody and iodine-131-labeled bivalent hapten dosimetry in patients with medullary thyroid or small-cell lung cancer. *J. Nucl. Med.* **37**: 1853-1859

Benhar, I., and Pastan, I., 1995, Characterization of B1(Fv)PE38 and B1(dsFv)PE38: single-chain and disulfide-stabilized Fv immunotoxins with increased activity that cause complete remissions of established human carcinoma xenografts in nude mice. *Clin. Cancer Res.* **1**: 1023-1029

Bardwell, J.C.A., 1994, Building bridges: disulphide bond formation in the cell. *Mol. Microbiol.* **14**: 199-205

Bebbington, C.R., Renner, G., Thomson, S., King, D., Abrams, D., and Yarranton, G.T., 1992, High-level expression of a recombinant antibody from myeloma cells using a glutamine synthetase gene as an amplifiable selectable marker. *Bio/Technology* **10**: 169-175

Bessette, P.H., Åslund, F., Beckwith, J., and Georgiou, G., 1999, Efficient folding of proteins with multiple disulfide bonds in the *Escherichia coli* cytoplasm. *Proc. Natl. Acad. Sci. USA* **96**: 13703-13708

Better, M., Bernhard, S.L., Lei, S-P., Fishwild, D.M., Lane, J.A., Carrol, S.F., and Horwitz, A.H., 1993, Potent anti-CD5 ricin A chain immunoconjugates from bacterially produced Fab' and F(ab')$_2$. *Proc. Natl. Acad. Sci. USA* **90**: 457-461

Bird, R.E., Hardman, K.D., Jacobson, J.W., Johnson, S., Kaufman, B.M., Lee, S.M., Lee, T., Pope, S.H., Riordan, G.S., and Whitlow, M., 1988, Single-chain antibody-binding sites. *Science* **242**: 423-426

Bolton, A.E., and Hunter, W.M., 1973, The labelling of proteins to high specific radioactivities by conjugation to a ^{125}I-containing acylating agent. *Biochem. J.* **133**: 529-539

Bothmann, H., and Plückthun, A., 1998, Selection for a periplasmic factor improving phage display and functional periplasmic expression. *Nature Biotechnol.* **16**: 376-380

Bothmann, H., and Plückthun, A., 2000, The periplasmic *Escherichia coli* peptidylprolyl *cis, trans*-isomerase FkpA. I. Increased functional expression of antibody fragments with and without *cis*-prolines. *J. Biol. Chem.* **275**: 17100-17105

Brown, B.A., Comeau, R.D., Jones, P.L., Liberatore, F.A., Neacy, W.P., Sands, H., and Gallagher, B.M., 1987, Pharmacokinetics of the monoclonal antibody B72.3 and its fragments labelled with either ^{125}I or ^{111}In. *Cancer Res.* **47**: 1149-1154

Buchegger, F., Pèlegrin, A., Delaloye, B., Bischof-Delaloye, A., and Mach, J-P., 1990, Iodine-131-labeled MAb F(ab')$_2$ fragments are more efficient and less toxic than intact anti-CEA antibodies in radioimmunotherapy of large human colon carcinoma grafted in nude mice. *J. Nucl. Med.* **31**: 1035-1044

Buchegger, F., Pèlegrin, A., Hardman, N., Heusser, C., Lukas, J., Dolci, W., and Mach, J-P., 1992, Different behaviour of mouse-human chimeric antibody F(ab')$_2$ fragments of IgG$_1$, IgG$_2$ and IgG$_4$ sub-class *in vivo*. *Int. J. Cancer* **50**: 416-422

Buist, M.R., Kenemans, P., den Hollander, W., Vermorken, J.B., Molthoff, C.J.M., Burger, C.W., Helmerhorst, T.J.M., Baak, J.P.A., and Roos, J.C., 1993, Kinetics and tissue distribution of the radiolabeled chimeric monoclonal antibody Mov18 IgG and F(ab')$_2$ fragments in ovarian carcinoma patients. *Cancer Res.* **53**: 5413-5418

Cao, Y., and Suresh, M.R., 1998, Bespecific antibodies as novel bioconjugates. *Bioconj. Chem.* **9**:635-634

Cabanes-Macheteau, M., Fitchette-Lainé, A.C., Loutelier-Bourhis, C., Lange, C., Vine, N.D., Ma, J.K.C., Lerouge, P., and Faye, L., 1999, N-Glycosylation of a mouse IgG expressed in transgenic tobacco plants. *Glycobiol.* **9**: 365-372

Carpenter, P.A., Pavlovic, S., Tso, J.Y., Press, O.W., Gooley, T., Yu, X-Z., and Anasetti, C., 2000, Non-Fc receptor-binding humanized anti-CD3 antibodies induce apoptosis of activated human T cells. *J. Immunol.* **165**: 6205-6213

Carter, P., Kelley, R.F., Rodrigues, M.L., Snedecor, B., Covarrubias, M., Velligan, M.D., Wong, W.L.T., Rowland, A.M., Kotts, C.E., Carver, M.E., Yang, M., Bourell, J.H., Shepard, H.M., and Henner, D., 1992, High level *Escherichia coli* expression and production of a bivalent humanized antibody fragment. *Bio/Technology* **10**: 163-167

Carter, P., 2001, Bispecific human IgG by design. *J. Immunol. Methods* **248**: 7-15

Carteron, N.L., Schimenti, C.L., and Wofsy, D., 1989, Treatment of murine lupus with F(ab')$_2$ fragments of monoclonal antibody to L3T4. *J. Immunol.* **142**: 1470-1475

Casey, J.L., Keep, P.A., Chester, K.A., Robson, L., Hawkins, R.E., and Begent, R.H.J., 1995, Purification of bacterially expressed single chain Fv antibodies for clinical applications using metal chelate chromatography. *J. Immunol. Methods* **179**: 105-116

Antibody Fragments

Chapman, A.P., 2002, PEGylated antibodies and antibody fragments for improved therapy: a review. *Adv. Drug Deliv. Rev.* **54**: 531-545

Champan, A.P., Antoniw, P., Spitali, M., West, S., Stephens, S., and King, D.J., 1999, Therapeutic antibody fragments with prolonged *in vivo* half-lives. *Nature Biotechnol.* **17**: 780-783

Chao, Y.P., Law, W.S., Chen, P.T., and Hung, W.B., 2002a, Stringent regulation and high level expression of heterologous genes in Escherichia coli using T7 system controllable by the araBAD promoter. *Biotechnol. Prog.* **18**: 394-400

Chao, Y.P., Law, W.S., Chen, P.T., and Hung, W.B., 2002b, High production of heterologous proteins in *Escherichia coli* using the thermo-regulated T7 expression system. *Appl. Microbiol. Biotechnol.* **58**: 446-453

Chong, S., Montello, G.E., Zhang, A., Cantor, E.J., Liao, W., Xu, M.Q., and Benner, J., 1998, Utilizing the C-terminal cleavage activity of a protein splicing element to purify recombinant proteins in a single chromatographic step. *Nucleic Acids Res.* **26**: 5109-5115

Choy, E.H.S., Hazleman, B., Smith, M., Moss, K., Lisi, L., Scott, D.G.I., Patel, J., Sopwith, M., and Isenberg, D.A., 2002, Efficacy of a novel PEGylated humanized anti-TNF fragment (CDP870) in patients with rheumatoid arthritis: a phase II double-blinded, randomised, dose-escalating trial. *Rheumatology* **41**: 1133-1137

Covell, D.G., Barbet, J., Holton, O.D., Black, C.D.V., Parker, R.J., and Weinstein, J.N., 1986, Pharmacokinetics of monoclonal Immunoglobulins G1, F(ab')$_2$, and Fab' in mice. *Cancer Res.* **46**: 3969-3978

Cranenburgh, R.M., Hanak, J.A., Williams, S.G., and Sherratt, D.J., 2001, *Escherichia coli* strains that allow antibiotic-free plasmid selection and maintenance by repressor titration. *Nucleic Acids Res.* **29**: e26

Derrick, J.P., and Wigley, D.B., 1992, Crystal structure of a streptococcal protein G domain bound to an Fab fragment. *Nature* **359**: 752-754

Dooley, H., Grant, S.D., Harris, W.J., and Porter, A.J., 1998, Stabilization of antibody fragments in adverse environments. *Biotechnol. Appl. Biochem.* **28**: 77-83

Dorai, H., McCartney, J.E., Hudziak, R.M., Tai, M-S., Laminet, A.A., Houston, L.L., Huston, J., and Oppermann, H., 1994, Mammalian cell expression of single-chain Fv (sFv) antibody proteins and their C-terminal fusions with interleukin-2 and other effector domains. *Bio/Technology* **12**: 890-897

Dove, A., 2000, Milking the genome for profit. *Nature Biotechnol.* **18**: 1045-1048

Eldin, P., Pauza, M.E., Hieda, Y., Lin, G., Murtaugh, M.P., Pentel, P.R., and Pennell, C.A., 1997, High-level secretion of two antibody single chain Fv fragments by *Pichia pastoris*. *J. Immunol. Methods* **201**: 67-75

Fahrner, R.L., Blank, G.S., and Zapata, G.A., 1999, Expanded bed protein A chromatography of a recombinant humanized monoclonal antibody: process development, operation, and comparison with a packed bed method. *J. Biotechnol.* **75**: 273-280

Fagnani, R., Halpern, S., and Hagan, M., 1995, Altered pharmacokinetic and tumour localization properties of Fab' fragments of a murine monoclonal anti-CEA antibody by covalent modification with low molecular weight dextran. *Nucl. Med. Communic.* **16**: 362-369

Faye, L., Johnson, K.D., Sturm, A., and Chrispeels, M.J., 1989, Structure, biosynthesis, and function of asparagine-linked glycans on plant glycoproteins. *Physiologia Plantarum* **75**: 309-314

Fiedler, M., and Skerra, A., 2001, *pro*BA complementation of an auxotrophic *E. coli* strain improves plasmid stability and expression yield during fermenter production of a recombinant antibody fragment. *Gene* **274**: 111-118

Firestone, R.A., Willner, D., Hofstead, S.J., King, H.D., Keneko, T., Braslawsky, G.R., Greenfield, R.S., Trail, P.A., Lasch, S.J., Henderson, A.J., Casazza, A.M., Hellström, I., and Hellström, K.E., 1996, Synthesis and antitumor activity of the immunoconjugate BR96-Dox. *J. Control. Release* **39**: 251-259

Fischer, R., and Emans, N., 2000, Molecular farming of pharmaceutical proteins. *Transgenic Res.* **9**: 279-299

Forsberg, G., Forsgren, M., Jaki, M., Norin, M., Sterky, C., Enhörning, A., Larsson, K., Ericcson, M., and Björk, P., 1997, Identification of framework residues in a secreted recombinant antibody fragment that control production level and localization in *Escherichia coli. J. Biol. Chem.* **272**: 12430-12436

Fuchs, C., Köster, D., Wiebusch, S., Mahr, K., Eisbrenner, G., and Märkl, H., 2002, Scale-up of dialysis fermentation for high cell density cultivation of *Escherichia coli. J. Biotechnol.* **93**: 243-251

Garnett, M.C., 2001, Targeted drug conjugates: principles and progress. *Adv. Drug Deliv. Rev.* **53**: 171-216

Gemmill, T.R., and Trimble, R.B., 1999, Overview of N- and O-linked oligosaccharide structures found in various yeast species. *Biochim. Biophys. Acta* **1426**: 227-237

Ghettie, V., and Ward, E.S., 2000, Multiple roles for the major histocompatibility complex class I-related receptor FcRn. *Annu. Rev. Immunol.* **18**: 739-766

Glennie, M.J., McBride, H.M., Worth, A.T., and Stevenson, G.T., 1987, Preparation and performance of bispecific F(ab'γ)₂ antibody containing thioether-linked Fab'γ fragments. *J. Immunol.* **139**: 2367-2375

Glockshuber, R., Malia, M., Pfitzinger, I., and Plückthun, A., 1990, A comparison of strategies to stabilize immunoglobulin Fv-fragments. *Biochemistry* **29**: 1362-1367

Goel, A., Beresford, G.W., Colcher, D., Pavlinkova, G., Booth, B.J.M., Baranowska, J., and Batra, S.K., 2000, Divalent forms of CC49 single-chain antibody constructs in *Pichia pastoris*: expression, purification, and characterization. *J. Biochem.* **127**: 829-836

Goldenberg, D.M., 2002, Targeted therapy of cancer with radiolabeled antibodies. *J. Nucl. Med.* **43**: 693-713

Goodwin, D.A., Meares, C.F., McCall, M.J., McTigue, M., and Chaovapong, W., 1988, Pre-targeted immunoscintigraphy of murine tumours with indium-111 labeled bifunctional haptens. *J. Nucl. Med.* **29**: 226-234

Grabherr, R., Nilsson, E., Striedner, G., Bayer, K., 2002, Stabilizing plasmid copy number to improve recombinant protein production. *Biotechnol. Bioeng.* **77**: 142-147

Grant, S.D., Cupit, P.M., Learmonth, D., Byrne, F.R., Graham, B.M., Porter, A.J.R., and Harris, W.J., 1995, Expression of monovalent and bivalent antibody fragments in *Escherichia coli. J. Hematotherapy.* **4**: 383-388

Greenwald, R.B., Conover, C.D., and Choe, Y.H., 2000, Poly(ethylene glycol) conjugated drugs and prodrugs: a comprehensive review. *Crit. Rev. Therap. Drug Carrier Syst.* **17**: 101-161

Guzman, L.M., Belin, D., Carson, M.J., and Beckwith J., 1995, Tight regulation, modulation, and high-level expression by vectors containing the arabinose P_{BAD} promoter. *J. Bacteriol.* **177**: 4121-4130

Hamann, P.R., Hinman, L.M., Beyer, C.F., Lindh, D., Upeslacis, J., Flowers, D.A., and Bernstein, I., 2002a, An anti-CD33 antibody-calicheamicin conjugate for treatment of acute myeloid leukaemia. Choice of linker. *Bioconj. Chem.* **13**: 40-46

Hamann, P.R., Hinman, L.M., Hollander, I., Beyer, C.F., Lindh, D., Holocomb, R., Hallett, W., Tsou, H-R, Upeslacis, J., Shochat, D., Mountain, A., Flowers, D.A., and Bernstein, I., 2002b, Gentuzumab ozogamicin, a potent and selective anti-CD33 antibody-calicheamicin conjugate for treatment of acute myeloid leukaemia. *Bioconj. Chem.* **13**: 47-58

Hamers-Casterman, C., Atarhouch, T., Muyldermans, S., Robinson, G., Hamers, C., Songa, E.B., Bendahman, N., and Hamers, R., 1993, Naturally occurring antibodies devoid of light chains. *Nature* **363**: 446-448

Hamilton, G.E., Morton, P.H., Young, T.W., and Lyddiatt, A., 1999, Process intensification by direct product sequestration from batch fermentations: application of a fluidised bed, multi-bed external loop contactor. *Biotechnol. Bioeng.* **64**: 310-321

Hamilton, G.E., Luechau, F., Burton, S.C., and Lyddiatt, A., 2000, Development of a mixed mode adsorption process for the direct product sequestration of an extracellular protease from microbial batch cultures. *J. Biotechnol.* **79**: 103-115

Hansen, M.B., Lihme, A., Spitali, M., and King, D.J., 1999, Capture of Human Fab fragments by expanded bed adsorption with a mixed mode adsorbent. *Bioseparation* **8**: 189-193

Hara, S., and Yamakawa, M., 1996, Production in *Escherichia coli* of moricin, a novel type antibacterial peptide from the silkworm, Bombyx mori. *Biochem. Biophys. Res. Communic.* **220**: 664-669

Harrison, J.S., Gill, A., and Hoare, M., 1998, Stability of a single-chain Fv antibody fragment when exposed to a high shear environment combined with air-liquid interfaces. *Biotechnol. Bioeng.* **59**: 517-519

Haught, C., Davis, G.D., Subramanian, R., Jackson, K.W., and Harrison, R.G., 1998, Recombinant production and purification of novel antisense antimicrobial peptide in *Escherichia coli. Biotechnol. Bioeng.* **57**: 55-61

Hexham, J.M., King, V., Dudas, D., Graff, P., Mahnke, M., Wang, Y.K., Goetschy, J.F., Plattner, D., Zurini, M., Bitsch, F., Lake, P., and Digan, M.E., 2001, Optimization of the anti-(human CD3) immunotoxin DT389-scFv(UCHT1) N-terminal sequence to yield a homogeneous protein. *Biotechnol. Applied Biochem.* **34**: 183-187

Holliger, P., Wing, M., Pound, J.D., Bohlen, H., and Winter, G., 1997, Retargeting serum immunoglobulin with bispecific diabodies. *Nature Biotechnol.* **15**: 632-636

Hollis, G.F., and Mark, G.E., 1995, Homologous recombination antibody expression system for murine cells. *WO Patent*-95/17516

Holms, W.H., 1986, The central metabolic pathways of *Escherichia coli*: relationship between flux and control at a branch point, efficiency of conversion to biomass, and excretion of acetate. *Curr. Topics Cell. Reg.* **28**: 69-105

Horn, U., Strittmatter, W., Krebber, A., Knüpfer, U., Kujau, M., Wenderoth, R., Muller, K., Matzku, S., Plückthun, A., and Riesenberg, D., 1996, High volumetric yields of functional dimeric miniantibodies in *Escherichia coli*, using an optimized expression vector and high-cell-density fermentation under non-limited growth conditions. *Applied Microbiol. Biotechnol.* **46**: 524-532

Horwitz, A.H., Chang, C.P., Better, M., Hellstrom, K.E., and Robinson, R.R., 1988, Secretion of functional antibody and Fab' fragment from yeast cells. *Proc. Natl. Acad. Sci., U.S.A* **85**: 8678-8682

Hu, S.Z., Shively, L., Raubitschek, A., Sherman, M., Williams, L.E., Wong, J.Y.C., Shively, J.E., and Wu, A.M., 1996, Minibody: a novel engineered anti-carcinoembryonic antigen antibody fragment (single-chain Fv-C_H3) which exhibits rapid, high-level targeting of xenografts. *Cancer Res.* **56**: 3055-3061

Humphreys, D.P., 2003, Production of antibodies and antibody fragments in Escherichia coli and a comparison of their functions, uses and modification. *Curr. Opin. Drug Discov. Develop.* **6**: 188-196

Humphreys, D.P., and Glover, D.J., 2001, Therapeutic antibody production technologies: molecules, applications, expression and purification. *Curr. Opin. Drug Discov. Develop.* **4**: 172-185

Humphreys, D.P., Carrington, B., Bowering, L.C., Ganesh, R., Sehdev, M., Smith, B.J., King, L.M., Reeks, D.G., Lawson, A., and Popplewell, A.G., 2002, A plasmid system for the optimisation of Fab' production in *Escherichia coli*: importance of balance of heavy chain and light chain synthesis. *Prot. Expr. Purif.* **26**: 309-320

Humphreys, D.P., Chapman, A.P., Reeks, D.G., Lang, V., and Stephens, P.E., 1997, Formation of dimeric Fabs in *Escherichia coli*: effect of hinge size and isotype, presence of interchain disulphide bond, Fab' expression levels, tail piece sequences and growth conditions. *J. Immunol. Methods* **209**: 193-202

Humphreys, D.P., King, L.M., West, S.M., Chapman, A.P., Sehdev, M., Redden, M.W., Glover, D.J., Smith, B.J., and Stephens, P.E., 2000, Improved efficiency of site-specific copper(II) ion-catalysed protein cleavage effected by mutagenesis of cleavage site. *Prot. Eng.* **3**: 201-206

Humphreys, D.P., Vetterlein, O.M., Chapman, A.P., King, D.J., Antoniw, P., Suiters, A.J., Reeks, D.G., Parton, T.A.H., King, L.M., Smith, B.J., Lang, V., and Stephens, P.E., 1998, F(ab')$_2$ molecules made from *Escherichia coli* produced Fab' with hinge sequences conferring increased serum survival in an animal model. *J. Immunol. Methods* **217**: 1-10

Huston, J.S., Levinson, D., Mudgett-Hunter, M., Tai, M.S., Novotný, J., Margolies, M.N., Ridge, R.J., Bruccoleri, R.E., Haber, E., Crea, R., and Oppermann, H., 1988, Protein engineering of antibody binding sites: recovery of specific activity in an anti-digoxin single-chain Fv analogue produced in *Escherichia coli*. *Proc. Natl. Acad. Sci., U.S.A* **85**: 5879-5883

Jefferis, R., Lund, J., and Pound, J.D., 1998, IgG-Fc-mediated effector functions: molecular definition of interaction sites for effector ligands and the role of glycosylation. *Immunol. Rev.* **163**: 59-76

Jung, S., and Plückthun, A., 1997, Improving *in vivo* folding and stability of a single-chain Fv antibody fragment by loop grafting. *Prot. Eng.* **8**: 959-956

Jung, M., 2001, Antibody directed enzyme prodrug therapy (ADEPT) and related approaches for anticancer therapy. *Mini Rev. Medicinal Chem.* **1**: 399-407

Jurado, P., Titz, D., Beckwith, J., de Lorenzo, V., and Fernández, L.A., 2002, Production of functional single-chain Fv antibodies in the cytoplasm of *Escherichia coli*. *J. Mol. Biol.* **320**: 1-10

Karreman, S., Karreman, C., and Hauser, H., 1997, Construction of recombinant cell lines with defined properties using FLP recombinase driven gene replacement. In: *Animal Cell Technology* (M.J.T. Carrondo *et al.*, eds.), Kluwer Academic Publishers, Dordrecht, pp.511-516

King, D.J., 1998, *Applications and Engineering of Monoclonal Antibodies*. Taylor and Francis, London

King, D.J., Adair, J.R., Angal, S., Low, D.C., Proudfoot, K.A., Lloyd, J.C., Bodmer, M.W., and Yarranton, G.T., 1992, Expression, purification and characterisation of a mouse-human chimeric antibody and chimeric Fab' fragment. *Biochem. J.* **281**: 317-323

King, D.J., Antoniw, P., Owens, R.J., Adair, J.R., Haines, A.M.R., Farnsworth, A.P.H., Finney, H., Lawson, A.D.G., Lyons, A., Baker, T.S., Baldock, D., Mackintosh, J., Gofton, C., Tarranton, G.T., McWilliams, W., Shocat, D., Leichner, P.K., Welt, S., Old, L.J., and Mountain, A., 1995, Preparation and preclinical evaluation of humanised A33 immunoconjugates for radioimmunotherapy. *Br. J. Cancer* **72**: 1364-1372

King, D.J., Byron, O.D., Mountain, A., Weir, N., Harvey, A., Lawson, A.D.G., Proudfoot, K.A., Baldock, D., Harding, S.E., Yarranton, G.T., and Owens, R.J., 1993, Expression, purification and characterization of B72.3 Fv fragments. *Biochem. J.* **290**: 723-729

King, D.J., Turner, A., Farnsworth, A.P.H., Adair, J. R., Owens, R.J., Pedley, B., Baldock, D., Proudfoot, K.A., Lawson, A.D.G., Beeley, N.R.A., Millar, K., Millican, T.A., Boyce,

B.A., Antoniw, P., Mountain, A., Begent, R.H.J., Shochat, D., and Yarranton, G.T., 1994, Improved tumor targeting with chemically cross-linked recombinant antibody fragments. *Cancer Res.* **54**: 6176-6185

Kipriyanov, S.M., Moldenhauer, G., Martin, A.C.R., Kupriyanova O.A., and Little, M., 1997, Two amino acid mutations in an anti-human CD3 single chain Fv antibody fragment that affect the yield on bacterial secretion but not the affinity. *Prot. Eng.* **10**: 445-453

Knappik, A., and Plückthun, A., 1994, An improved affinity tag based on the FLAG epitope for detection and purification of recombinant antibody fragments. *Biotechniques* **17**: 754-761

Knappik, A., and Plückthun, A., 1995, Engineered turns of a recombinant antibody improve its *in vivo* folding. *Prot. Eng.* **8**: 81-89

Koelemij, R., Kuppen, P.J., van de Velde, P.J., Fleuren, G.J., Hagenaars, M., and Eggermont, A.M., 1999, Bispecific antibodies in cancer therapy, from the laboratory to the clinic. *J. Immunotherapy* **22**: 514-524

Koumenis, I.L., Shahrokh, Z., Leong, S., Hsei, V., Deforge, L., and Zapata, G., 2000, Modulating pharmacokinetics of an anti-interlukin-8 F(ab')$_2$ by amine-specific PEGylation with preserved bioactivity. *Int. J. Pharmaceutics* **198**: 83-95

Lee, M-H., Park, T-I., Park, Y-B., and Kwak, J-W., 2002, Bacterial expression and *in vitro* refolding of a single-chain Fv antibody specific for human plasma apolipoprotein B-100. *Prot. Expr. Purif.* **25**: 166-173

Lee, S.Y., 1996, High cell-density culture of *Escherichia coli. Trends Biotechnol.* **14**: 98-105

Leong, S.R., DeForge, L., Presta, L., Gonzalez, T., Fan, A., Reichert, M., Chuntharapai, A., Kim, K.J., Tumas, D.B., Lee, W.P., Gribling, P., Snedecor, B., Chen, H., Hsei, V., Schoenhoff, M., Hale, V., Deveney, J., Koumenis, I., Shahrokh, Z., McKay, P., Galan, W., Wagner, B., Narindray, D., Hébert, C., and Zapata, G., 2001, Adapting pharmacokinetic properties of a humanized anti-interleukin-8 antibody for therapeutic applications using site-specific PEGylation. *Cytokine* **16**: 106-119

Levy, R., Weiss, R., Chen, G., Iverson, B.L., and Georgiou, G., 2001, Production of correctly folded Fab antibody fragment in the cytoplasm of *Escherichia coli trxB gor* mutants *via* the coexpression of molecular chaperones. *Prot. Expr. Purif.* **23**: 338-347

Lu, D., Jiminez, X., Zhang, H., Bohlen, P., Witte, L., and Zhu, Z., 2002, Fab-scFv fusion protein: an efficient approach to production of bispecific antibody fragments. *J. Immunol. Methods* **267**: 213-226

Lihme, A., Hansen, M., Olander, M., and Zafirakos, E., 2000, Expanded bed adsorption in the purification of biomolecules. In *Methods in Biotechnology, Vol. 9: Downstream Processing of Proteins: Methods and Protocols* (M.A. Desai, ed.), Humana Press, Totowa, NJ, pp.121-139.

Lyddiatt, A., 2002, Process chromatography: current constraints and future options for the adsorptive recovery of bioproducts. *Curr. Opin. Biotechnol.* **13**: 95-103

Mallender, W.D., and Voss, E.W., 1994, Construction, expression, and activity of a bivalent bispecific single chain antibody. *J. Biol. Chem.* **269**: 199-206

Maynard, J., and Georgiou, G., 2000, Antibody Engineering. *Annu. Rev. Biomed. Eng.* **2**: 339-376

McConnell, S.J., Dinh, T., Le, M.H., Brown, S.J., Becherer, K., Bluymeyer, K., Kautzer, C., Axelrod, F., and Spinella, D.G., 1998, Isolation of erythropoietin receptor agonist peptides using evolved phage libraries. *Biol. Chem.* **379**: 1279-1286

Melton, R.G., and Sherwood, R.F., 1996, Antibody-enzyme conjugates for cancer therapy. *J. Natl. Cancer Inst.* **88**: 153-165

Mikolajczyk, S.D., Meyer, D.L., Fagnani, R., Hagan, M.S., Law, K.L., and Starling, J., 1996, Dextran modification of a Fab'-β-lactamase conjugate modulated by variable pre-treatment of Fab' with amine-blocking reagents. *Bioconj. Chem.* **7**: 150-158

Milenic, D.E., Yokota, T., Filpula, D.R., Finkelman, A.J., Dodd, S.W., Wood, J.F., Whitlow, M., Snoy, P., and Schlom, J., 1991, Construction, binding properties, metabolism, and tumor targeting of a single-chain Fv derived from the pancarcinoma monoclonal antibody CC49. *Cancer Res.* **51**: 6363-6371

Missiakas, D., and Raina, S., 1997, Protein folding in the bacterial periplasm. *J. Bacteriol.* **179**: 2465-2471

Müller, K.M., Arndt, K.M., Strittmatter, W., and Plückthun, A., 1998, The first constant domain (C_H1 and C_L) of an antibody used as heterodimerization domain for bispecific miniantibodies. *FEBS Letters* **422**: 259-264

Murray, A., Sekowski, M., Spencer, D.I.R., Denton, G., and Price, M.R., 1997, Purification of monoclonal antibodies by epitope and mimotope affinity chromatography. *J. Chromatography A* **782**: 49-54

Ng, H.C., and Khoo, H.E., 2002, Cancer-homing toxins. *Curr. Pharmaceut. Design* **8**: 1973-1985

Nieba, L., Honegger, A., Krebber, C., and Plückthun, A., 1997, Disrupting the hydrophobic patches at the antibody variable/ constant domain interface: improved *in vivo* folding and physical characterization of an engineered scFv fragment. *Prot. Eng.* **10**: 435-444

O'Shannessy, D.J., and Quarles, R.H., 1987, Labeling of the oligosaccharide moieties of immunoglobulins. *J. Immunol. Methods* **99**: 153-161

Pack, P., and Plückthun, A., 1992, Miniantibodies: use of amphipathic helices to produce functional, flexibly linked dimeric Fv fragments with high avidity in Escherichia coli. *Biochem.* **31**: 1579-1584

Peakman, T.C., Worden, J., Harris, R.H., Cooper, H., Tite, J., Page, M.J., Gewert, D.R., Bartholemew, M., Crowe, J.S., and Brett, S., 1994, Comparison of expression of a humanized monoclonal antibody in mouse NS0 myeloma cells and chinese hamster ovary cells. *Human Antibod. Hybridomas* **5**: 65-74

Pedley, R.B., Boden, J.A., Boden, R., Dale, R., and Begent, R.H.J., 1993, Comparative radioimmunotherapy using intact or F(ab')$_2$ fragments of ^{131}I anti-CEA antibody in a colonic xenograft model. *Br. J. Cancer* **68**: 69-73

Peeters, K., De Wilde, C., De Jaeger, G., Angenon, G., and Depicker, A., 2001, Production of antibodies and antibody fragments in plants. *Vaccine* **19**: 2756-2761

Pollock, D.P., Kutzko, J.P., Birck-Wilson, E., Williams, J.L., Echelard, Y., and Meade, H.M., 1999, Transgenic milk as a method for the production of recombinant antibodies. *J. Immunol. Methods* **231**: 147-157

Potter, K.N., Li, Y., and Capra, D., 1996, Staphylococcal protein A simultaneously interacts with framework region 1, complementarity-determining region 2, and framework region 3 on human V_H3-encoded Igs. *J. Immunol.* **157**: 2982-2988.

Powers, D.B., Amersdorfer, P., Poul, M-A., Nielson, U.B., Shalaby, M.R., Adams, G.P., Weiner, L.M., and Marks, J.D., 2001, Expression of single-chain Fv-Fc fusions in *Pichia pastoris*. *J. Immunol. Methods* **251**: 123-135

Presta, L.G., 2002, Engineering antibodies for therapy. *Curr. Pharmaceut. Biotechnol.* **3**: 237-256

Proba, K., Ge, L., and Plückthun, A., 1995, Functional antibody single-chain fragments from the cytoplasm of *Escherichia coli*: influence of thioredoxin reductase (TrxB). *Gene* **159**: 203-207

Proudfoot, K.A., Torrance, C., Lawson, A.D.G., and King, D.J., 1992, Purification of recombinant chimeric B72.3 Fab' and F(ab')$_2$ using Streptococcal protein G. *Prot. Expr. Purification* **3**: 368-373

Prinz, W.A., Åslund, F., Holmgren, A., and Beckwith, J., 1997, The role of the thioredoxin and glutaredoxin pathways in reducing protein disulfide bonds in the *Escherichia coli* cytoplasm. *J. Biol. Chem.* **272**: 15661-15667

Raag, R., and Whitlow, M., 1995, Single-chain Fvs. *FASEB J.* **9**: 73-80

Racher, A.J., Tong, J.M., and Bonnerjea, J., 1999, Manufacture of therapeutic antibodies. In *Recombinant proteins, monoclonal antibodies, and therapeutic genes. Vol 5a of Biotechnology, 2nd edition* (A. Mountain, U. Ney and D. Schomberg, eds.), Wiley-VCH, Weinheim pp.245-274

Ramm, K., and Plückthun, A., 2000, The periplasmic *Escherichia coli* peptidylprolyl *cis, trans*-isomerase FkpA. II. Isomerase-independent chaperone activity *in vitro*. *J. Biol. Chem.* **275**: 17106-1713

Ramm, K., and Plückthun, A., 2001, High enzymatic activity and chaperone function are mechanistically related features of the dimeric *E. coli* peptidyly-prolyl-isomerase FkpA. *J. Mol. Biol.* **310**: 485-498

Reddy, M.P., Kinney, C.A., Chaikin, M.A., Payne, A., Fishman-Lobell, J., Tsui, P., Dal Monte, P.R., Doyle, M.L., Brigham-Burke, M.R., Anderson, D., Reff, M., Newman, R., Hanna, N., Sweet, R.W., and Trunch, A., 2000, Elimination of Fc receptor-dependent effector functions of a modified IgG4 monoclonal antibody to human CD4. *J. Immunol.* **164**: 1925-1933

Riechman, L., Foote, J., and Winter, G., 1988, Expression of an antibody Fv fragment in myeloma cells. *J. Mol. Biol.* **203**: 825-828

Riechmann, L., and Muyldermans, S., 1999, Single domain antibodies: comparison of camel vH and camelised human vH domains. *J. Immunol. Methods* **231**: 25-38

Riesenberg, D., Schulz, V., Knorre, W.A., Pohl, H.D., Korz, D., Sanders, E.A., Ross, A., and Deckwer, R.A., 1991, High cell density cultivation of *Escherichia coli* at a controlled specific growth rate. *J. Biotechnol.* **20**: 17-27

Rodrigues, M.L., Shalaby, M.R., Werther, W., Presta, L., and Carter, P., 1992, Engineering a humanized bispecific F(ab')$_2$ fragment for improved binding to T cells. *Intl. J. Cancer Suppl.* **7**: 45-50

Rodrigues, M.L., Snedecor, B., Chen, C., Wong, W.L.T., Garg, S., Blank, G.S., Maneval, D., and Carter, P., 1993, Engineering Fab' fragments for efficient F(ab')$_2$ formation in *Escherichia coli* and for improved in vivo stability. *J. Immunol.* **151**: 6954-6961

Rodwell, J.D., Alvarez, V.L., Lee, C., Lopes, A.D., Goers, J.W.F., King, H.D., Powsner, H.J., and McKearn, T.J., 1986, Site-specific covalent modification of monoclonal antibodies: *in vitro* and *in vivo* evaluations. *Proc. Natl. Acad. Sci. USA* **83**: 2632-2636

Rudolph, N., 1999, Biopharmaceutical production in transgenic livestock. *Trends Biotechnol.* **17**: 367-374

Saga, T., Neumann, R.D., Heya, T., Sato, J., Kinuya, S., Le, N., Paik, C.H., and Weinstein, J.N., 1995, Targeting cancer micrometastases with monoclonal antibodies: a binding-site barrier. *Proc. Natl. Acad. Sci. USA* **92**: 8999-9003

Sandén, A.M., Prytz, I., Tubulekas, I., Försberg, C., Le, H., Hektor, A., Neubauer, P., Pragai, Z., Harwood, C., Ward, A., Picon, A., de Mattos, J.T., Postma, P., Farewell, A., Nyström, T., Reeh, S., Pederson, S., and Larsson, G., 2003, Limiting factors in *Escherichia coli* fed-batch production of recombinant proteins. *Biotechnol. Bioeng.* **81**: 158-166

Schmidt, T.G.M., and Skerra, A., 1994, One-step affinity purification of bacterially produced proteins by means of the strep-tag and immobilized recombinant core streptavadin. *J. Chromatography A:* **676**: 337-343

Segal, D.M., Weiner, G.J., and Weiner, L.M., 1999, Bispecific antibodies in cancer therapy. *Curr. Opin. Immunol.* **11**: 558-562

Schott, M.E., Frazier, K.A., Pollock, D.K., and Verbanac, K.M., 1993, Preparation, characterization, and *in vivo* biodistribution properties of synthetically cross-linked multivalent antitumour antibody fragments. *Bioconj. Chem.* **4**: 153-165

Sharkey, R.M., Karacay, H., Griffiths, G.L., Behr, T.M., Blumenthal, R.D., Mattes, M.J., Hansen, H.J., and Goldenberg, D.M., 1997, Development of a streptavadin-anti carcinoembryonic antigen antibody, radiolabeled biotin pretargeting method for radioimmunotherapy of colorectal cancer. Studies in a human xenograft model. *Bioconj. Chem.* **8**: 595-604

Shusta, E.V., Raines, R.T., Plückthun, A., and Wittrup, K.D., 1998, Increasing the secretory capacity of *Saccharomyces cerevisiae* for production of single-chain antibody fragments. *Nature Biotechnol.* **16**: 773-777

Simmons, L.C., Reilly, D., Klimowski, L., Raju, T.S., Meng, G., Sims, P., Hong, K., Shields, R.L., Damico, L.A., Rancatore, P., and Yansura, D.G., 2002, Expression of full-length immunoglobulins in *Escherichia coli*: rapid and efficient production of aglycosylated antibodies. *J. Immunol. Methods* **263**: 133-147

Skerra, A., 1994, Use of the tetracycline promoter for the tightly regulated production of a murine antibody fragment in *Escherichia coli*. *Gene* **151**: 131-135

Smith, B.J., Popplewell, A., Athwal, D., Chapman, A.P., Heywood, S., West, S.M., Carrington, B., Nesbitt, A., Lawson, A.D.G., Antoniw, P., Eddleston, A., and Suiters, A., 2001, Prolonged *in vivo* residence times of antibody fragments associated with albumin. *Bioconj. Chem.* **12**: 750-756

Sproule, K., Morrill, P., Pearson, J.C., Burton, S.J., Hejnaes, K.R., Valore, H., Ludvigsen, S., and Lowe, C.R., 2000, New strategy for the design of ligands for the purification of pharmaceutical proteins by affinity chromatography. *J. Chromatography B.* **740**: 17-33

Stan, A.C., Radu, D.L., Casares, S., Bona, C.A., and Brumeanu, T-D., 1999, Antineoplastic efficacy of doxorubicin enzymatically assembled on galactose residues of a monoclonal antibody specific for carcinoembryonic antigen. *Cancer Res.* **59**: 115-121

Studier, F.W., Rosenberg, A.H., Dunn, J.J., and Dubendorff, J.W., 1990, Use of T7 RNA polymerase to direct expression of cloned genes. *Methods Enzymol.* **185**: 60-89

Tacon, W.C.A., Bonass, W.A., Jenkins, B., and Emtage, J.S., 1983, Expression plasmid vectors containing *Escherichia coli* tryptophan promoter transcriptional units lacking the attenuator. *Gene* **23**: 255-265

Teng, S.F., Sproule, K., Husain, A., and Lowe, C.R., 2000, Affinity chromatography on immobilized "biomimetic" ligands. Synthesis, immobilization and chromatographic assessment of an immunoglobulin G-binding ligand. *J. Chromatography B.* **740**: 1-15

Todorovska, A., Roovers, R.C., Dolezal, O., Kortt, A.A., Hoogenboom, H.R., and Hudson, P.J., 2001, Design and application of diabodies, triabodies and tetrabodies for cancer targeting. *J. Immunol. Methods* **248**: 47-66

Trepod, C.M., and Mott, J.E., 2002, A spontaneous runaway vector for production-scale expression of bovine somatotropin from *Escherichia coli*. *Appl. Microbiol Biotechnol.* **58**: 84-88

van Spriel, A.B., van Ojik, H.H., and van de Winkel, J.G.J., 2000, Immunotherapeutic perspective for bispecific antibodies. *Immunol. Today* **21**: 391-397

Venturi, M., Seifert, C., and Hunte, C., 2002, High level production of functional antibody Fab fragments in an oxidizing bacterial cytoplasm. *J. Mol. Biol.* **315**: 1-8

Verma, R., Boleti, E., and George, A.J.T., 1998, Antibody engineering: comparison of bacterial, yeast, insect and mammalian expression systems. *J. Immunol. Methods* **216**: 165-181

Wall, J.G., and Plückthun, A., 1999, The hierarchy of mutations influencing the folding of antibody domains in *Escherichia coli*. *Prot. Eng.* **12**: 605-611

Weir, A.N.C., and Bailey, N.A., 1994, Process for obtaining antibodies utilizing heat treatment. *US Patent* 5665866

Weir, A.N.C., Nesbitt, A., Chapman, A.P., Popplewell, A.G., Antoniw, P., and Lawson, A.D.G., 2002, Formatting antibody fragments to mediate specific therapeutic functions. *Biochem. Soc. Transactions* **30**: 512-516

Wentworth, P., Datta, A., Blakey, D., Boyle, T., Partridge, L.J., and Blackburn, G.M., 1996, Toward antibody-directed "abzyme" prodrug therapy, ADAPT: carbamate prodrug activation by a catalytic antibody and its *in vitro* application to human tumor cell killing. *Proc. Natl. Acad. Sci. USA* **93**: 799-803

Werlen, R.C., Lankinen, M., Offord, R.E., Schubiger, P.A., Smith, A., and Rose, K., 1996, Preparation of a trivalent antigen-binding construct using polyoxime chemistry: improved biodistribution and potential for therapeutic application. *Cancer Res.* **56**: 809-815

Willner, D., Trail, P.A., Hofstead, S.J., King, H.D., Lasch, S.J., Braslawsky, G.R., Greenfield, R.S., Kaneko, T., and Firestone, R.A., 1993, (6-Maleimidocaprolyl)hydrazone of doxorubicin – a new derivative for the preparation of immunoconjugates of doxorubicin. *Bioconj. Chem.* **4**: 521-527

Wood, C.R., Dorner, A.J., Morris, G.E., Alderman, E.M., Wilson, D., O'Hara Jr., R.M., and Kaufman, R.J., High level synthesis of immunoglobulins in chinese hamster ovary cells. *J. Immunol.* **145**: 3011-3016

Wörn, A., and Plückthun, A., 2001, Stability engineering of antibody single-chain Fv fragments. *J. Mol. Biol.* **305**: 989-1010

Xu, G., and McLeod, H.L., 2001, Strategies for enzyme/prodrug cancer therapy. *Clin. Cancer Res.* **7**: 3314-3324

Yee, L., and Blanch, H.W., 1992, Recombinant protein expression in high cell density fed-batch cultures of *Escherichia coli*. *Bio/Technology* **10**: 1550-1556

Young, W.W., Tamura, Y., Wolcock, D.M., and Fox, J.W., 1984, Staphylococcal protein A binding to the Fab fragments of mouse monoclonal antibodies. *J. Immunol.* **133**: 3163-3166

Zalipsky, S., 1995, Functionalized poly(ethylene glycol) for preparation of biologically relevant conjugates. *Bioconj. Chem.* **6**: 150-165

Zapata, G., Ridgway, J.B.B., Mordenti, J., Osaka, G., Wong, W.L.T., Bennett, G.L., and Carter, P., 1995, Engineering linear F(ab')$_2$ fragments for efficient production in *Escherichia coli* and enhanced antiproliferative activity. *Prot. Eng.* **8**: 1057-1062

Zhu, Z., Zapata, G., Shalaby, R., Snedecor, B., Chen, H., and Carter, P., 1996, High level secretion of a humanized bispecific diabody from *Escherichia coli*. *Bio/Technology* **14**: 192-196

Zhu, Z., Presta, L.G., Zapata, G., and Carter, P., 1997, Remodeling domain interfaces to enhance heterodimer formation. *Prot. Sci.* **6**: 781-788

Zwick, M.B., Shen, J., and Scott, J.K., 1998, Phage-displayed peptide libraries. *Curr. Opin. Biotechnol.* **9**: 427-436

Chapter 3

LARGE-SCALE PRODUCTION OF THERAPEUTIC ANTIBODIES: CONSIDERATIONS FOR OPTIMIZING PRODUCT CAPTURE AND PURIFICATION

Glen Kemp[a] and Paul O'Neil[b]
[a]Millipore (UK) Ltd. Consett, County Durham UK., [b]Euroflow (UK) Ltd. Stratham, NH, USA.

1. INTRODUCTION

The first therapeutic proteins produced by fermentation of genetically engineered bacteria emerged two decades ago. With the notable exception of insulin, most of the initial wave of biotechnology products launched in the 1980s and 1990s were peptide hormones and enzymes licensed for indications with relatively small patient populations and for short–term rather than chronic use. Consequently, the market requirement for these products was frequently in the low kilogram range.

Products based on monoclonal antibody technology have now reached the market and are creating new pressures for production technology. Two factors combine to increase product requirements significantly – larger patient populations and long term use in chronic indications. There are now several monoclonal therapeutics both on the market and in clinical trials for which the requirements are at or approaching hundreds of kilograms. This has had ramifications across the industry and has impacted all aspects of drug development. Most notably, this demand has spurred drug developers to dramatically expand fermentation capacity, locate capacity at contract manufacturers or explore alternatives such as microbial expression or transgenic technology. Fermentation groups are reporting expression levels into the gram range by different techniques, and drug developers are exploring ways to boost the potency of antibodies with directed evolution or by coupling with cytotoxins or radiochemicals, indirectly reducing requirements for bulk product. Despite these measures, pressure will continue to be placed on the downstream process to cope with ever-larger amounts of antibody.

The requirement for an ever-increasing mass of antibody is only part of the story. The key driver before product approval is the 'time to market'. It is critical to get product in time and in sufficient amounts and with high enough purity for clinical trials to take place. Once product approval has been gained, there is usually a fundamental shift in emphasis towards a reduced cost of goods and increased process efficiency, both in terms of yield and reliability. This has occurred in several companies with large scale antibody products on the market and will undoubtedly occur for many more companies when they too reach this stage of growth. One of the key lessons to be learned from this is that the 'product' from a pilot scale group should not only be clinical trial material but also a process that is robust, scalable and cost effective. In order to achieve this, process optimization should be considered from the very earliest stages in the pilot plant.

Well designed processes will not only yield sufficiently pure protein but will also maximize throughput and minimize process costs. Efficient processes can decrease the requirement for fermentation capacity significantly, with a direct impact on capital resources for the size of the recovery operations and facilities, and further savings in cost of goods once a plant comes online. There is of course a compromise in terms of time to market, but investment in intensive process development can lead to eventual savings in capital costs and cost of goods sold.

Recent developments in process design and implementation have focused on strategies to improve overall economics. These include: *improvements in throughput*, which decrease scale of individual process steps, shorten turnaround times and improve utilization of equipment, and *process compression* to combine one or more steps into a smaller unit area and decrease raw material consumption, hardware requirements and overall footprint. These approaches have been used both in isolation and in combination.

In this chapter we discuss strategies for increasing process throuhout and examine how these improvements can be applied to large-scale antibody purification, focussing particular attention on optimizing product capture and trace contaminant removal. We then review a series of new or emerging methodologies being applied to enhance process efficiency and improve economics.

Large-scale production of therapeutic antibodies 77

2. PURIFICATION PROCESSES

2.1 Production/Purification Goals and Challenges

Modern therapeutic monoclonal antibodies and their derivatives are produced as recombinant proteins most often via mammalian cell fermentation. These production systems are capable of relatively high levels of product expression and with a degree of glycosylation sufficient to enhance biological activity at the therapeutic application. Relative to more physically stable microbial cultures, mammalian cell fermentation results in somewhat more challenging feed streams due in large part to host cell-derived contaminants liberated by cell attrition. In addition to host cells and cell debris, contaminants include host cell proteins, media additives (serum supplements or protein/other additives such as growth promoters or stabilizers), adventitious agents such as viruses and bacterial pathogens or breakdown products of same (e.g., endotoxins), and any potential leachates from contact surfaces of equipment. Impurities may include incompletely expressed product, remnants of proteolysis of target or other proteins, and aggregates of the target product. Increasingly, there is a trend towards higher expression levels resulting in a lower relative content of impurities. However the higher stress placed on the cells can result in a change in the profile of the contaminants which may in turn increase stress on the downstream purification process.

Table 3.1. Common process compounds and methods of removal or purification

Component	Culture harvest level	Final product level	Conventional method
Therapeutic Antibody	0.1-1.5 g/l	1-10 g/l	UF/Cromatography
Isoforms	Various	Monomer	Chromatography
Serum and host proteins	0.1-3.0 g/l	< 0.1-10 mg/l	Chromatography
Cell debris and colloids	10^6/ml	None	MF
Bacterial pathogens	Various	$<10^{-6}$/dose	MF
Virus pathogens	Various	$<10^{-6}$/dose (12 LRV)	virus filtration
DNA	1 mg/l	10 ng/dose	Chromatography
Endotoxins	Various	<0.25 EU/ml	Chromatography
Lipids, surfactants	0-1 g/l	<0.1-10 mg/l	Chromatography
Buffer	Growth media	Stability media	UF
Extractables/leachables	Various	<0.1-10 mg/l	UF/ Chromatography
Purification reagents	Various	<0.1-10mg/l	UF

Conventionally, a combination of several filtration and chromatographic methods are employed and work in aggregate and, ideally, in concert, to improve the purity and maintain the quality of the target biotherapeutic. Table 3.1 lists the downstream processing method that is primarily responsible for achieving reduction of each contaminant class.

2.2   Generic processing

The current practice of large-scale monoclonal purification, with protein A affinity capture as the cornerstone, represents perhaps the closest the industry comes to a generic downstream process. In addition to reducing development costs, it simplifies manufacturing implementation and enhances reliability at all phases of manufacturing. Applying a generic approach for similar molecules also simplifies some of the regulatory considerations. For example, while the effectiveness of a given processing step must be proven for each therapeutic and each facility, development of the protocols and systems employed to generate validation data need only occur once.

For the purposes of this discussion, processes are divided into the following general phases: (1) *initial capture*, in which the harvested culture is clarified and the target product is rapidly isolated and concentrated on an adsorbing medium, and (2) *contaminant removal*, in which contaminants remaining at sub parts per hundred are removed by a series of purification and finishing or polishing steps.

A summary of methods developed to address the downstream processing needs of monoclonal antibody production is provided in Table 3.2. Most of these are applied today in conventional large scale processing, but others that are not yet fully employed are listed for completeness. A more thorough description of the most widely used of these methods and the relative effectiveness and practicality of each is discussed below.

Table 3.2. Commonly used downstream processing methods

Processing method	Attributes	Benefits	Limitations
Clarification:			
Sedimentation based clarification	Continuous centrifugation	Capable of handling very large harvest volumes	Open process- contamination and safety issues
Normal flow Filtration	Microporous		Volume and throughput limited
	Charged filter media		
	Cellulose pads		
Tangential flow filtration	Contained systems	Capable of handling large harvest volumes	

Large-scale production of therapeutic antibodies 79

Processing method	Attributes	Benefits	Limitations
Capture: Chromatography	Protein A Affinity	High throughput, high purity	High initial cost
	Other affinity ligands	High throughput	Purity, regulatory acceptance
	Cation exchange	Low cost media	Low throughput, feedstock preconditioning
Simultaneous clarification and capture	Expanded bed adsorption (EBA)	Reduces unit operations	Sensitive to feed variations and fouling. Challenge for sanitization
Purification: Chromatography	Ion exchange, HIC, hydroxyapatite, IMAC	Variety of selectivities, high capacity, robust	Often flow rate limited
Adsorptive membrane	Charged membranes	High throughput, contained, suited to trace contaminant removal	Low capacities

2.3 Initial Capture (clarification and initial recovery)

The initial steps after fermentation are designed to remove solids and particulates, to reduce volumes and to bring product to a stable holding point as quickly as possible. In practice, this means harvesting a 10,000-liter fermenter and processing product through at least the first recovery step to prevent degradative exposure to proteolytic enzymes and/or product breakdown due to instability.

Centrifugation can be used to clarify cell culture feedstocks. Stacked disk centrifuges are capable of handling large volumes of liquid and are well suited to removal of cells; however, there may be disruption of the cells during the process, increasing the burden placed on the subsequent downstream step. It can be a challenge to maintain sterility within a stacked disk centrifuge and pre- and post-use preparation of the equipment is laborious. More recently developed formats for large scale spinning bowl centrifuges are now available which are designed for use in a clean environment and offer significant advantages over disk stack centrifuges for clarification. Advances include automated semi-continuous operation and programmable cleaning cycles.

A number of filtration approaches are possible to achieve clarification of mammalian cell harvest. At industrial scale, a succession of methods are employed, grouped within 3 stages: primary, secondary and sterilizing. Primary clarification removes whole cells and large particles by centrifugation or microfiltration in either the tangential or normal flow mode. Secondary clarification clears colloidal particulate and any other material that can shorten the life of finer filters downstream. The sterilizing filter, frequently 0.22 um pore size, eliminates bacteria and other remaining bioburden prior to the first chromatography unit operation.

2.4 Clarification Process Compression

Traditionally, secondary filtration has been accomplished with a series of depth filters of diminishing pore size, typically in two or three stages (e.g., 1 um followed by 0.2 um, etc.). Considerable development/optimization can be required, as efficient pre-filtration must be achieved to ensure adequate capacity at each subsequent filtration step. This has been especially problematic for mammalian cell cultures both because they are more costly to produce than other systems and they tend to carry higher colloid loads.

The excessive consumption of facility floor space and the inevitable loss of yield at each step have motivated several suppliers to design advanced composite, multi-layered alternatives for increased filter capacity. These composite membranes, with biphasic characteristics, incorporate an initial charged depth filter to remove coarse particulates, followed by a finer filtration surface within the same device. Further development has resulted in devices which also include a charge on one of the coarse filter layers to act as a further pre-conditioning step prior to downstream purification (Figure 3.1). The incorporation of the coarse elements protect the finer filter and prolong usage while the integration into a single device reduces the amount of handling required at this process stage. The result is compression of the process train and highly effective protection of the sterilizing filter.

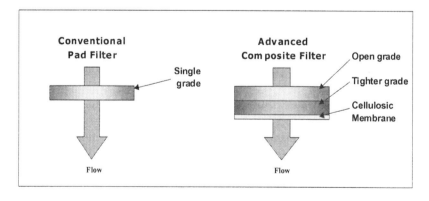

Figure 3.1 Composite membrane construction of Millistack HC+ (Millipore).

3. CAPTURE CHROMATOGRAPHY

Affinity chromatography using immobilized Protein A provides the foundation for all current large scale antibody processes due to its exquisite selectivity, an ability to load/bind product with minimal pre-treatment of the feed, and relatively simple and generic protocols. Such highly selective initial capture steps can be scaled for the target compound and need not have significant excess capacity to handle additional material in the sample. Some of the largest columns installed today range up to several hundred liters in scale, but the alternatives using ion exchange would be an order of magnitude larger. Protein A capture achieves removal of bulk contaminants (host cell protein, DNA, virus, and elements of the cell culture medium) resulting in a purity of >95% and product concentration in a single step. An additional benefit of the use of protein A affinity capture is the integrated hold in low pH elution buffer, providing partial compliance with product safety requirements of two orthogonal methods/steps to accomplish virus clearance (as discussed in section 3.4.4).

3.1 Protein A Affinity chromatography process considerations

Increasing productivity by good process design has become a significant area of research (Kamiya *et al.* 1990, Yamamoto and Sano 1992, Kemp *et al.* 2001). The rate limiting parameter of initial capture chromatography is traditionally the flow rate capability of the capture media at a point in the process in which process volumes are greatest, and the potential for product loss via proteolytic degradation is highest. Process economics for the capture step at commercial scale are dictated by the rate at which the target product is isolated (*productivity*), the media and buffer volumes consumed, and the footprint or plant area occupied by the operation.

Over recent years, increases in antibody expression levels have been shifting the bottleneck in affinity protein A capture from volume limitation to time limitation. As seen in Table 3.3, a 10-fold increase in antibody expression level from 100mg/litre to 1000mg/litre will be accompanied by a 10-fold decrease in the volume of loading material. In such cases, very high flow rate media offer less of an advantage over moderate flow rate media. Thus it can be seen that a reduction from a 20 hour load to a 7 hour load is highly desirable, but a reduction from 2 hours to 40 minutes, although useful, is less dramatic. Hence, for high concentrations of IgG, the emphasis is placed on high capacity media over high flow ratecapabilities. However, for expression levels of IgG below 1g/litre, which is still commonly the case, especially in the early development phases, high flow rate operation will still confer a significant throughput advantage. New versions of the two most widely used industrial scale protein A affinity media have recently been introduced (MabSelect, Amersham Biosciences, PROSEP Ultra, Millipore) which offer both high capacity and increased flow capability compared to previous media.

Table 3.3. Effect of expression levels on process parameters and throughput

Expression level:	100mg/litre	100mg/litre	1000mg/litre	1000mg/litre
Media:	PROSEP A HC	FF Sepharose A	PROSEP A HC	FF Sepharose A
Operating flow velocity	600 cm/hr	200 cm/hr	600 cm/hr	200 cm/hr
Column size	250mm diameter x 200mm bed	250mm diameter x 200mm bed	250mm diameter x 200mm bed	250mm diameter x 200mm bed
Dynamic binding capacity	20 mg/ml	20 mg/ml	20 mg/ml	20 mg/ml
Load volume	2000 litres	2000 litres	200 litres	200 litres
Load time	6.8 hours	20.4 hours	0.68 hours	2 hours
Wash/elute/regen time	0.68 hours	2 hours	0.68 hours	2 hours
Cycle time (hrs)	7.5	22.4	1.4	4
IgG Throughput	26.8 g /hr	8.9 g/hr	147 g/hr	50 g/hr

3.2 Optimizing Protein A media for maximal productivity

3.2.1 Throughput and productivity

The key parameters to consider when optimizing a protein A capture step are throughput, defined as: the mass of antibody produced per unit time, and productivity, defined as: the throughput per litre of media per unit cost. Throughput is relatively easy to determine. First, the optimum combination of dynamic binding capacity and flow rate should be established. In general, as the flow rate is increased, the dynamic binding capacity will decrease; clearly these two parameters are in conflict. A common mistake in optimizing the protein A capture process is to try and achieve the highest dynamic binding capacity possible. This can only happen at low flow rates, i.e. long residence times for the antibody within the packed bed. However, long residence times will result in long cycle times which are inefficient in terms of throughput (mass of antibody *per unit time*). From a plot of residence time versus dynamic binding capacity (Figure 3.2) for variants of

Large-scale production of therapeutic antibodies 83

PROSEP A affinity media (Millipore), it can be seen that, for residence times above 3 minutes, the relative increase in binding capacity is disproportionate to the time this will add to the process cycles. Similarly, decreasing the residence time too far will require a larger number of very short cycles. The practical considerations of equipment capabilities and QC burden generally make the use of very large numbers of short cycles less economically efficient, even though they may be very efficient in terms of throughput.

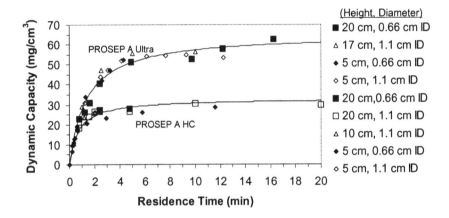

Figure 3.2. Effect of residence time on dynamic binding capacity for hIgG.

The relationship between flow rate and capacity can be modeled. Several authors have reported using eqn 1 or close derivations to characterize the performance of media. The values of Qmax and tau will be specific for each media. It can also be seen that flow rate is expressed indirectly, in terms of residence time (eqn 2). This allows the flow rate to be normalized to any column bed height. In practice, very short beds (<5cm) tend to show distribution anomalies, whereas very long beds (>60cm) will require unreasonably high flow rates to achieve even modest residence times; thus operation tends to remain within these nominal boundaries

$$Q_d = \frac{Q_{max} \times t_r}{\tau + t_r}$$ eqn 1

Q_d is the dynamic capacity (mg/ml or g/l)
Q_{max} is the theoretical maximum dynamic capacity
t_r is the residence time (in minutes or seconds)
τ (tau) is the residence time required for $Q_d = 1/2 \times Q_{max}$

$$t_r = \frac{60 \times CSA \times h}{U} \quad \text{eqn 2}$$

t_r = Residence time in seconds
CSA = cross section area of the column in cm^2
h = bed height in cm
U = Flow rate in ml per minute

High throughput and favorable process economics in process-scale antibody purification trains are achieved through the use of chromatography media possessing high capacity, high permeability, and good chemical stability (i.e. re-usable for multiple cycles). A fully rigid matrix clearly offers high flow rate capability but, in order for this to translate into higher productivity, the adsorptive media must also allow rapid mass transfer of target solutes to and from available binding sites to enable high dynamic capacity. When extremely high capture rates are enabled by these media properties, then very large fermenter harvest volumes (>10,000 l) can be accommodated economically by rapid cycling of the protein A capture step using a proportionately reduced capture column size (Table 3.4). The use of smaller columns offers capital cost savings via both by reducing equipment costs and by minimizing the space consumed in the purification suite. Since the column will experience more frequent use, the immediately obvious savings in media costs must be substantiated by proving long media lifetime (expressed as usable cycle #).

Table 3.4. Productivity and scheduling

Parameter	Case 1	Case 2
Sample volume (litres)	10,000	10,000
Sample concentration (g/l)	1	1
Loading flow velocity (cm/hr)	500	750
Elution regeneration flow (cm/hr)	500	1000
Column diameter (cm)	80	60
Bed height (cm)	20	25
Column volume (litres)	100	71
Number of cycles	5	6
Time (hours)	7.8	7.7

Production rates in the protein A capture step have been the focus of several recent studies (Fahrner *et al*. 1999b, H. Iyer 2002, Garcia *et al*. 2003). Iyer *et al*. demonstrated that a capture affinity medium enabling 2.5-fold higher processing rate offset that medium's lower adsorption capacity and provided higher productivity and reduction in overall processing costs for the purification of a humanized monoclonal antibody. The above authors all point to the ultimate importance of considering productivity (mass of IgG x h^{-1} x L bed volume^{-1}), rather than dynamic binding capacity (mass IgG/ L bed volume) alone, when establishing overall processing costs. In studies comparing productivity within the permeability-dependent flow constraints of various protein A media, Fahrner, et al. (1999a). showed that the highest productivity resulted from use of rigid media. Production rates (P_r) for different human IgG feed concentrations and residence times were determined for PG 700 and PG 1000 using equation 3 adopted from Fahrner et al. (1999b):

$$P_r = \frac{1}{1000\left(\frac{1}{C_o U_L} + \frac{N}{Q_d U_E}\right)} \qquad \text{eqn 3}$$

where production rate is a function of five parameters: dynamic capacity (Q_d), protein concentration in the feed (C_o); number of column volumes for product recovery and column regeneration for repeat cycling, including wash, elute, clean and equilibration steps (N), load velocity (U_L), and regeneration velocity (U_E). Twenty (N=20) column volumes were assumed for recovery and regeneration.

Having determined the relationship between residence time and dynamic binding capacity, and knowing the permeability (pressure drop) of a media it is possible to use this equation to model the productivity over a range of flow rates and bed heights. Limits can be set to reflect maximum pressure capabilities of the system -- either the media or the hardware, whichever is the lower -- and also by selecting a maximum cycle time beyond which the process would be deemed uneconomical. Such a plot provides an indication of the envelope of operation for a given media. It can be seen from Figure 3.3 that a rigid permeable media with efficient mass transfer properties will afford the process developer a much greater scope of operation, allowing taller packed beds and faster flow rates to be fully exploited.

As noted above, the trend towards higher expression levels in mammalian fermentation systems is changing the optimal performance window for capture media. To address this, manufacturers have developed higher capacity media which are still capable of operating at high flow rates. One such media is PROSEP A Ultra. This is based on a controlled pore glass as is the case for standard PROSEP A HC but, in order to achieve a higher capacity, a controlled pore glass bead with a smaller pore diameter was selected. The pore size was reduced from 1000A down to 700A (Figure 3.4). This resulted in an increase in surface area from 23m^2/ml to 35m^2/ml. The glass beads were activated and protein A immobilized using the same chemistry as PROSEP A HC. Dynamic binding capacity tests were performed to confirm that the additional capacity was available for binding.

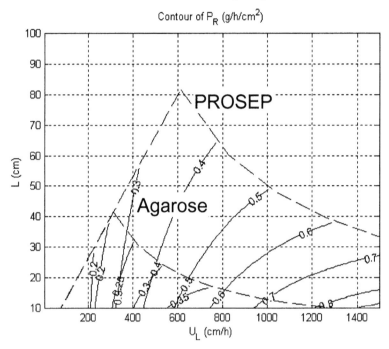

Figure 3.3. Productivity profiles

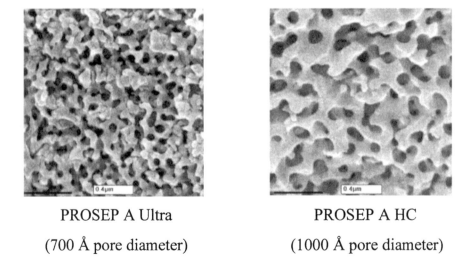

PROSEP A Ultra

(700 Å pore diameter)

PROSEP A HC

(1000 Å pore diameter)

Figure 3.4. Scanning electron micrographs of 700A and 1000A pore size glass beads.

The productivity models discussed above were then used to determine the effect, if any, of this increase in available binding capacity.

Plotting production rates obtained for a range of feed concentrations and load residence times showed that PROSEP A Ultra and PROSEP A HC achieved similar production rates at hIgG feed concentrations ≤ 1.0 mg/cm^3. However, as the hIgG feed concentration increased, the production rate for PROSEP A Ultra became greater than for PROSEP A HC. The reason for this is that, at lower expression levels, the greater volume required to saturate the PROSEP A Ultra media cancels out the benefits of higher capacity by requiring a significantly longer time to load. However, as the concentration of antibody increased, the relative impact of load time was reduced and the productivity increased. This is in agreement with the trends shown in Table 3.3.

Additional studies conducted by the authors have shown a similar trend for the purification of an Fc fusion protein. It is possible, however, that for antibody constructs that are larger than IgG (e.g., conjugates or high MW fusion proteins), the PG 1000 medium would exhibit higher productivity than the PG 700, due to greater accessibility to internal pore surface area and binding sites.

3.3 Scaling-up by changing bed height

A consensus practice has formed which teaches scale up of the protein A capture step based on residence time, rather than by holding velocity and bed height constant (Malmquist at al. 2000, Kemp *et al.* 2001). This is in contrast to the conventional scale-up procedure in which the bed height is held constant and scale up is by increasing the column diameter alone (Figure 3.5). In this latter case, the volumetric flow rate is adjusted according the to the ratio of cross sectional areas of the columns. When scaling up by increasing bed height, the important parameter to maintain constant is the residence time within the column for a notional IgG molecule. It can be seen that scale up by diameter is, in effect, a special subset of scale up by maintaining residence time. Conceptually linked to this practice is an understanding that flexibility in column geometry delivers measurable economic benefit by the use of smaller diameter, taller beds. Savings are derived from lower equipment costs and facility space savings. Taller columns of smaller diameter, which nevertheless are of the same bed volume, can cost half as much as wider, shorter alternatives, and can occupy one half the space required for packing and operating.

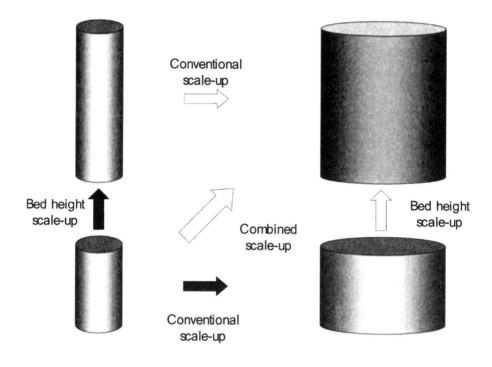

Figure 3.5 Scale-up options for protein A affinity chromatography

When scaling up by increasing bed height, care should be taken not to exceed the pressure limits of the equipment or media. In the case of compressible media such as agarose, the limiting factor will usually be the mechanical strength of the media itself. With rigid media the maximum operating pressure will usually be dictated by the pressure limitation of the column.

3.4 Other considerations for the Protein A capture step

3.4.1 Elution conditions

Antibody fragmentation and aggregation can be significant contributors to product yield loss. The harshness of acidic elution conditions is one of the most common causes for aggregation. Therefore, thorough methods development should include establishing the minimum pH required to recover product and to optimize its isolation from aggregates, contaminating antibodies, or antibody fragments.

3.4.2 Media lifetime

When considering the cost impact of the protein A capture step, a key factor is the lifetime of the media. This should always be considered in conjunction with the initial acquisition of the media when making comparisons against other methods. As the number of use cycles increases, the initial media purchase cost becomes much less significant in proportion to other process costs such as labour, process buffers and plant overheads. Often these costs are not obvious during development stages.

Protein A is a robust protein capable of withstanding exposures to pH as low as 1.5. However, it is less stable in high pH environments. Although immobilization increases the alkaline stability of protein A, the use of high concentrations of NaOH sufficient to sanitize the media are still not feasible. This means that, unlike ion-exchange media and hydrophobic interaction media, cleaning and sanitizing methods using 0.5-1.0M NaOH are not appropriate. A common cleaning procedure is to use a very low pH wash of pH1.5 acid, usually phosphoric or hydrochloric, after each elution. This is complemented by a more rigorous cleaning step, using 4-6M guanidine hydrochloride, at the end of each batch or prior to storage in 20% ethanol or 0.1% benzyl alcohol. Production processes using such cleaning regimes have been validated to 400 purification cycles and are routinely used in excess of 200 cycles. However, the efficacy of cleaning will always be dependent upon the feedstock and it is essential to perform lifetime studies on each product and for the specific media to be used. Agarose media have lower chemical stability at low pH (<2.0) compared to polymeric resins or controlled pore glass. While very dilute solutions of NaOH (0.01M) have been advocated recently as cleaning agents (Amersham Biosciences) for agarose-based protein A media, these should be accompanied by at least 2.0M NaCl to afford some protection to the protein A. Even under these conditions, some inactivation of the protein A is to be expected. Moreover, hydroxide at this relatively low concentration is not effective as a sanitant.

3.4.3 Intermediate washing

Once sample has been loaded onto the protein A column, an intermediate wash step is included to remove any feedstock in the interstitial spaces between the chromatography beads or remaining within the pores of the beads. This is also an opportunity to reduce any non-specific binding which occurs. The main contaminating group in any feedstock is usually host cell proteins. These represent a diverse range of proteins with an equally diverse range of physicochemical properties. Non-specific binding can occur due to interaction between host cell proteins and the protein A ligand, the activation chemistry, or the base media itself. Non-specific binding can also occur between the chromatography media and non-protein constituents such as DNA, endotoxin or culture media additives. All modern media are treated during manufacture to minimize non-specific binding. However, the incorporation of specific wash steps between loading and elution can reduce the load of non-specifically bound contaminants even further. Typical washes may include NaCl (1.0M) or organic modifiers such as tetramethyl ammonium chloride (Sulkowski 1987) and may have to be fine tuned for the specific impurity binding.

3.4.4 Virus removal

Protein A chromatography provides a very effective step for virus removal (Brorson et al. 2003). Two mechanisms are used which will provide clearance of virus particles. The first is the physical separation of viruses from the antibody by partition on the column. The second is through chemical inactivation during the low pH elution. By using PCR to monitor the reduction in virus nucleic acid in conjunction with enumeration of viable virus particles, it is possible to quantify and validate each of these components separately and present evidence for two orthogonal virus removal steps. When used in combination with a physical method of removal, such as a virus filtration membrane, this provides sufficient validatable virus removal to satisfy the regulatory authorities.

3.4.5 Ligand leaching

It is a fact of chemistry that all protein A affinity media will leach to some extent (Fuglistaller 1989, Fahrner 1999b). The amount of leaching can be affected by several factors: the physical and chemical strength of the backbone support, the method of immobilization and the presence of proteases. The assay of leached protein A is made more difficult by the fact that it is in the presence of a large excess of IgG which can also bind to the protein A and interfere with detection. In general, the assay system of choice is an enzyme-linked immunosorbent assay (ELISA). Several ELISA kits are now available which are specifically designed to quantify residual levels of protein A in the presence of human IgG. For each ELISA, the nature of the protein A itself – e.g., natural, full recombinant, truncated recombinant - will affect the assay methodology. As a general rule, the control protein A used for the assays of leached protein A should always be from the same source as the protein A used to manufacture the affinity media.

4. POST AFFINITY PURIFICATION STEPS

4.1 Contaminant removal

While dramatically enriched for the product antibody, the eluted pool from the protein A capture step requires additional processing to remove remaining trace contaminants -- including and residual host cell protein, DNA, virus and endotoxin -- before it can be administered parenterally. As discussed above, there will also probably be trace levels of leached protein A ligand present with antibody at a relative concentration of 10-100 PPM antibody. A number of methods may be used to remove these trace impurities. The most common are discussed below. One method not covered here, but often mentioned in older literature, is size exclusion chromatography. While this method can give excellent result in the lab and at pilot scale, it is usually deemed too slow and cumbersome for use at very large scale use.

4.2 Ion exchange

Ion exchange chromatography, immediately following protein affinity capture, is generally regarded as the most effective orthogonal means of achieving significant reduction in remaining trace contaminants. It is typically preferred at commercial scale because it is largely non-denaturing and, with sufficient methods development, offers a robust, flexible, and reasonably selective purification tool. As the majority of monoclonal antibodies are basic proteins (pI >7) and predominating contaminants are acidic, cation exchange media represents a better choice for the second purification column. While anion exchange media may be operated under conditions that bind MAb, capacity co-consumption by the mostly acidic contaminants would necessitate larger columns than desired. Instead, anion exchange functionality is better applied downstream for IgG flow-through steps for removal of trace remaining contaminants, typically clearing 2-5 logs endotoxin and 3-5 logs DNA.

Table 3.5. Typical contaminant clearance values

Contaminant	Affinity load	Intermediate purification load	Polishing load
Host cell protein (ng/ml)	10^5	10^3	10
Endotoxin (EU/ml)	10^6	10	<1
DNA (pg/ml)	10^6	10^3	10^2

Chromatographic selectivity, defined here as the degree to which soluble protein A and host cell protein are resolved from the antibody, is a major focus of methods optimization. When optimizing the cation exchange step, the factors to take into account include the loading conditions, the elution method and the rate of operation.

Ideally, the loading conditions should allow the IgG eluted from the protein A column to be loaded directly, with no pre-conditioning. In practice, this is not always possible. The low pH elution buffer may be too low for long term stability of the IgG activity. Although a hold period at low pH for virus inactivation is common after elution from the protein A column, the buffer pH is then usually adjusted up to nearer neutral pH. The conductivity of the feed for the cation exchange column is also critical to the performance of the media and so limits should be tested during process development. Usually the feed should have conductivity in the range of 4-10mS. Below this value, precipitation of the immunoglobulins can occur; above this conductivity, the binding capacity of the media may be adversely affected.

4.3 Other Chromatographic Purification Methods

Although ion exchange is the most common chromatography method used following protein A affinity, two other alternative methods have been widely exploited: hydrophobic interaction chromatography (HIC) and hydroxyapatite chromatography. These are especially useful when the isoelectric point of the monoclonal antibody is lower than pH 6. When this is the case, the monoclonal antibody and many of the host cell proteins and leached protein A will tend to co-elute from ion exchange media. Hydroxyapatite itself is a crystalline form of calcium phosphate. In this form it is friable and not suited to large scale chromatography. However, it is also available commercially in a ceramic bead form which confers sufficient mechanical robustness to make large scale use possible. The separation is based on a combination of cation, anion and calcium-induced interactions. The novel selectivity of hydroxyapatite makes it difficult to predict optimal operating conditions without recourse to direct experimentation (Stapleton *et al.* 1996, Aoyama and Chiba 1993).

Hydrophobic interaction chromatography is somewhat under-utilized at an industrial scale, yet it is capable of very effective purification of monoclonal antibodies. Perhaps the main disadvantage of HIC is the requirement to add lyotropic salts to promote binding. This can present significant problems at large scale due to the quantity, expense and handling difficulties involved with high purity ammonium or sodium sulphate solutions. In the lab, HIC has traditionally been used as the step following initial precipitation since this reduces the amount of feedstock conditioning required. The use of hydrophobic interaction for the purification of monoclonal antibodies has been well reviewed by Gagnon (1996).

5. POLISHING

Following one or two intermediate purification steps, a common orthogonal method applied for final trace contaminant removal is anion exchange chromatography operated in the flow through mode. As DNA, endotoxin, many viruses, and a large percentage of host cell proteins are negatively charged at neutral pH, they are bound while the typically basic (i.e. positively charged at neutral pH) antibody species is not. Adsorptive membranes provide an alternative to conventional strong anion exchange beaded media but with three primary advantages: they are less kinetically limited (i.e., permit rapid mass transfer), less hydraulically limited, and imminently more convenient to install. When utilizing conventional packed-

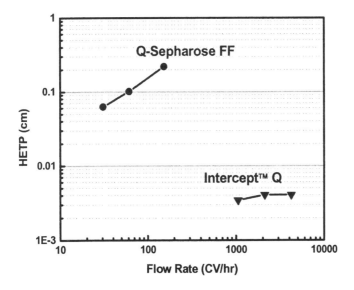

Figure 3.6. Comparison of anion exchange membrane and chromatography media performance.

bed chromatography, columns of very large diameter are required to permit high volumetric flow rates in order to prevent a process bottleneck at the polishing step. As proper flow distribution in production columns requires minimum bed depths of approximately 10 cm, bed volume becomes significant. The result is that such columns are dramatically under-utilized.

In comparison, the capacity of an adsorptive membrane presented in a multi-layered cartridge format is more completely utilized. The physical nature of such devices also lends itself to rapid processing (Figure 3.6). While device integrity testing is advisable, one avoids the manually intensive tasks of packing and testing for flow dispersion properties (e.g., measurement of HETP, asymmetry).

6. OTHER PURIFICATION METHODS

6.1 Crystallization

Crystallization and liquid-solid separation is considered a possible means of addressing future production requirements for monoclonal antibodies (Harris 1995, Visuri 2002). Some precedent exists for the partial purification of IgG by this method as an element of the Cohn plasma fractionation scheme and in the preparation of IgG and antibody fragments for x-ray diffraction structural studies. As the flexibility of the whole IgG molecule imparted by the hinged regions of the heavy chains is thought to challenge the reproducible recovery of stable and active antibody by this method, it may be more practical for isolating subunits such as Fab fragments than for whole IgG. Practical, large-scale purification of therapeutic monoclonal antibodies by crystallization has not yet been reported. Among the issues warranting more study is the process-friendliness of the required salts or organic modifiers, their contributions to cost at large scale, and overall process economies in the face of unknown recoveries/yields, the possible need for costly temperature controls and other equipment requirements.

6.2 Enhanced Ultrafiltration (EUF)

Novel approaches have been applied to improve process economy of tangential flow ultrafiltration steps. In all ultrafiltration there is a trade-off between product yield and throughput that affects the economics of the unit operation. While a lower molecular weight cut-off membrane is more retentive for the target product, and thereby permits higher yield, the permeability of such membranes is typically low. The price for that higher yield is paid in the form of increased membrane area requirements and longer processing times. Similarly, use of a higher molecular weight membrane offers higher flux but at the cost of product yield.

Large-scale production of therapeutic antibodies 95

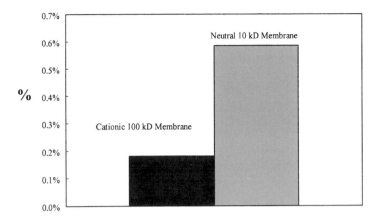

Figure 3.7 – Difference in percent sieving of IgG for neutral and charged 100KkDa membrane

The relationship between yield and permeability can be favorably impacted with the use of charged membranes (Van Reis 1999, Christy *et al.* 2002). The presence of a diffuse counter-ion cloud layered around the charged protein makes it effectively larger in size than if uncharged. If it is then presented to a membrane that has the same charge, the membrane's permeability for that species is reduced both because of its larger effective size and because of electrostatic repulsion from the membrane and its pores. As a result, a membrane having a MW cut-off much closer to that of the retained species can be used, thereby permitting higher flux rates without sacrificing retention and yield. This effect has been demonstrated for IgG using a cationic membrane of a nominal MW cut-off of 100kD (Figure 3.7). Typically, it would be advisable to employ a 30 kD MWCO membrane to achieve the best retention and yield of IgG. However, as a result of the phenomena described above, retention of IgG with the charged 100kD membrane was greater than for an uncharged 30 kD version.

The effects are most evident when the antibody is in a buffer having low ionic strength to minimize the potential that other ions present dampen repulsion effects by means of ion pairing (e.g., below 50mM buffer and other salts). Also, enhancement is greatest at low concentration of charged protein impurities, to avoid loss of membrane permeability by the fouling effects of oppositely charged impurities. Therefore, enhanced ultrafiltration (UEF) will be most practically applied following one or more post-clarification purification steps. It is ideally suited for post-polishing diafiltration operations just preceding product formulation.

6.3 Expanded Bed Adsorption (EBA)

An approach which continues to show promise is the use of stabilized expanded beds. The system is based on adsorption media that are considerably more dense than conventional media. It is contained in suspension in a chromatography column with certain design modifications to vary bed height/expansion volume and to allow one to monitor the height of the expanded bed. The unprocessed fermentation broth is applied directly through this device and the sample of interest is retained as other materials pass through to waste. The potential benefits lie in removing one or more filtration or centrifugation steps, improving yields and lowering costs.

In principle, expanded beds allow the operator to ignore bioburden. However, in practice it is not quite so simple and the overall bioburden can have a significant impact in the life length of the gel, so conditions must be optimized carefully to minimize binding of contaminants (Thommes et al. 1996, Feuser et al. 1999, Fernandez-Lahore et al. 2000). Another factor that has limited the application of EBA is that the density of agarose based materials (in composite with quartz particles) available for expanded bed use is not significantly greater than the buffers used, so the allowable flow rate range is typically limited to 200-300 cm/h. Such flow velocities are at least half of those that can be achieved using a conventionally packed bed of controlled pore glass based media. The use of significantly more dense base media such as zirconia or stainless steel particles may permit flow rates an order of magnitude higher. Equipment design also has had a significant impact on the successful implementation of the technique, and although there are quite useful designs at pilot scale, the cost of similar designs at full scale can be 2-3 times that of a conventional column. Lastly, the material eluting form an expanded bed column still must undergo sterile filtration.

Notwithstanding these challenges, there are several cases where expanded bed processes have been scaled up successfully to production scale with products purified to homogeneity. In such examples, it is appropriate to examine process economy and other benefits. In the case of monoclonal antibody purification, workers at Genentech have compared EBA to conventional processes (Fahrner et al. 1999c). They showed that contaminant profiles varied and that, although yields were better after the first step, contaminants were also present at greater levels. This could result in the need for an additional purification step later in the train in certain situations. A separate study concerning media lifetime showed that EBA media lifetimes were considerably lower than would be expected for a conventional process. As these authors point out, the development of robust, selective ligands, which can withstand extensive cleaning, would greatly assist the widespread utilization of expanded bed technology.

6.4 Future directions

Despite the strong position of protein A affinity chromatography within the monoclonal antibody industry there is still intensive research to find lower cost, more robust alternatives. Some of these stem from work previously carried out on thiophilic media (See Boschetti 2001 for a review of thiophilic chromatography). The basis of thiophilic media is that a small discrete chemical ligand can have an unexpectedly specific interaction with immunoglobulins. Further work in this field has identified some alternative small chemical ligands, which also have high specificity towards immunoglobulins. The general mode of action for the ligands had been described as hydrophobic charge induction (Schwartz et al. 2001, Boschetti 2002). So far, these ligand have proved to be interesting but their general applicability is reduced by the degrees of non-specific binding they can show, especially towards hydrophobic contaminants -- such as cellular lipid and antifoams -- and their poor performance at the flow rates required for high throughput processes.

The search for alternative ligands to Protein A has also utilised methods more commonly applied to drug discovery, such as phage display screening (Erlich 2001) or protein engineering (Gülich 2000), in addition to the increased research into alternative bacterial proteins such as Protein L (Graille 2001). However, the weight of regulatory compliance, accepted practice and accumulated knowledge still makes protein A the ligand of choice.

As expression levels increase and growth media become better defined and free of animal products, alternative paradigms may be required for the purification for monoclonal antibodies. The emphasis will move away from capture in the first instance, towards clarification and concentration. Subsequent purification steps will be more analogous to polishing whereby trace impurities are removed from the product stream, often by negative, or flow-through, chromatography. In such a case, the absolute capacity will not need to be as high as for capture steps and the use of charged membranes may become favoured. As noted in the introduction, there is a significant pressure on process developers to meet the requirement for ever-increasing amounts of antibodies. There is also strong cost pressure on monoclonal therapeutics. It can be expected that these pressures will drive monoclonal production towards still higher throughputs more commonly achieved in the conventional pharmaceutical and fine chemical industry. Early research is already under way underway on forms of simulated moving bed (SMB) chromatography which may yield pseudo-continuous processes for antibody purification. SMB processes have already gained acceptance in the chemical industry and may prove to be the future direction of the biotechnology industry too.

7. CONCLUSION

The fundamental goal of process validation is to ensure that the detailed quality specifications of the product are consistently met, even in the face of variability in the process inputs. Inputs include raw materials, such as the many elements of the fermentation system (cell line, media components), and resulting harvest, as well as any in-process materials contacting the product. The latter includes all chromatographic media, filter media, and equipment.

It is worth noting that a process can be robust and validated without necessarily being cost effective. In general, purification processes will be fixed before producing Phase III clinical trial material. This process will then remain fixed until after product approval is gained. Even after product approval, there is inevitably great reluctance to implement process changes. Although the approach of the FDA is becoming more amenable to scale-up and post-approval changes (SUPAC) of complex biologicals, such changes still tend to be fraught with difficulty and uncertainty and usually prove to be both time consuming and expensive. In short, it is important to appreciate that the successful validation of a cost-*in*efficient process will greatly impact future returns on investment and may prove difficult to change. Hence the requirement for process efficiencies in terms of throughput and cost of goods produced to be factored in from the earliest stages of process development.

ACKNOWLEDGEMENTS

The Authors would like to thank the following Millipore colleagues for their input and discussions on many of the topics discussed above: Igor Quinones-Garcia, Fred Mann, Duncan Low, Linda Taylor, Herb Lutz, Justin McCue, Ralf Kuriyel, Glen Bolton, Michael Phillips

REFERENCES

Aoyama, K., Chiba, J., (1993) Separation of different molecular forms of Mouse IgA and IgM monoclonal antibodies by High-performance liquid chromatography on spherical hydroxyapatite beads. *J. Immunol.methods* **162**, pp 201-210

Boschetti, E., (2001) The use of thiophilic chromatography for antibody purification: a review, *Journal of Biochemical and Biophysical Methods,* **49**, pp 361-389

Boschetti, E., (2002) Antibody separation by hydrophobic charge induction chromatography, *Trends in Biotechnology,* **20**, pp 333-337

Brorson, K., Brown, J., Hamilton, E., Stein, K.E., (2003) Identification of protein A media performance attributes that can be monitored as surrogates for retrovirus clearance during extended re-use, *J. Chromatog. A*, **989**, pp 155-163

Christy, C., Adams, G,. Kuriyel, R., Bolton, G., Seilly, A., (2002). High-performance tangential flow filtration: a highly selective membrane separation process, *Desalination*, **144**, pp 133-136

Ehrlich, G.K., Bailon, P., (2001) Identification of model peptides as affinity ligands for the purification of humanized monoclonal antibodies by means of phage display, *Journal of Biochemical and Biophysical Methods*, **49**, pp443-454

Fahrner, R., Iyer, H.V., Blank, G.S., (1999a) The optimal Flow Rate and Column Length for maximal Production rate of Protein A Affinity Chromatography. *Bioprocess Engineering*, **21** pp287-292

Fahrner, R., Whitney, D.H., Vanderlaan, M., Blank, G.S., (1999b) Performance Comparison of Protein A Affinity Chromatography Sorbents for Purifying Recombinant Monoclonal Antibodies. *Biotechnol. Appl. Biochem*. **30** pp121-128

Fahrner, R.L., Blank, G. S., Zapata, G.A., (1999c) Expanded bed protein A affinity chromatography of a recombinant humanized monoclonal antibody: process development, operation, and comparison with a packed bed method, *J. Biotech.*, **75**, pp273-280

Fernández-Lahore, H,M,. Geilenkirchen, S., Boldt, K., Nagel, A., Kula, M. -R., Thömmes, J., (2000) The influence of cell adsorbent interactions on protein adsorption in expanded beds, *J. Chromatog. A*, **873**, pp 195-208

Feuser, J., Halfar, M., Lütkemeyer, D,, Ameskamp, N., Kula, M.-R., Thömmes, J., (1999) Interaction of mammalian cell culture broth with adsorbents in expanded bed adsorption of monoclonal antibodies, *Process Biochemistry*, **34**, pp 159-165

Fuglistaller, P. (1989) Comparison of immunoglobulin binding capacities and ligand leakage using eight different protein A affinity chromatography matrices. *J. Immunol. Methods*, **124**, pp. 171-177.

Gagnon, P. (1996) Purification tools for monoclonal antibodies. Validated Biosystems, Tucson, Arizona

Graille, M., Stura, E.A., Housden, N.G., Beckingham, J.A., Bottomley, S.P., Beale, D., Taussig, M.J., Sutton, B.J., Gore, M.G., Charbonnier, J-B. (2001) Complex between Peptostreptococcus magnus Protein L and a Human Antibody Reveals Structural Convergence in the Interaction Modes of Fab Binding Proteins, *Structure*, **9**, pp 679-687

Gülich, S., Linhult, M., Nygren, P-A., Uhlén, M., Hober, S. (2000) Stability towards alkaline conditions can be engineered into a protein ligand, *J. Biotechnol*, **80**, pp169-178

Harris, L.J., Skaletski, E., McPherson, A., (1995) Crystallization of Monoclonal antibodies. *Proteins: Struct. Funct. Genet*. **23**: pp285-289

Iyer, H., Henderson, F., Cunningham, E., Webb, J., Hanson, J., Bork, C., Conley, L. (2002) Considerations during development of a Protein A based antibody purification process. *Biopharm* **Jan 2002** pp 14-20

Kamiya, Y., Majima, T., Sohma, Y., Katoh, S. and Sada, E. (1990). Effective purification of bioproducts by fast flow affinity chromatography. *J. Ferment. Bioeng*. **695**, pp. 298-301

Kemp, G., Hamilton, G., Mann, A,F., O'Neil, P. (2001) Increasing Throughput in Affinity Applications by Increasing Bed Height – An Alternative Approach to Process Scale-up. Poster presentation *IBC Conference on Antibody Engineering*, Feb 2001, San Diego.

McCue, J.T., Kemp, G.D., Low, D., Garcia, I.Q. (2003) Evaluation of Protein A Chromatography Media *J.Chromatog. A* **989** pp139-153

Malmquist, G., Lindberg, U., Bergenstrahle A., Lindahl, P. (2000) Differences in the effect of sample residence time on the dynamic binding capacity of Protein A Media. Poster presentation *GAb2000*, Barcelona.

van Reis, R., Leonard, L.C., Hsu, C.C., Builder, S.E. (1991). Industrial scale harvest of proteins from mammalian cell culture by tangential flow filtration. *Biotechnol. Bioeng*. **38**, pp. 413-422.

van Reis, R., Brake, J.M., Charkoudian. J., Burns. D.B., Zydney. A.L. (1999) High-performance tangential flow filtration using charged membranes, *Journal of Membrane Science*, **159**, pp 133-142

Thömmes, J., Bader, A., Halfar, M., Karau, A., Kula, M -R. (1996) Isolation of monoclonal antibodies from cell containing hybridoma broth using a protein A coated adsorbent in expanded beds, *J. Chromatogr. A*, **752**, pp111-122

Schwartz,W., Judd,D., Wysocki M., Guerrier,L., Birck-Wilson E., Boschetti. E. (2001) Comparison of hydrophobic charge induction chromatography with affinity chromatography on protein A for harvest and purification of antibodies, *J. Chromatogr. A*, **908**, pp 251-263

Stapleton, A., Zhang, X., Petrie, H., Machamer, J.E. (1996) Evaluation of different approaches for the chromatographic purification of monoclonal antibodies. *Tech Note 2026*. BioRad Laboratories,

Sulkowski, E. (1987) Controlled pore glass chromatography of proteins: Protein purification micro to macro; *Proceedings of a Cetus-UCLA symposium*. Richard Burgess, New York AR Liss, Vol 68 pp177-195

Visuri, K. ((2002) Potential use of crystallisation in purification of antibodies, 8th *International Antibody Production and Downstream Processing conference*, San Diego CA

Yamamoto, S., Sano, Y. (1992) Short cut method for predicting the productivity of affinity chromatography.
J. Chromatogr. **597** pp173-179

Chapter 4

SCALE-UP OF ANTIBODY PURIFICATION
From laboratory scale to production

Lothar R. Jacob and Matthias Frech
Merck KGaA, Germany

1. INTRODUCTION

Recent developments of highly specific biotherapeutics are mainly based on immunoaffinity mechanisms. After ups and downs of monoclonal antibodies (mAb) these molecules are now gaining respect again. Among the "Top Twenty" biopharmaceuticals the number of antibodies and related products is increasing. In the pipeline of new biological entities most of the molecules either are murine monoclonal antibodies, chimeric monoclonal antibodies, humanized monoclonal antibodies, or human monoclonal antibodies. Examples of approved monoclonal antibodies which have already a multi-million dollar market volume are the chimeric monoclonal antibodies ReoPro and Remicade (Johnson & Johnson/Centocor), Simulect (Novartis), and IDEC's Zevlin, the human or humanized antibodies Humira (Abbott), Herceptin (Genentech/Roche), Zenapax (Roche/PDL), Mylotarg (Celltech/Wyeth), Campath (Ilex/Schering), Xanelim (Genentech/Xoma) and Avastin (Genentech) or the murine derived antibodies Bexxar (Corixa/GSK), Rituxan (IDEC/Genentech) and Orthoclone (Johnson & Johnson).

In contrast to well-characterized chemical drugs, biotherapeutics are derived from living cells. Thus, their characteristics cannot be completely predicted and variances in post-translational modifications might result in an inhomogeneous mixture of antibodies. In addition, due to slightly different conditions during cell growth, the concentration of the antibody in the starting material can be different. But not only the concentration of the antibody can vary, the impurity profile could also be changed resulting in different levels of existing impurities and even new ones. Because all medical applications require a very high purity of the corresponding antibody, any impact of the manufacturing process and such small batch-to-batch variations from the cell culturing process on the final purity of the monoclonal antibody have to be avoided. Therefore, the whole production process defines the product and a validation of each individual step is essential. This chapter gives an overview of the current strategies to manufacture monoclonal antibodies. The main focus is the scale-up procedure of chromatographic techniques from laboratory bench to production scale. Compared to the countless papers describing laboratory scale monoclonal antibody purifications, only very few papers are available showing large-scale purifications. Most of the manufacturers' strategies of mAb production are confidential and it is very difficult to get an overview at one glance. All information presented here is based on published data and our own results. Also our experience and some assumptions contributed to create a more detailed analysis of current antibody production schemes. However, there is no claim of completeness and one knows, that even if a process was shown during a scientific conference there is no evidence that this is exactly the way the presenting company is manufacturing the antibody.

2. DESIGN OF DOWNSTREAM PROCESSES

The aim of any downstream process is to use the shortest way from the starting material to the specified final product. During this procedure the yield has to be maximized while at the same time maintaining biological activity. In addition, all safety aspects have to be fulfilled to guarantee a production, which ends always with an antibody with the same high purity (CBER, 1997). Process development should be done by design rather than by trial and error.

Downstream processing generally consists of various filtration steps followed by chromatographic unit operations. Among the different separation methods, it is important to know their value regarding large-scale antibody production. To obtain the final purity, several orthogonal chromatographic steps are necessary. Between these steps two virus removal or inactivation steps have to be incorporated. As a general guideline these two steps should be based on different mechanisms and must be robust. Effective steps are able to provide virus reduction factors larger than log 4, moderately effective steps reduction factors log 2 – log 4. Less than log 2 is not considered a removal step. For the complete process, the sum of the individual steps has to be considered. It should be prohibitive to use reagents or other compounds derived from animal sources. Compared to small scale purification performed in laboratories, large-scale production is mostly driven by economic aspects. In order to minimize the costs of downstream processing it is often necessary to make compromises. Not every chromatographic resin that gives the highest resolution or the best result in lab-scale columns will be transferable to production scale, if the costs are too high. On the other hand, as a portion of the overall manufacturing costs, the costs for chromatographic media are less significant. To make the complete process more economical, important points to consider are the protein binding capacity for the particular antibody at high flow rate and the re-use of resins. Therefore, the protein binding capacity has to be analyzed carefully under process conditions. Also, the number of cycles has to be checked experimentally for each antibody manufacturing process. In general, the mAb production scheme can be divided into three parts, the capture step, one or two intermediate steps and a final polishing and formulation step. Although there is no generic downstream process available for all the different antibodies, a template process as given in Figure 4.1 could be considered as a general recommendation.

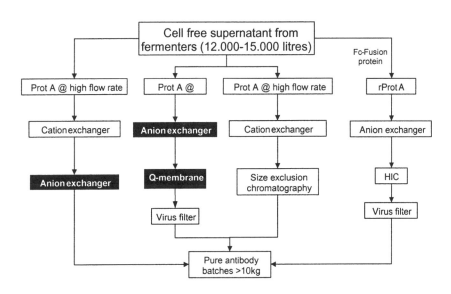

Figure 4.1. Flow chart of downstream processing for monoclonal antibodies. Four different possibilities for the purification of monoclonal antibodies are illustrated. Negative purification steps where the antibody of interest is not bound to the resin are marked by black boxes. More details are explained in this chapter.

3. CAPTURE OF ANTIBODIES

If one assumes that the fermentation is done in 2000-15000 litre reactors this translates into approximately 0.5-22.5 kg of crude product depending on the cell culture (average yield is about 0.25 g/L, maximum yield 1.5 g/L). This amount has to be processed at once or in several batches. If the output of the bioreactor has to be processed in small batches the yield goes down from 70-80% to about 40%, which will negatively affect the economics.

For any given protein purification strategy, the less specific methods like ion exchange chromatography are used first, followed by higher resolution techniques. However, as reported during all recent conferences, monoclonal antibodies are first bound onto a protein A affinity column (Iyer et al., 2002, Cahill et al., 2000, Francis, 1999, McCue et al., 2003). Protein A is a well-characterized cell-wall protein from *Staphylococcus aureus* that binds to the constant region of antibodies. Either the native protein A or its recombinant form is covalently coupled to different types of matrices. Recombinant protein A is genetically modified to remove the albumin binding region of the native molecule and is produced without any contact with mammalian products during fermentation and purification. Before sample loading, the cell culture fluid has been treated with different filtration units like microfiltration, ultra- or diafiltration and the salt concentration has to be adjusted. In some cases treatment with Benzonase® endonuclease, by digesting viscous DNA, facilitates downstream processing of the supernatant. Applying optimum binding conditions, final immunoglobulin (IgG) fractions with a purity of more than 95% of monomeric IgG can be obtained. At the same time, by using a high salt wash to disrupt electrostatic interactions, efficient endotoxin removal occurs. Significant DNA and virus clearance can be obtained using protein A affinity chromatography (Tauer et al., 1995; Brorson et al., 2003). However, protein A is an expensive product, whose isolation involves complex and labour intensive procedures. Due to the fact that protein A is a high molecular weight biomolecule, the efficiency of the separation can be very susceptible to changes in chromatographic conditions like temperature, pH, ionic strength, and/or buffer additives. Because ligand leakage from affinity supports occurs, time consuming analytical controls are required to detect the presence of contaminants associated with the isolated IgG prior to its use for therapeutic purposes in humans. In addition it has to be considered that protein A leakage causes a reduction of binding capacity of the column. This has to be addressed during process validation studies.

Reduction of process volume and the rapid separation from proteases is an important function of this step. High throughput and an efficient cleanability of the resin is also desirable. Both parameters are usually the most critical ones when protein A media are used. Although new techniques utilizing synthetic affinity ligands to mimic the interaction between the IgG and protein A became available years ago, to date, no industrial scale application has been reported. A review of conventional and novel isolation techniques used in industrial applications for the downstream processing of protein molecules was published by Desai (2000).

4. INTERMEDIATE PURIFICATION

The intermediate step is performed to remove most of the remaining host cell proteins (hcp). Final removal of DNA, viruses, and endotoxins is performed in this step. Ion exchange chromatography (IEC) is the method of choice for the intermediate purification of mAbs. IEC is based on the interaction between charged ligands, fixed on the chromatographic support, and the opposite charged areas on the surface of the target molecule. In contrast to purification strategies for plasma derived antibodies, where weak ion exchangers are widely used, strong ion exchangers are preferred if mAbs have to be manufactured. As shown by Necina et al. (1998), mAbs bind also to weak cation exchangers carrying a carboxy group. However, the main ligand for cation exchange chromatography is the sulfo group, whereas for anion exchange chromatography quaternary amines are used. Both belong to the class of strong ion exchangers, which can be used over a wide pH range. In contrast, weak ion exchangers have changing degrees of ionisation depending on pH. Cation exchangers are able to remove unfolded forms of the mAb as well as aggregates of the mAb and small molecular weight impurities (Iyer et al., 2002). Both modes of IEC are able to separate protein A leakage products. Also HIC was reported to contribute to the final purity when implemented at this level.

5. POLISHING STEP

Polishing steps are designed to remove small amounts of oligomers of the antibody, traces of DNA, and remaining host cell proteins, as well as protein A leakage products. In addition, polishing can be used to exchange the product into formulation buffer. In most cases, strong anion exchangers are used to remove traces of DNA. The final polishing of antibodies can also be achieved by size exclusion chromatography (SEC). SEC is not only a powerful tool for the quality control of antibodies because this method shows a broad fractionation range especially for antibodies and their aggregates, but can also be utilized for larger applications (Walter, 1999).

SEC is the only biochromatographic method in which no interaction between the chromatographic support and the molecules takes place. Thus, the buffer system can be adapted to the final formulation conditions.

6. OTHER METHODS FOR MAB PURIFICATION

A review published by Huse et al. (2002) focuses on other different affinity techniques in addition to protein A as a ligand. Protein G, another bacterial cell wall protein with an affinity to antibodies, can be used for the isolation of antibodies when immobilized on a chromatographic support (Bill et al., 1995). Though the conditions used to purify antibodies with Protein G are less harsh, the high price of the reagent prevents its use in production. Alternative techniques like thiophilic adsorption chromatography and immobilized metal ion affinity chromatography might be of interest because of their higher stability compared to Protein A and Protein G.

6.1 Thiophilic adsorption chromatography

Salt promoted thiophilic adsorption chromatography, especially designed for antibody separation (Belew et al., 1987), is based on an electron donor-acceptor mechanism between the covalently attached ligand and tryptophan residues on the surface of the antibody. Albumin is not adsorbed on thiophilic media, which often simplifies the effective separation of antibodies. Thiophilic adsorption chromatography on Fractogel® EMD TA was used successfully for the isolation of recombinant antibodies, which cannot be purified on Protein A or Protein G resins (Schulz et al., 1994). In addition, yolk immunoglobulins from chicken, human IgG_3, mouse IgG_3 and rat IgGs can be isolated using thiophilic adsorption chromatography. Although there are some advantages, this method still lacks wide acceptance. One reason besides its lack of specifity is the need to handle the mAb at high ammonium sulphate or sodium sulphate concentrations.

6.2 Affinity chromatography on immobilized metal ions

Affinity chromatography on immobilized metal ions (IMAC) is another method, which can be exploited for antibody purification, especially the purification of recombinant single chain Fv antibodies with histidine C-terminal tails (Casey et al., 1995). IMAC eliminates the harsh conditions required to elute antibodies from protein A columns. The mild elution conditions and the ease of regeneration make this technique an interesting alternative. Good results can be obtained for example on resins with iminodiacetic acid (*e.g.* Chelating Sepharose® fast flow; Amersham Biosciences, Fractogel® EMD Chelate; Merck KGaA) saturated with copper(II), nickel(II), or cobalt(II) ions prior to the loading of antibody. The level of Cu^{2+} leaching which can be achieved with IMAC columns can be below the recommended level given in routine intravenous nutrition (5-10 µM/day) (Casey et al., 1995). For monoclonal antibodies IMAC can be used, but up to now no published data have been available concerning production scale columns.

6.3 Hydrophobic Interaction Chromatography

Hydrophobic Interaction Chromatography (HIC) is rarely considered to be an efficient separation technique in spite of the fact that this column chromatography separation can be optimally integrated into a purification scheme after an ammonium sulphate precipitation step. However, at very large scale any precipitation of the antibody has to be avoided. Thus, HIC can only be used for the removal of certain impurities like viruses and DNA. Without changing the column geometry HIC processes can be scaled-up by keeping constant the linear flow rate, the bed height and the ratio of gradient volume and total column volume. The sample load has to be constant with respect to the amount of protein loaded per millilitre of gel. Sometimes it is also recommended to keep the height to diameter ratio of the column constant (Vorauer et al., 1992).

Efficient harvest and recovery of high-purity monoclonal antibodies using hydrophobic charge induction chromatography (HCIC) was described by Schwartz et al. (2001). This method is based on the pH-dependent behaviour of a dual-mode, ionisable ligand. Despite the fact that HCIC could be a cost-effective, process-compatible alternative to protein A affinity chromatography, no large-scale application has been published up to now.

6.4 Chromatography on hydroxyapatite

The miscellaneous chromatographic mode of hydroxyapatite can be considered to be a special case of an ion exchange separation in which negatively charged phosphate residues as well as positively charged calcium ions of the column matrix interact with the antibody. Recent developments introduced mechanically stable hydroxyapatite supports with larger particle sizes. In principle, such media allow faster separation and can be used with a high reproducibility. However, no large-scale mAb process has been published yet.

7. SCALE-UP STRATEGIES

Scale-up is not a simple increase in the size and volume of the laboratory equipment. During the screening of antibodies the most important task is to deliver small quantities of many different antibodies for the very first biological tests. At this stage, where high throughput of many samples is required, purity, safety, and economical aspects are often neglected. After a specific antibody has been identified to become a potential drug, the first material for the clinical development is made in bioreactors containing a few hundreds of litres. Many approaches that will result in a pure antibody preparation at small scale, cannot be transferred even to pilot scale. Finally, the fermentation will be increased to several thousands of litres and huge volumes have to be handled. For example, the mAb Synagis® from MedImmune was scaled-up from 20 litres to 10.000 litres as an equivalent molecule (Schenerman et al., 1999). Another production related detail was published by Cahill et al. (2000), showing an isolation of a therapeutic mAb that was produced at 15,000 litre scale. Columns containing several hundreds of litres of resin and thousands of litres of buffer have to be used. The scale-up starts from the mg-level and ends up at the kg scale.

The transfer of a method from laboratory through to production scale is also affected by the switch to large equipment. Initially, every chromatographic separation is developed at laboratory scale and the resin is packed in small columns. Larger piping dimensions, larger dead volumes, larger column diameters, and different kinds of pumps will introduce new factors for consideration. System factors can be avoided using the optimal system configuration and selecting optimal equipment. From our experience a careful selection of suitable small-scale equipment is essential. For example, method development should start with columns of 16 mm inner diameter if enough sample material is available. Due to increased wall support, scale-up from smaller columns would predict lower back pressures than those observed at manufacturing scale.

After all the parameters are fixed for the process at the final scale, certain validation steps can be performed at small scale again (down-scale) under identical process conditions. Most of the virus- and DNA-removal/clearance as well as the lifetime of the resin can be validated in smaller columns. Also process loading studies can be made at small scale when testing the total amount of protein to be loaded.

7.1 Scale-up affinity chromatography on protein A

The production rate, which gives the amount of mAb, purified per unit of time and per unit of column volume should be the main focus during process development. Although effects of temperature, flow rate and composition of binding buffer on adsorption of mouse monoclonal IgG$_1$ antibodies to protein A were described by van Sommeren et al. (1992), process operating conditions for protein A steps can be fairly generic. Equilibration is usually done at pH 7 and, after the addition of an appropriate amount of sodium chloride, a direct load of harvest fluid is desirable. After a wash step with equilibration buffer and an intermediate pH wash, the final elution takes place at low pH conditions (pH 3-4). Before the column run, tests have to be done to show that the buffer system, pH, conductivity and temperature are not affecting the biological activity of the antibody.

As described by Kang and Ryu (1991) the capacity of Protein A resins show a clear relationship with the amount of immobilized protein A. In order to optimise the downstream process, the capacity of protein A media has improved during the last decade. But the economics of the manufacturing process depends not only on the capacity of the sorbent. High throughput has to be achieved to process the large sample volume in a short period of time. Because labour costs and especially night shifts have a negative effect on the manufacturing costs, process time should be minimised. On the other hand, the capture step should not be the bottleneck of the downstream process, which limits the fermentation frequency. Therefore, protein A resins providing high dynamic binding capacities that can be operated at low back pressure due to high permeability are required.

Usually, when the column diameter is increased, the capacity of the protein A column increases with the ratio of the cross-sectional area of the column. In contrast to ion exchange chromatography, protein A affinity columns provide increased IgG binding capacity when the column increases in the axial direction. However, gel compression increases linearly with the increase in height. As a result, the productivity will go down if the flow rate has to be reduced. It was also shown that the concentration of the desorbed IgG depends on the column geometry. Whereas the influence of the buffer composition can be checked at small scale, the impact of column dimensions is part of the scale-up studies.

Among the media for protein A affinity chromatography that are commercially available only very few are used at large scale (Table 4.1). They differ according to the chemical structure of the support, their pore and particle size. The obtained purities using any of these protein A resins are more or less comparable, thus, the productivity and cost considerations become much more important. Fahrner et al. (1999) investigated five commercial protein A media (using recombinant protein A as ligand) with respect to capacity, yield, purity, and pressure drop. They reported significant differences between the protein A sorbents with respect to capacity and pressure drop. Although the saturation capacities (at 50%

breakthrough at a flow rate of 500 cm/hr) were in the range from 24-38 mg of antibody per millilitre of gel, the dynamic capacities measured at 1% breakthrough vary from 7.5-17.5 mg/ml. As a consequence, in conjunction with the pressure drop, the production rates were quite different. The most critical parameter is the flow rate and column length, which together determine the residence time. Similar observations were found by Hahn et al. (2003) when comparing 15 different protein A resins. Agarose based media gave the best results in terms of dynamic capacity at residence times longer than three minutes. The residence time is equal to the bed height (cm) divided by the fluid velocity (cm/hr) applied during mAb loading and has to be kept constant during scale-up. The higher the flow rate the shorter the processing time will be. As a prerequisite, protein A has to be immobilized onto matrices providing high permeability and high mechanical stability.

Table 4.1. Main packings commercially available for protein A affinity chromatography at large scale

Name	Manufacturer	Chemical structure	Ligand
Prosep rA High Capacity	Millipore	controlled pore glass	recombinant protein A
Prosep A High Capacity	Millipore	controlled pore glass	native protein A
Protein A Sepharose 4 Fast Flow	Amersham Biosciences	highly cross-linked 4% agarose	native protein A
rProtein A Sepharose 4 Fast Flow	Amersham Biosciences	highly cross-linked 4% agarose	recombinant protein A
MabSelect	Amersham Biosciences	HF agarose, highly cross-linked	recombinant protein A
Streamline rProtein A	Amersham Biosciences	highly cross-linked 4% agarose, with metal core	recombinant protein A
Poros 50 A High Capacity	Perseptive Biosystems	cross-linked poly(styrene-divylbenzene)	recombinant protein A

There are many other protein A resins available for laboratory scale and pilot plant

Typically mAb downstream processing uses columns containing 50-300 litres of affinity resin that are loaded several times to purify a single batch. Due to the costs of protein A resins, a column providing the total capacity to bind mAb from one 12,000 litre fermentation is extremely expensive. This cycling of the capture step increases the total production time and has to be optimised. As reported by Iyer et al. (2002), the substitution of the compressible protein A Sepharose® FF with the more rigid Prosep®-rA resin increased the fluid velocities during column loading. As a result, the overall process time could be significantly reduced. Protein A Sepharose® 4 Fast Flow with a dynamic binding capacities up to 20 mg of mAb per millilitre of gel can be loaded at less than 200 cm/hr, the Prosep®-rA resin can be operated at 500 cm/hr. The relation of the production rate of protein A affinity chromatography to flow rate and column length was calculated by Fahrner et al. (1999). Because the height of the packed bed and the flow rate can easily be varied, these parameters should be used to find the optimal conditions. The only empirical data needed for this approach is the relationship of dynamic capacity to flow rate and column length. Table 4.2 shows the impact of the bed height on the total binding capacity of a column packed with 60 litres of a protein A resin at a fixed linear flow rate. One important limitation is the mechanical stability of the chromatographic support. The longer the column the longer the residence time with a corresponding increase in dynamic capacity. However, at the same time pressure drop also increases and, as a consequence, the flow rate has to be reduced. The net result is a decrease in throughput.

Table 4.2. Calculated binding capacities for 60 litre of protein A resin at different bed heights

Column height	10 cm	20 cm	30 cm	40 cm
Column diameter	87 cm	62 cm	51 cm	44 cm
Dynamic capacity	11 mg/ml	18 mg/ml	23 mg/ml	27 mg/ml
Residence time	1.2 min	2.4 min	3.6 min	4.8 min
Column capacity	660 g	1080 g	1380 g	1620

Linear flow rate: 500 cm/hr

Together with the costs of the affinity matrix, the optimum compromise has to be identified for the specific mAb. Before scaling up, the column volume according to the required binding capacity has to be calculated and the optimum bed height has to be determined. The protein load must be constant at all different scales. The column diameter has to be selected to obtain a bed height that allows high flow rates and high dynamic capacities. The actual dimensions depend on the affinity resin used for production; the operating flow rate should not exceed more than 70% of the maximum flow rate given by the resin's supplier (Amersham Biosciences, 2001). For rProtein A Sepharose® FF a bed height of 5-15 cm is recommended by the manufacturer. MabSelect® can be packed to bed heights of 27-30 cm at column diameters of 45 and 60 cm, respectively. However, as the pressure drop increases, the highest amount of mAb in the shortest time with the highest recovery can be obtained at 20 cm bed height (Amersham Biosciences, 2001). Even if a protein A resin is much more expensive but provides higher throughput, it can make the process more economic because less processing time for is needed. Another approach to increasing throughput was introduced about ten years ago using an expanded bed for the adsorption (EBA). Several examples were published demonstrating the proof of principle at least up to the pilot scale (Lutkemeyer et al. 2001; Barnfield Frej et al., 1997; Ameskamp et al., 1999). A separation of a murine monoclonal antibody by rProtein A using expanded bed adsorption chromatography is shown in Fig. 4.2.

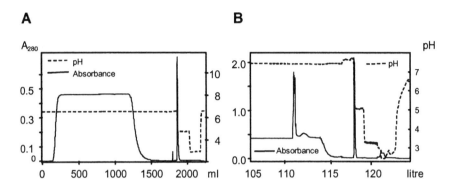

Figure 4.2. A. Chromatography using EBA rProtein A. 1100 ml of the protein solution was loaded onto the column at pH 7 in the presence of 0.5 M NaCl. Decreasing the pH to a value of 5 eluted the target antibody. B. Upscale to 110 litre hybridoma supernatant using EBA rProtein A. 110 litres of the protein solution was loaded onto the column at pH 7 in the presence of 0.5 M NaCl. Again the target antibody was eluted by decreasing the pH to 5.

In a small scale experiment 1.1 litre of the hybridoma supernatant was used to establish the chromatography over Streamline® rProtein A. Chromatography was done using a Streamline® 25 column (25 mm inner diameter; Amersham Biosciences). The NaCl concentration of the hybridoma supernatant was adjusted to 0.5 M NaCl, the pH of the buffer was adjusted to 7.0. The bed volume was expanded with an upward flow by a factor of 2.3. The protein sample was loaded at pH 7.0 onto the column. The antibody was eluted with a pH shift to pH 5.0 using 0.1 M citrate buffer. The chromatography efficiently captured the murine mAb from the hybridoma supernatant. The content of bovine immunoglobulin from cell culture, which contained 2% fetal calf serum, dropped by a factor of 6 and was about hundred times less than the target murine antibody. The DNA amount as measured by the Pico Green (Molecular Probes) assay was reduced 1000-fold (Tab. 4.3). Protein concentrations were measured by the BCA Method. The concentration of the murine mAb and the bovine immunoglobulins were determined using the appropriate specific ELISA test. Subsequently, the separation was increased and transferred to a Streamline® 50 column (bed volume 300 ml, expansion factor 2.5) and 110 litre of hybridoma supernatant

Scale-up of antibody purification 113

was applied. The elution profile is very similar and no significant change in the chromatographic behaviour was observed (Fig. 4.2 B).

Table 4.3. Removal of DNA and bovine compounds during protein A affinity chromatography.

	Total amount of protein	Amount of murine antibody	Amount of bovine immunoglobulin	DNA
Starting material	2266 mg	27 mg	1.7 mg	860200 ng
Pass through	2189 mg	0.3 mg	0.9 mg	n. d.
Eluted protein	34 mg	29 mg	0.28 mg	82 ng

n. d. = not determined

In the scale up the most critical sources of variation in expanded bed adsorption are related to the feed material. These parameters and their critical process limits have to be examined very carefully. For scale up, the strategy is to maintain all the parameters that are related to the chromatographic and hydrodynamic performance, such as sedimented bed height, expanded bed height, flow velocity, volume of process buffers. Typically the Streamline® 25 is used for method optimisation experiments whereas the Streamline® 50 or larger diameters are used for the final process.

7.2 Stability and re-use of protein A media

The stability of different protein A affinity matrices was compared by Füglistaller (1989). The lowest leakage is associated with affinity resins in which protein A was bound by an alkylamine or ether linkage. Although he reported a significant leakage of protein A of 1.8 up to 88 ppm (weight/weight), many validation studies showed the repeated use of protein A resins for more than 100 cycles without any changes in the purification results. However, appropriate column hygiene is necessary.

For column hygiene of protein A resins caustic and acidic steps as well as treatment with detergents are recommended (e. g. about 0.4 M acetic acid, 0.5 M NaCl and 0.1% Tween 20). For cleaning the affinity resin, usually short time washing (contact time 15 min) with 50 mM NaOH and 1 M NaCl is performed. Columns have to be cleaned every 1-10 runs and a sanitization step is needed between individual batches. Exact details on used reagents and exposure times have been determined in the development of the down stream process. An estimation of the actual cycle number of column runs was published by O'Leary et al. (2001). The protein A affinity step had a useful lifetime of 225 cycles at production scale. The corresponding resin was still able to reduce the level of host cell proteins and DNA without any apparent trend. As far as the removal of viruses, which has to be maintained for all production runs, is considered it became obvious that the IgG binding performance on protein A Sepharose® FF deteriorates long before there is a change in viral clearance.

7.3 Scale-up of ion exchange chromatography

Antibodies have been reported to have isoelectric points between 5 and 8 and, therefore, can be purified at pH<pI on cation exchangers (Bai et al., 2000; Necina et al., 1998, Denton et al., 2001). High purities and high recoveries can be obtained. IEC is robust and scales-up efficiently from laboratory to production. Among more than 70 different media for IEC which are commercially available for low and medium pressure applications (Levison et al., 1997), the most efficient one has to be chosen for each individual separation by screening procedures prior to scale-up. But only chromatographic media that are uniform and have no anomalous properties can be utilized. When choosing the media, long-term availability of the required amounts of media, lot-to-lot consistency, resin lifetime, and supporting documentation have to be considered. The most relevant batch related data, which characterize media, are summarized in Table 4.4.

Table 4.4.

To be specified	Information value
Appearance, microscopic evaluation,	Foreign material check
Particle size distribution	Flow characteristics, permeability
Pressure drop	Flow characteristics, permeability
Protein binding capacity	Number of functional groups
Microbial contamination	Bioburden
Endotoxins	Pyrogen check
Functional test	Type of functional groups

The easiest way to scale-up the procedure is to change the column dimensions by keeping the height of the gel bed constant and increasing the column diameter. In many biotech companies large ion exchange columns can be found containing several hundreds of litres of media. Column diameters usually are in the range between 60 and 160 cm. The scale-up is typically done in two steps, the first step from laboratory to pilot plant is on the order of 50- to 100-fold. The final scale-up from pilot plant to full-scale manufacturing is 10- to 50-fold (Rathore and Velayudhan, 2003).

A typical 60-fold scale up on an anion exchanger is shown in Figure 4.3. To demonstrate the similarity of the chromatogram obtained from a 20 cm inner diameter column the scale up of a therapeutic protein was used as an example. In contrast to an antibody elution profile with only one peak, this separation is more complex. During scale-up, the total load of protein per millilitre of resin should be identical and the linear flow rate has to be maintained.

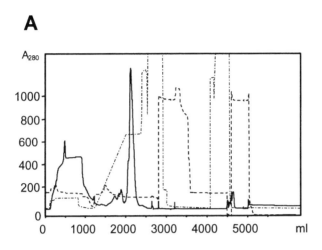

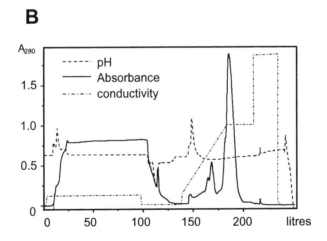

Figure 4.3. To demonstrate the similarity of the chromatograms from a scale up experiment a separation of a therapeutic protein is shown using a lab-scale column (A) and a pilot-scale column (B). **A.** Fractogel® EMD DEAE (M) (Merck KGaA), packed in a 2.6 cm inner diameter column, was loaded with a total protein amount of 1.3 g (sample volume: 815 ml) at a flow rate of 13.3 ml/min. **B.** About 155 g of protein (sample volume: 96 L) loaded onto a 20 cm inner diameter column containing the same type of resin gave nearly the same elution profile. The volumetric flow rate was adjusted to 47.1 l/hr. The linear flow rate was 150 cm/hr; bed height of both columns was about 26 cm (Buffer A: 50 mM Na-P pH: 6.3; Buffer B: 50 mM Na-P, 1 M NaCl pH: 6.3).

In order to achieve higher flow rates and more profitability, synthetic polymers are advantageous. Chromatographic media based on carbohydrates like cellulose or agarose provide lower flow rates and lower throughputs. As many downstream process media as possible should be tested. The chosen matrix is the key to the success of chromatography and to process robustness. In contrast to the protein binding capacities given by the suppliers of media, in the case of monoclonal antibodies some types of ion exchangers provide unexpected high binding capacities.

7.4 Capacity of ion exchangers for mAbs

Because there are only very few comparative studies available and the results are not always transferable, one has to undertake experiments using various strong cation-exchangers to select the most suitable one for the process to be developed. Many different, commercially available gels are able to bind IgG under process conditions, but the amount of bound IgG per millilitre of gel varies often significantly. Figure 4.4 summarises the results from a survey, which was designed to identify resins for the isolation of a mAb. (Gottschalk et al., 1997). The binding capacities clearly depend on the amount of sample load and were found to be at the highest level when tentacle-type strong cation exchangers (Fractogel® EMD SO$_3$ or Fractogel®

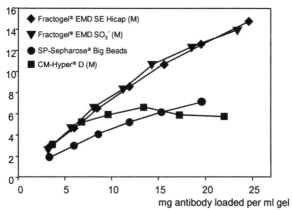

Figure 4.4. Binding of diafiltered antibody concentrate onto different cation exchange gels. Adsorption was achieved using buffer A (0.03 M sodium phosphate, 0.03 M NaCl, pH 6.5), for elution 0.03 M sodium phosphate containing 1 M NaCl (pH 6.5) was used; the linear flow rate was 400 cm/hr.

EMD SE Hicap) were used. Normally up to ten resins are tested, in order to find a material which is capable of binding the particular mAb in a sufficient amount per millilitre of gel and which gives a high yield of purified product. The media described here should be regarded as more or less suitable for a specific purpose, and only testing for the specific application will determine which one is the optimal resin.

7.5 New models for the antibody binding mechanism

As reported by Hubbuch et al. (2002) the adsorption profiles of single- and two-component mixtures during packed bed cation-exchange chromatography appear to exhibit different transport characteristics. As analysed by confocal laser scanning microscopy, for BSA a classical "shrinking core" behaviour could be described, whereas IgG_{2a} adsorption cannot be explained by pure diffusional transport. The adsorption of IgG_{2a} is rather a fast migration of the adsorbed molecule to the centre of the bead. While the IgG_{2a} molecules move to the inside of the support, newly arriving proteins bind to the outer part of the chromatographic bead. Although there are no models for multi-component systems up to now, at least for a mixture of two proteins (BSA and IgG_{2a}) a superposition of the single-component profiles combined with a classical displacement probably takes place during the adsorption step. We have found that binding of the mAb on the cation exchange resin should not be too strong, because then the binding capacity is reduced. As shown in Figure 4.5, the binding capacity for antibodies is

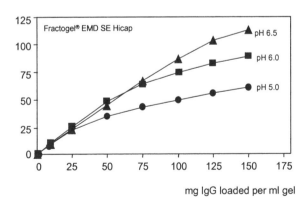

Figure 4.5. Impact of pH of the loading buffer on the antibody binding capacity of cation exchange resin Fractogel® EMD SE Hicap (Merck KGaA).

decreased, if the pH of the loading buffer is too far away from pI. The most important key structural characteristic of the chromatography media seems to be the surface charge density. According to Dziennik et al. (2003) there is a significant non-diffusive contribution to protein transport in ion exchange chromatography. The rapid uptake transport implicates electrostatic effects that might be influenced by the binding strength and, thus, by the pH of the loading buffer.

7.6   Screening of cation exchange resins

A comparative study has been undertaken by Shukla et al. (2002), on eight different cation-exchangers to investigate the binding capacity of chromatographic resins. The resins tested included: SP Sepharose® FF, SP Sepharose® XL, CM Sepharose® FF, Toyopearl® CM, Toyopearl® SP, Fractogel® EMD SO_3, Fractogel® EMD SE Hicap and Macro-Prep® High S (BioRad). Batch binding experiments were conducted over a range of salt concentrations and pHs to rapidly evaluate these resins for IgG binding. Fractogel® EMD SO_3 and Fractogel® EMD SE Hicap were found to have the highest overall binding capacity for the tested mAb. More than 30 mg of the mAb could be bound per ml of gel in the batch capacity experiment (Figure 4.6). The mAb binding capacity was also determined dynamically at 5% breakthrough. The results were similar, but slightly higher binding capacities could be obtained with the dynamic test possibly due to sampling variations with the batch experiments. The dynamic capacity of Fractogel® cation exchangers was at least two times higher compared to other methacrylate derived cation exchangers. The batch incubation mode was also used to evaluate various additives to a wash buffer following protein loading on the Fractogel® EMD SO_3 resin. This technique can potentially form the basis of a high throughput screening technique for ion-exchangers. To maximize the host cell protein clearance a combination of 50 mM NaCl and 5 mM DTT gave the best results. This can be potentially ascribed to the association of host cell protein contaminants to the target protein by both electrostatic and covalent disulfide linkages.

Another practical approach was investigated by Gottschalk et al. (1997) to identify the resin providing the highest binding capacity at high ionic strength. The property of the Fractogel® cation exchange media persisted when the comparison was carried out under varied conditions, *e.g.* for different buffer concentrations in the column feed stream as is shown in Figure 4.7 for two of the gels with high binding capacity. Further optimisation of the cation exchange step showed that Fractogel® EMD SE Hicap could bind approximately 18 of applied 20 mg of IgG in the presence of 30 mM salt and 30 mM phosphate buffer at pH 6.5, conditions which

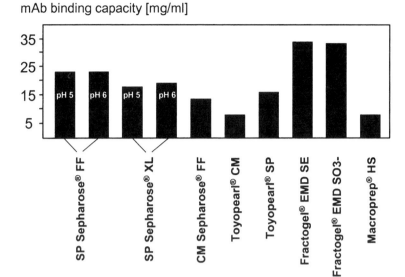

Figure 4.6. Comparison of different cation exchange resins with respect to their antibody binding capacity. Tests were performed in a batch mode. Depending on the chemistry of the media different antibody binding capacities were obtained.

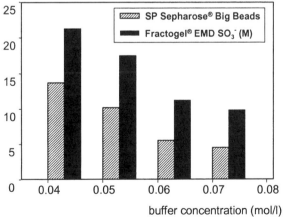

Figure 4.7. Binding of diafiltered antibody concentrate at pH 6.5 onto cation exchange resins at different buffer concentrations The total antibody binding capacity decreases at high salt concentrations at different degrees for SP-Sepharose® Big Beads and Fractogel® EMD SO_3.

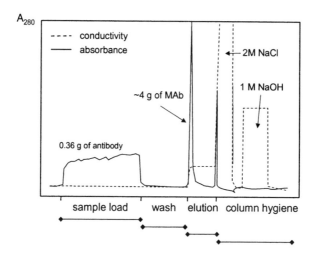

Figure 4.8. Sample chromatogram for the capturing of monoclonal affinity antibody on a column packed with Fractogel® EMD SE Hicap. Column: 5.0 x16.8 cm (c.v. = 330 ml) Sample: 4.6 g antibodies from 40 l fermentation broth Flow rate: 60 ml/min. The breakthrough contained 0.36 g of protein, whereas 3.97 g were eluted in the step gradient. The NaCl wash following the elution step contained less than 1% of the total protein load. With the NaOH wash only traces of residual material were eluted from the column.

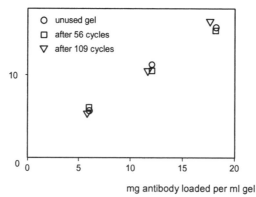

Figure 4.9. Stability of Fractogel®EMD SE Hicap to treatment with 1 M sodium hydroxide. The long-term stability of the gel against repeated clean-in-place (CIP) cycles was examined by measuring the antibody binding capacity at different levels of protein loading in a packed column after the individual cycles. Each alkaline cleaning step was performed with eluent C for 1 h. Column: 1.0 x 3.8 cm (c.v. = 2.98 ml gel) Flow rate: 3 ml/min; eluent A: 0.03 M Na-phosphate, 0.03 M NaCl, pH 6.5; eluent B: 0.03 M Na-phosphate, 1 M NaCl, pH 6.5; buffer C: 1 M NaOH (Gottschalk et al., 1997).

proved to give satisfactory results with respect to recovery of protein and biological activity of the purified product. The recovery of this step was about 88%. In conclusion, methacrylate based strong cation exchangers were considered as successful candidates for the large-scale purification of mAbs. The chromatogram of the pilot scale column is shown in Figure 4.8. Although in all manufacturing schemes anion exchange columns are used, the mAb binding characteristics are less important because in most cases this step is used as a negative purification method for the removal of specific contaminants. Strong anion exchange chromatography can efficiently remove DNA and, in addition, was described to contribute to viral clearance (Walter et al., 1998). Endotoxin reduction is another purpose of this chromatographic mode.

7.7 Stability and re-use of ion exchange media

One very important parameter for process applications is column re-use. Chromatographic media must be evaluated to see whether multiple cycle use has changed its ability to purify the antibody and to remove the specific contaminants. In general, the studies should assure adequacy of the column and integrity of the product. For example, the endotoxin and contaminant protein levels on the product lot made using regenerated resin must be checked. Validation studies should exceed the number of expected production lots. The validation studies can be performed in laboratory scale columns; however, scale-down chromatography must accurately represent full-scale production. Regarding re-use of the resin, chemical stability as well as the protein binding capacity is of interest. The functional performance after storage in different solutions at ambient temperature indicates chromatographic stability. It has been shown that media for analytical-scale separations can be used for 1000 repetitive runs or more (Tice et al., 1987). The longevity of preparative columns is more likely affected by irreversibly adsorbed contaminants due to the use of high sample concentration and large sample mass applied. Different protein aggregates and lipoproteins can physically coat the column surface during the chromatographic separations. This leads to changes in the surface chemistry and the total available surface for separation can be markedly reduced. On the other hand, substances can bind to active sites on the matrix and interfere with analyte binding. Thus, preparative-scale separations require very efficient washing and regenerations steps between every run in order to maintain optimum product quality. O'Leary et al. (2001) showed a useful lifetime of 50 cycles for the intermediate cation exchange step without any reduction in host cell protein, DNA, and protein A removal. The same number of cycles was given for the final anion exchange step. The result of more than 100 repeated injections of approximately 4 g of antibodies from a

40 litre fermentation onto a 5.0 x 16.8 cm Fractogel® EMD SE Hicap column (column volume 330 ml) is shown in Figure 4.9.

This study included clean-in-place steps with 1M NaOH/NaCl after each run. The resin proved to be highly stable and no changes of the column parameters of chromatographic results could be observed.

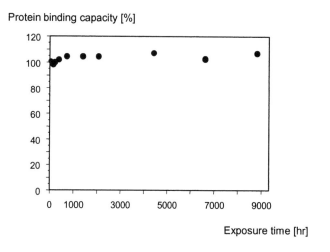

Figure 4.10. Fractogel® EMD SO$_3$ (Merck KGaA) does not loose protein binding capacity even after exposure to 1 M sodium hydroxide solution for several months at room temperature

Although each validation study is linked to the actual production process, some general data should be provided by suppliers with the resins. Such data comprises stability of the resin under clean-in-place (CIP) and storage conditions. Normally, treatment with sodium hydroxide is recommended for clean-in-place and sanitization. CIP protocols are specifically designed to remove feed stream impurities that remain bound to the column after the product was eluted, and should render the column ready for the next purification cycle. The aim of any sanitization protocol is to reduce the number of microbial contaminants to acceptable levels. If a resin is not caustic resistant, alternative methods have to be developed and validated.

Data showing the stability of resins in the presence of ethanol (20%), sodium hydroxide (0.1 M up to 1 M), acetic acid (1.1 M up to 1 M), urea and/or guanidine hydrochloride are available from media suppliers (Lagerlund et al., 1998). The expected number of regeneration cycles for a given column can be estimated from manufacturers' data. For example, stability data for a cation exchanger stored in a sodium hydroxide solution under ambient temperature for several months is illustrated in Figure 4.10. The results show that the adsorbent is chemically stable and that the chromatographic properties are retained under the tested conditions. Thus, the number of possible regeneration cycles can be estimated. The chemical stability can be monitored as the carbon leakage from the matrix to the storage solution at different, process related conditions. The carbon content in the supernatant can be determined with Total Organic Carbon (TOC) technique. A typical result of a blank run without any protein should show no TOC during the re-equilibration after the clean-in-place procedure. Of course, during the sodium hydroxide step at a very high pH, traces of leakage might be detectable (Andersson et al., 1998).

For Macroprep® High-S (BioRad) a validation study demonstrated that the resin can be used for at least 42 runs. The re-use study showed that Macroprep® High-S continues to perform after 42 runs and was not affected by any regeneration or sanitization procedure. For this experiment, yield, host cell protein and DNA clearance were also determined (Breece et al., 2002).

During these experiments, any protein precipitation and subsequent clogging of the top filter has to be avoided in order to exclude such effects as the reason for the observed changes in the elution profile. For example, for Q-Sepharose® HP a test under analytical- and preparative-scale conditions showed protein clogging of the top filter. This was the main reason for the observed decrease in retention volume, gel bed height and peak height during 300 analytical separations of a standard protein mixture. Different washing procedures proved that adsorbed protein molecules decreased the column performance. As reported by Kundu et al. (2001) the same effect was visible even after 25 cycles when ion exchange chromatography was used for simultaneous 60-fold concentration and purification from a clarified cell culture harvest.

7.8   Scale-up size exclusion chromatography

As a rule the volume of the loaded sample should not exceed 5% of the column volume. The productivity of size exclusion chromatography is best optimised by choosing the highest possible linear flow rate, a protein concentration as high as possible, and reducing the sample volume to obtain the required purity. SEC allows the rapid preparation of homogeneous antibodies. At least pilot plant columns can provide an efficient purification of mAbs. However, since the separation mode is based on the differential penetration of molecules of different size and shape into the pores of the stationary phase, long columns have to be packed. Then, from a technical point of view, some limitations will occur. An example of scale up from 5 cm to 10 cm id SEC columns is shown in Fig. 4.11.

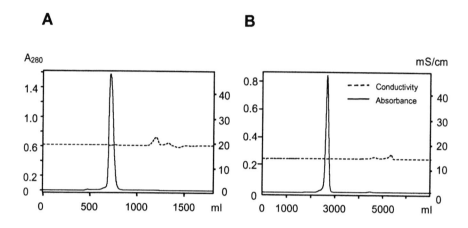

Figure 4.11. Size exclusion chromatography of a monoclonal antibody using Fractogel® EMD BioSEC (S) (Merck KGaA). A. Sample containing 40 ml of protein (12.8 mg/ml) was loaded onto a 1000 x 50 mm inner diameter column (bed volume: 1.806 litre, bed height 920 mm) at a flow rate of 5ml/min. B. Separation was transferred to a 100 mm inner diameter column with the same bed height (column volume 7.225 litre). The sample volume was 124 ml corresponding to 2.778 g of protein, a flow rate of 20 ml/min was applied with PBS, pH 7.4 as eluent.

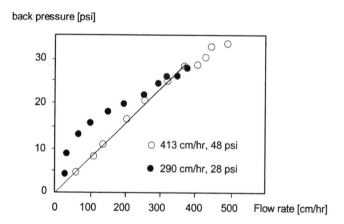

Figure 4.12. Pressure flow curves of Fractogel® EMD TMAE flow packed at different flow rates in a column with an inner diameter of 100 mm. A linear relation between the backpressure and flow rates up to 400 cm/hr can be achieved if the packing was done using a high flow rate. If the flow rate is too low, the column will show gap formation during the separation or the subsequent cleaning procedure.

This step represents an important contribution to the removal of viruses and endotoxins. For production scale separations, column diameters up to 30 cm are recommended and can be managed technically. Usually the length of the column is in the range of 60 - 100 cm for smaller column diameters (less than 50 mm). Columns with larger diameters can be packed up to 90 cm. It always should be kept in mind that the column length will influence the resolution of any size exclusion column. Although the viscosity of the sample solution may affect the resolution, for practical reasons highly concentrated antibody samples will give the best separations in the case of SEC with respect to the process economy. This has to be combined with steps to concentrate the protein solution, which could lead to loss of protein or in some cases to aggregation problems. The actual loading capacity always depends on the sample composition and the separation problem. Because in SEC no adsorption takes places, the accumulation of contaminants can rather be neglected and many cycles can be run. However, when carbohydrate based resins are used, any microbial growth has to be avoided. This might be a potential source of endotoxin contamination of the final product. As the fermentation volume will be increased SEC does not meet the need of an economical processing of large quantities.

8. LARGE SCALE COLUMN PACKING

Optimal separation performance can be achieved by selecting the right combination of media characteristics and column properties. The pressure/flow properties of chromatographic media have an impact on their behaviour when packed into large columns where no column wall effects help to stabilize the packed bed. On the other hand, the column should be constructed with consideration to the properties of the intended media. Because the packing of large columns can be particularly tedious, a reliable packing method resulting in consistent performance through scale-up has to be set up. Packing methods developed at lab-scale columns may not be applicable at large scale due to differences in column design. Therefore, a robust method for column packing has to be established in advance. All production columns should be packed only as easily as it is achieved in manufacturing environment. For example, the height equivalent to a theoretical plate (HETP) is at commercial scale often less than 0.05 mm and the asymmetry (A_s) between 0.7 and 1.3 (Sofer, 1996). The technical instructions of the columns have to be considered and each resin has to be packed according to the manufacturer's instructions to avoid problems. Availability of pressure-flow relationships, column efficiency and peak asymmetry values at different scales are helpful. A collection of commercially available columns for production is listed in Table 4.5.

These columns provide manual variable adapters or hydraulic assisted adapters. Columns, which have to be packed to a fixed bed size without any adjustable adapter, are less convenient to pack. A variable height adapter allows axial pressure packing, the recommended packing method for most media, which should be packed in a one step procedure. Unfortunately, due to the costs of packing studies, only a few papers were published showing operating parameters of production scale columns. Williams et al., (2002), described packing and maintenance of a 40 cm inner diameter and a 200 cm inner diameter Chromaflow® column (Amersham Biosciences), Moscariello et al., (2001) showed some packing studies using an IsoPak column (Millipore) with an inner diameter of 44 cm. An empirical model has been developed that allows prediction of pressure-flow curves in packed beds of compressible media based on experiments done with columns less than 5 cm in inner diameter by Stickel and Fotopoulos (2001). The results indicate that it is not possible to operate a rProtein A Sepharose® column with a bed height of 20 cm at flow velocities of 100 cm/hr. In order to operate a production column at 100 cm/hr, the bed height has to be reduced to 15 cm and a larger diameter is required to meet capacity requirements.

Table 4.5. Commercially available production scale columns for biochromatography

Manufacturer	Product Name	Maximum diameter	Maximum pressure
Amersham Biosciences (Sweden)	BPG	450 [mm]	2.5 [bar]
	Danprocess	1200 [mm]	up to 6 [bar]
	Chromaflow	2000 [mm]	3 [bar]
Millipore Corporation (USA)	IsoPak	1000 [mm]	Customer specified
	Vantage	250 [mm]	3 [bar]
	Moduline	630 [mm]	3 [bar]
Eastern Rivers, Inc. (Chattanooga, TN, USA)	customized	2000 [mm]	3 [bar]

There are many other columns available for laboratory scale and pilot plant

In general, semi-rigid synthetic polymers provide higher pressure stability than soft gels. Furthermore, high mechanical stability is necessary for packing large production-size columns. Pressure drop across chromatography beds can cause significant problems in the operation of large-scale preparative columns, if the scale-up procedure does not reflect the production column. For example, biphasic pressure versus flow rate curves were seen for Fractogel® EMD TMAE (Merck KGaA) that was flow packed at a slow flow rate (Fig. 4.12). If resins are not packed to sufficient density with a minimum of interstitial volume (i.e. the volume between the

Scale-up of antibody purification

porous particles), gap formation between the top adapter and the packed bed will be observed, as the flow rate approaches the packing velocity.

Column cleanliness can be monitored by yield losses in the eluate or increases in target protein in flowthrough fraction. On the other hand an increase of the pressure drop can be used as marker for cleaning efficiency. Nitrate ion capacity is a useful orthogonal test for column cleanliness.

9. SUMMARY

The rapidly growing market for mABs is very promising for biotech companies. However, compared to chemical drugs, the manufacturing of biotherapeutics is more sophisticated. Today the worldwide fermentation capacity is too small to meet the growing demand within the next years. Due to the fact that the upstream fermentation is limited, it becomes increasingly more important to make the complete downstream processing as fast as possible. However, this should be done without any additional risk regarding the safety of the biotherapeutic substance. To avoid any bottlenecks in production every step has to be optimised. One prerequisite is "state of the art equipment" for the plant. Also separation media providing all the necessary properties are needed to capture and purify the target antibody with a high recovery in a short period of time.

Table 4.6. Process steps and their main purpose.

Protein A affinity chromatography	Cation exchange chromatography	Anion exchange chromatography	Size exclusion chromatography
capture of Mab	separation of protein A leakage products	negative purification step of mAb	adjustment of final mAb concentration
recovery >90% of mAb	removal of hcp	removal of hcp	transfer to final formulation buffer
>60-fold concentration	removal of culture additives	removal of proteases removal of DNA	removal of mAb - aggregates
endotoxin removal	removal of aggregates	viral clearance	removal of traces of DNA
viral clearance	reduction of volume	endotoxin removal	
	separation of DNA	separatation of protein A leakage products	
	viral clearance		
	removal of endotoxins		

As a result of resin screening, it is possible to design a robust process with only two or three chromatographic steps consisting of protein A for capture and ion exchange for subsequent purification in addition to ultrafiltration steps. At each step, different goals can be defined and validated (Table 4.6). Effects of different process parameters such as the gradient slope, pH, flow velocity and protein loading on the mAb's purity, including removal of certain contaminants, have to be evaluated before scaling up.

The most important parameter for the scale-up of the affinity step is residence time, which has to be kept constant as well as the protein load. The back pressure of the media at large bed heights often restricts production scale applications. It has to be considered that the same amount of affinity gel will provide different productivities if the column geometry is varied. Especially buffer pH for the cation exchanger can affect protein binding capacity and, thus, has to be determined experimentally at laboratory scale. Ion exchange chromatography can easily be transferred to large scale by maintaining the bed height, linear flow, protein load and increasing the diameter of the column. Taking into account all the regulatory, commercial, and manufacturing requirements a rework of the process entails, it should be avoided unless absolutely necessary.

Based on small-scale studies, optimum operating conditions should be chosen. Then the purification process can be successfully scaled-up to a large-scale robust process with step yields and product quality that were better than those at the small scale.

10. OUTLOOK

There are now technologies evolving to screen for chromatographic conditions rapidly at small scale. Coupling for example the affinity baits as protein A or protein G on the biosensor surface of BIACORE allows one to study the interaction of proteins with that surface. This gives information concerning the kinetics and stability of the interaction. Screening of binding and elution conditions is fast and might lead to improved purification protocols for the protein.

Some mass spectrometry methods could be used for rapid screening of binding and elution condition for the target protein. In the surface enhanced laser desorption ionization time-of-flight mass spectrometry (SELDI-TOF-MS) ProteinChip® system (Ciphergen Biosystems) approach, the target protein is bound on a surface with the appropriate functional groups used for chromatography. The binding and the elution with various conditions can be easily monitored by mass analysis.

On the other hand, new developments like expanded bed adsorption as well as membrane chromatography might contribute to successful purification schemes. Also designed peptides or dye-derived ligands could replace protein A during the capture step providing more robustness. However, there is still a lot of manual experimental work to establish all relevant process parameters.

ACKNOWLEDGEMENTS

The authors would like to thank Abhinav Shukla (Amgen, Product Recovery, Seattle WA), Tessa Chao (EMD Chemicals, Gibbstown, NJ) and Winfried Linxweiler (Merck KGaA, Germany) for providing scientific results.

REFERENCES

Amersham Biosciences, 2001, MabSelect®, data file 71-5020-91 AA, and Protein A Sepharose® Fast Flow, data file 18-1125-19

Ameskamp, N., Priesner, C., Lehmann, J., and Lutkemeyer, D., 1999, Pilot scale recovery of monoclonal antibodies by expanded bed ion exchange adsorption. *Bioseparation* **8**:169-188

Andersson, M., Ramberg, M., and Johansson, B-L., 1998, The influence of the degree of cross-linking, type of ligand and support on the chemical stability of chromatography media intended for protein purification. *Process Biochemistry* **33**:47.55

Bai, L., Burman, S., Gledhill, L, 2000, Development of ion exchange chromatography methods for monoclonal antibodies. *J. Pharm. Biomed. Anal.* **22**:605-611

Barnfield Frej, A.-K., Johansson, H.J., Johansson, S., Leijon, P., 1997, Expanded bed adsorption at production scale: scale-up verification, process example and sanitization of column and adsorbent. *Bioprocess Eng.* **16**:57—63

Belew, M., Juntti, N., Larsson, A., and Porath, J., 1987, A one-step purification method for monoclonal antibodies based on salt-promoted adsorption chromatography on a "thiophilic" adsorbent. *J. Immunol Methods* **102**:173-182

Bill, E., Lutz, U., Karlsson, B.M., Sparrman, M., and Allgaier, H., 1995, Optimization of protein G chromatography for biopharmaceutical monoclonal antibodies. *J. Mol. Recognit.* **8**:90-94

Breece, T.N., Gilkerson, E., and Schmelzer, C., 2002, Validation of large-scale chromatographic processes, part II; Results from the case study of neuleze capture on Macroprep High-S. *BioPharm* **July 2002**:35-42

Brorson, K., Brown, J., Hamilton, E., and Stein, K., 2003, Identification of protein A media performance attributes that can be monitored as surrogates for retrovirus clearance during extended re-use. *J. Chromatogr. A* **989**:155-163

Casey, J.L., Keep, P.A., Chester, K.A., Robson, L., Hawkins, R.E., and Begent, R.H.J., 1995, Purification of bacterially expressed single chain Fv antibodies for clinical applications using metal chelate chromatography. *J. Immunol. Methods* **179**:105-116

Cahill, M., Macniven, R., Hawkins, K., Gallo, C., Sernatinger, J., Myers, J., and Notarnicola, S., 2000, Viral Clearance by Protein A Affinity and Anion Exchange Chromatography.

Downstream GAb abstracts "Reports from GAb 2000" Amersham Biosciences, Code number, **18-1150-47**:24-26

Center for Biologics Evaluation and Research, 1997, Points to consider in the manufacture and testing of monoclonal antibody products for human use; Food and Drug Administration, U. S. Department of Health and Human Services, Rockville, MD

Denton, G., Murray, A., Price, M.R., and Levison, P.R., 2001, Direct isolation of monoclonal antibodies from tissue culture supernatant using the cation-exchange cellulose Express-Ion S. *J. Chromatogr. A*, **908**:223-234

Desai, M.A., 2000, Methods in Biotechnology Vol 9, Downstream Processing of Proteins, Methods and Protocols. Humana Press Inc., Totowa, New Jersey

Dziennik, S.R., Belcher, E.B., Barker, G.A., DeBergalis, M.J., Fernandez, S.E., Lenhoff, A.M., 2003, Nondiffusive mechanisms enhance protein uptake rates in ion exchange particles. *Proc. Natl. Acad. Sci. USA*, **21**:420-425.

Fahrner, R.L. Iyer, H.V., Blank, G.S., 1999, The optimal flow rate and column length for maximum production rate of protein A affinity chromatography. *Bioprocess Engineering* **21**:287-292

Fahrner, R., Blank, G.S., and Zapata, G., 1999, Expanded bed protein A affinity chromatography of a recombinant humanized monoclonal antibody: process development, operation, and comparison with a packed bed method. *J. Biotechnol.* **75**:273-280

Füglistaller, P., 1989, Comparison of immunoglobulin binding capacities and ligand leakage using eight different protein A affinity chromatographic matrices. *J. Immunol. Meth.* **124**:171-177

Francis, R., 1999, Intensification of a large scale commercial monoclonal antibody purification process. paper presented at the "The Fourth Waterside Monoclonal Conference, 14-17 April, 1999, Norfolk, Virginia, USA". *Downstream* **30**:22-23

Gottschalk, U., Rosenkranz, E., and Britsch, L., 1997, Preparative capturing of mouse monoclonal antibodies from cell culture supernatant by cation exchange chromatography. *Bio World* **3**:42-44

Hahn, R., Schlegel, R., and Jungbauer, A., 2003, Comparison of Protein A affinity sorbents. *J. Chromatogr. B* **790**: 35-51

Hubbuch, J., Linden, T., Knieps, E., Thömmes, J., and Kula, M-R., 2002, Dynamics of protein uptake within the adsorbent particle during packed bed chromatography. *Biotechnol. Bioeng.* **80**:359-368

Huse, K., Bohme, H.J., and Scholz, G.H., 2002, Purification of antibodies by affinity chromatography. *J. Biochem. Biophys. Methods* **51**:217-31

Iyer, H., Henderson F., Cunningham E., Webb J., Hanson J., Bork C., and Conley L. 2002, Considerations during development of a protein A-based antibody purification process. *Biopharm* **January 2002**:14-20

Kang, K.A. and Ryu, D.D., 1991, Studies on scale-up parameters of an immunoglobulin separation system using protein A affinity chromatography. *Biotechnol. Prog.* **7**:205-212

Kundu, A., Allen, K., Carrillo R., Snyder M., and Burton, G., 2001, Development of a regeneration protocol for anion-exchange resins presented at the Recovery of Biological Products X in Cancún (Mexico; 2001)

Lagerlund, I., Larsson, E., Gustavsson, J., Färenmark, J., and Heijbel, A., 1998, Characterisation of ANX Sepharose® 4 Fast Flow media. *J. Chromatogr. A* **769**:129-140

Levison, P.R., Mumford, C., Streater, M., Brandt-Nielson, A., Pathirana, N.D., and Badger, S.E. 1997, Performance comparison od low-pressure ion-exchange chromatography media for protein separation. *J. Chromatogr. A* **760**:151-158

Lutkemeyer, D., Ameskamp, N., Priesner, C., Bartsch, E.M., and Lehmann, J., 2001, Capture of proteins from mammalian cells in pilot scale using different STREAMLINE® adsorbents. *Bioseparation* **10**:57-63

McCue, J.T., Kemp, G., Low, D. and Quinones-Garcia, I., 2003, Evaluation of protein A chromatography media. *J. Chromatogr. A* **989**:136-153

Moscariello, J., Purdom, G., Coffman, J., Root, T.W., and Lightfoot, E.N., 2001, Characterizing the performance of industrial-scale columns. *J. Chromatogr. A* **908**:131-41

Necina, R., Amatschek, K., and Jungbauer, A., 1998, Capture of Human Monoclonal Antibodies from Cell Culture Supernatant by Ion Exchange Media Exhibiting High Charge Density. *Biotechnol. Bioeng.* **60**:689-698

O'Leary, R.M., Feuerhelm, D., Peers, D., Xu, Y., and Blank, G., 2001, Determining the useful lifetime oc chromatographic resins. *BioPharm* **September 2001**:10-18

Rathore, A. and Velayudhan, A., 2003, Guidelines for optimization and scale up in preparative chromatography. *BioPharm* **January 2003**:34-42

Schulze, R., Kontermann, R., Queitsch, I., Dübel, S., and Bautz, E., 1994, Thiophilic adsorption chromatography of recombinant single-chain antibody fragments. *Analytical Biochemistry* **220**:212-214,

Schenerman, M.A., Hope, J.N., Kletke, C., Singh, J.K., Kimura, R., Tsao, E.I., and Folena-Wasserman, G., 1999, Comparability testing of a humanized monoclonal antibody (Synagis) to support cell line stability, process validation, and scale-up for manufacturing. *Biologicals* **27**:203-15

Schwartz, W., Judd, D., Wysocki, M., Guerrier, L., Birck-Wilson, E., and Boschetti, E., 2001, Comparison of hydrophobic charge induction chromatography with affinity chromatography on protein A for harvest and purification of antibodies. *J. Chromatogr A.* **908**:251-63

Shukla, A., Hinckley, P., Gefroh, E., Priyanka, G., and Hubbard, B., 2002, Generic purification processes for monoclonal antibodies and Fc fusion proteins; presented at IBC's Scaling-Up from Bench to Clinic & Beyond conference 14-16 August, 2002, San Diego, USA

Sofer, G., 1996, Validation: Ensuring the accuracy of scaled-down chromatography models. *BioPharm* **October 1996**:51-54

Stickel, J.J. and Fotopoulos, A., 2001, Pressure-flow relationship for packed beds of compressible chromatography media at laboratory and production scale, *Biotechnol. Prog.* **17**:744-751

Tauer, C., Buchacher, A., and Jungbauer, A., 1995, DNA clearance in chromatography of proteins, exemplified by affinity chromatography. *J. Biochem. Biophys. Methods* **30**:75-78

Tice, A., Mazsaroff, I., Lin, N.T., and Regnier, F.E., 1987, Effects of large sample loads on column lifetime in preparative-scale liquid chromatography. *J. Chromatogr.* **410**:43-51

van Sommeren, A.P., Machielsen, P.A., and Gribnau, T.C., 1992, Effects of temperature, flow rate and composition of binding buffer on adsorption of mouse monoclonal IgG1 antibodies to protein A Sepharose® 4 Fast Flow. *Prep Biochem.* **22**:135-149

Vorauer, K., Skias, M., Trkola, A., Schulz, P. and Jungbauer, A., 1992, Scale-up of recombinant protein purification by hydrophobic interaction chromatography. *J. Chromatogr.* **625**:33-39

Walter, J., 1999, Scale-up of downstream processing. In *Protein Liquid Chromatography (Journal of Chromatography Library vol. 61)* (M. Kastner, ed.), Elsevier, Amsterdam, pp. 765-783.

Walter, J.K., Nothelfer, F., and Werz, W., 1998, Virus Removal and Inactivation. *ACS Symp.Series 698, Validation of Biopharm. Manufac. Processes, Am.Chem.Soc, pp. 114-124.*

Williams, A., Taylor, K., Dambuleff, K., Persson, O., and Kennedy, R.M., 2002, Maintenance of column performance at scale. *J. Chromatogr. A* **944**:69-75

Chapter 5

PURIFICATION OF ANTIBODIES BY CHROMATOGRAPHIC METHODS

Caroline Vandevyver* and Ruth Freitag*[§]
* Laboratory of Chemical Biotechnology, Faculty of Basic Science, Swiss Federal Institute of Technology, Lausanne, Switzerland; § present address: Chair for Bioprocess Engineering, University of Bayreuth, Germany

1. INTRODUCTION

Antibodies belong to the immunoglobulin family, i.e. a class of proteins that constitute the so-called humoral branch of the immune system. They represent approximately 20 % of the proteins in human blood plasma. Besides their physiological function, antibodies are also important tools for general research as well as for the diagnosis and treatment of a vast array of diseases. This is largely due to the fact that antibodies can be purposedly raised against many natural and synthetic molecules, which they later recognize in a highly specific way, even in very complex matrices.

In bioseparation immobilized antibodies are, e.g., used for the specific isolation of their corresponding "antigens", both on the laboratory and on the large industrial scale. Immunochemical *in vitro* diagnostic procedures, such as the enzyme-linked immunosorbent assay (ELISA), the radioimmunoassay (RIA), or the many blot techniques employing antibodies linked to radioactive isotopes, enzymes, fluorescence or other markers allow the efficient detection of minute amounts of analytes such as individual proteins, nucleic acids, complex carbohydrates, or lipids with a high degree of specificity. Therapeutically, antibodies have been used *in vivo* for many years, e.g., for passive immunization or the prevention of hemolytic disease of the newborn. Recently, the high specificity of antibodies and the development of novel techniques for their production by chemical and biological means (e.g., hybridoma cells or transgenic animals for monoclonal antibodies and recombinant technologies for genetically engineered antibodies, Siegel DL, 2002), have led to the development of immunotherapies were (radio)labeled monoclonal antibodies ("monoclonals") specific for certain tumor-associated antigens are used to target the malignant cells *in vivo* and thereby deliver a diagnostic or even cytotoxic agent to them. At present, several of these monoclonals are in the pipeline and awaiting FDA approval. Together they represent almost 30 % of the biotechnology-derived drugs under development (Berger M et al., 2002).

As mentioned before, today many techniques exist for the production of antibodies and the sources from which these proteins may have to be isolated are no longer limited to the typical natural sources such as body fluids (blood, ascites) of immunized animals or human beings. Recombinant sources, such as cultures of engineered cells, like hybridoma and CHO cells, or phage display libraries, also represent major sources of commercially available antibodies. The purification of antibodies from crude feedstocks is usually a lengthy, multi-step process, especially in the case of therapeutic antibodies. A combination of methods is used, involving most often operations such as salting-out, ion-exchange chromatography and affinity chromatography. However, the purification of antibodies remains a problem for which no general solution can be proposed, due to the large variety of different antibody species, sources they derive from, and intended applications. It is quite possible that an established purification scheme that has already been successful in the case of several antibody species fails when applied to a certain new antibody. In addition, the multifunctional property of antibodies – antigen binding and effector functions – makes it more difficult to develop purification protocols in which both features remain unaffected. Finally, the choice of source material can affect the selection of techniques suitable for isolation and purification as a function of the presence of typical impurities in the matrix (Table 5.1) and the antibody concentrations reached in that particular source. Due to these difficulties, it is still quite common for many – even some established therapeutic – applications to use not a purified antibody preparation, but rather the whole serum or cell culture supernatant. However, it is clear that for some applications purified antibodies are needed, for example most therapeutic uses, or when antibodies are to be labeled or subjected to proteolytic fragmentation.

During the last 20 years, a plethora of protocols for the purification of antibodies has been reported by numerous authors (reviewed, e.g., by Grandics P, 1994). The present chapter focuses on the chromatographic methods for antibody purification with a special emphasis on novel (synthetic) ligands for affinity-chromatographic purification and the development of new chromatographic modes.

2. CHROMATOGRAPHIC PURIFICATION OF ANTIBODIES

A significant advantage when working with native or recombinant antibodies or fragments is that there is considerable information available about the product and its likely contaminants/impurities as shown in Tables 5.1 and 5.2 below.

Table 5.1. Antibody sources and their associated contaminants/impurities

	Molecular Type	Significant contaminants/impurities
Source: native		
Human serum	Polyclonal IgG, IgM, IgA, IgD, IgE	Albumin, transferrin, $\alpha 2$-macroglobulin, other serum proteins
Hybridoma: cell culture supernatants[1] with 10 % foetal calf serum	Monoclonal	Phenol red, water, albumin, transferrin, bovine IgG, $\alpha 2$-macroglobulin, other serum proteins, viruses
Hybridoma: cell culture supernatants serum free	Monoclonal	Albumin, transferrin (often added as supplements)
Ascites fluid[2]	Monoclonal	Lipids, albumin, transferrin, lipoproteins, endogenous IgG, other host proteins
Egg yolk	IgY	Lipids, lipoproteins and vitellin
Source: recombinant		
Extracellular protein expressed into supernatant	Recombinant antibodies, tagged antibodies, antibody fusion proteins, Fab or F(ab')$_2$ fragments	Proteins from the host. e.g. *E. coli.*, CHO cells, general low level of contamination
Intracellular protein expression		Proteins from the host, e.g. *E. coli*, phage

[1] An advantage of cell culture systems is the –theoretically - unlimited volume and quantity of material that can be produced.
[2] For ascites, the production volume is limited and in certain countries their production is subject to significant legal restrictions.

Table 5.2. Antibody characteristics

Molecular weight	M_r 150 000 – 160 000 (IgG)
	M_r 900 000 (IgM)
Isoelectric point (pI)	4-9, most > 6.0, often more basic than other serum proteins
Hydrophobicity	IgG is more hydrophobic than many other proteins and so precipitates more readily in ammonium sulfate
Solubility	IgG is very soluble in aqueous buffers. Lowest solubility (specific to each antibody) near pI or in very low salt concentration
Temperature stability	Relatively stable at room temperature (deviations from this rule must be expected in individual cases)
pH stability	Often stable over a wide pH interval, but unstable in very acidic buffers (specific to each antibody)
Carbohydrate content	2-3 % for IgG, higher for IgM (12 %), most carbohydrate is associated with the Fc region of the heavy chain

With this information a purification strategy can be developed. A shortcut purification sequence for therapeutic antibodies should consist of three steps: capture, purification and polishing (Figure 5.1). This generic approach is used in both the pharmaceutical industry and in the research laboratory to ensure fast method development, a short time to pure product and economic feasibility.

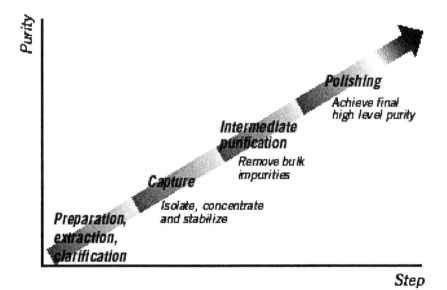

Figure 5.1. Multi-step purification strategy for antibody production (Reproduced by kind permission of Amersham Biosciences AB)

2.1 Affinity chromatography

2.1.1 Introduction

Affinity chromatography is a powerful tool for protein purification and not surprisingly plays an important role in the purification of antibodies as well. The method is based on the possibility of a highly specific, typically non-covalent interaction (binding) of an immobilized ligand with the target molecule, i.e. in our case the recombinant, monoclonal or polyclonal antibody (retention or capturing step). Affinity chromatography is particularly valuable in cases where the target molecule has to be separated from a matrix, which contains components of similar physical characteristics, e.g. other proteins. Under binding conditions, the target protein (antibody) forms a complex with the affinity ligand, while the other matrix components pass unretained through the column. The specifically bound protein can be eluted competitively, i.e. by adding the affinity ligand in unbound form to the elution buffer or - more commonly - by low or high pH buffers, which serve to dissociate the target protein/ligand complexes. Over the last 20 years, over 27'000 articles have been published that describe or discuss affinity chromatography techniques. There have also been many significant developments in the technique, such as the introduction of new and improved solid support materials (see below), accessory equipment leading to the maturation of the technique from a research tool to a widely used, industrial scale biopurification method (Godfrey MAJ et al., 1993, Goward CR, 1995).

Often, affinity purification strategies for antibodies are in fact multi-step approaches that take advantage of the structure of these target molecules. The first step may thus make use of the specific antigen of this particular antibody (binding to the variable region of the antibody), while the second one targets the constant part of the antibody, the F_c fragment, which varies only according to antibody class. Recent advances in the production of genetically engineered antibodies and antibody fragments have opened up many possibilities, not only to manipulate the biological properties of these compounds, but also to facilitate their purification. For example, tags can be introduced into such antibodies and antibody fragments and target molecules for which no affinity ligand was previously available may thus become eligible to effective affinity purification.

2.1.2 Ligands for affinity purification of antibodies

The effectiveness of affinity purification of antibodies relies on the availability of suitable affinity ligands, which can be immobilized efficiently and in highly active form on the chromatographic stationary phase. Several reviews addressing the development and evaluation of new ligands for affinity-chromatography of antibodies can be found in the literature (Huse K et al., 2002, Fassina G et al. 2001, Gaberc-Porekar V et al., 2001, Boschetti E, 2001, Lowe CR et al. 2001).

2.1.2.1 Antigens

Antibodies can be purified by using - if known - the corresponding antigen or a fragment thereof as affinity ligand (Fleminger G et al., 1990, Santucci A et al., 1988, Murray A et al., 1997). In a typical scheme a mixture of antibodies specific for human albumin and transferrin was to be separated from the γ-globulin fraction of goat antiserum by passing the mixture through a column carrying either immobilized albumin or transferrin (Wheatly JB, 1992). In a more ingenious, sequential affinity scheme, bispecific antibodies were extracted from a mixture containing also monospecific monoclonal antibodies. In particular, a bispecific monoclonal antibody, specific for methotrexate (MTX) and a tumor-associated antigen (gp72) was separated from monospecific anti-MTX and anti-gp72 antibodies in the hybridoma culture supernatant by a combination of affinity chromatography on a MTX-agarose immunoadsorbent and step-wise elution with acid from Sepharose-Protein A (Pimm MV et al., 1990). While these are interesting strategies, the problem remains that the binding strength of proteineous antigen-antibody complexes is typically very high; K_d of 10^{-11} M or smaller are not uncommon (Kristiansen T, 1978). This may make the elution of the antibody from the immunoaffinity sorbent rather difficult. Therefore, it is often desirable to modulate the strength of the antibody-antigen complex. This can be done by changing the ability for conformational rearrangements, e.g. by multipoint linkage, during the immobilization of a proteineous antigen. For example, when the antigen D-glyceraldehyde-3-phosphate dehydrogenase (GAPDH) was immobilized on Sepharose, it was possible to achieve preparations that where completely deprived of enzyme activity. The amount of antibody bound by the resulting matrix was similar as when the native forms of the enzyme was used, but the elution of the antibody was greatly facilitated (Cherednikova TV et al., 1980, 1981).

2.1.2.2 F_c receptors

The majority of therapeutic antibodies under development belong to the immunoglobulin G class. Purification of this type of monoclonal antibody is often based on the use of generic Fc receptors as affinity ligand in a first step for capturing and concomitant concentrating the immunoglobulin from the diluted feeds.

Such immunoglobulin-binding proteins have been found at the surface of numerous cells and viruses. Typically, they bind to the F_c part of the antibody, hence their classification as F_c receptors. Several bacterial F_c receptors have been studied in this context, most prominently Protein A from *Staphylococcus aureus* (Forsgen A et al., 1966) and (the more expensive) Protein G from *Streptococcus spp.* (Raeder R and Boyle MD, 1995). Both will bind IgG from different sources, although some differences exist in subtype specificity. Table 3 shows a comparison of the relative binding strengths of Protein A and Protein G towards their putative target molecules that has been compiled from various publications.

Another type of group specific ligand, namely Protein L *(Peptostreptococcus magnus)* (Bjorck L, 1988) has been introduced more recently for the purification of whole antibodies and antibody fragments (Nilson BH et al., 1993, Vola R et al., 1995). This ligand binds to an eventually present κ-light chain in the antibody molecule (Akerstram B et al., 1989, Nilson BH et al., 1992).

Protein A–affinity chromatography is probably the most common method for antibody purification (Langone JJ, 1982a). The fact that Protein A is by now an extremely well-characterized molecule (Deisenhofer J, 1981, Langone JJ, 1982b) that can be obtained in native or recombinant form and in large quantities from microorganisms or genetically modified bacteria, assures its continuing popularity. The molar dissociation constant of an Protein A–IgG complex is at about 10^{-7}, which reflects a high affinity of the Protein A for the F_c region of the immunoglobulins. Protein A contains four binding sites, two of which are able to interact with the F_c part of an antibody at the same time.

Protein G, a cell surface protein from Group G *streptococci*, is a type III F_c receptor. Like Protein A, it binds specifically to the F_c region of IgG by a non-immune mechanism. Compared to Protein A, Protein G binds more strongly to several polyclonal IgGs (Table 5.3) and to human IgG_3. From the bioseparation point of view, Protein G had the inherent disadvantage to interact not with antibodies but also with albumin and α2-macroglobulin, i.e. some typical major compounds in antibody cell culture media (Table 5.1). Some companies offer a recombinant form of Protein G from which the albumin- and/or α2-macroglobulin binding region(s) of the native molecule have been genetically deleted, thereby avoiding undesirable retention of these molecules. Recombinant G contains two F_c binding regions.

Protein A and G are very effective tools in the large-scale purification of monoclonal IgG antibodies. The capacity of Protein A/Protein G-activated chromatographic supports can reach up to 30-40 mg IgG/ml of affinity sorbent under optimized conditions. Many monoclonal antibodies currently on the market for therapy or diagnostics are purified by processes involving these affinity ligands. However, easy as it may appear, purifying antibodies with bacterial F_c receptors has some limitations, especially in the case of human therapeutics. First, the biological origin itself is the cause of some concern, and the absence of any residual affinity ligand molecules (caused e.g. by column "bleeding") in the final antibody preparation has to be assured, making the utilization of the ligands at large scale complex and expensive.

Table 5-3. Relative binding strengths of Protein A and Protein G

Species	Subclass	Protein A binding	Protein G binding
Human	IgA	Variable	-
	IgD	-	-
	IgE	-	-
	IgG_1	++++	++++
	IgG_2	++++	++++
	IgG_3	+	++++
	IgG_4	++++	++++
	IgM	variable	-
Chicken	IgY	-	-
Avian egg yolk	IgY	-	-
Cow	IgG	++	++++
Dog		++	+
Goat	IgG	+	++
Guinea pig	IgG_1	++++	++
	IgG_2	++++	++
Hamster		+	++
Horse	IgG	++	++++
	IgM	-	-
Koala		-	+
Lama		-	+
Monkey (rhesus)		++++	++++
Mouse	IgG_1	+	++++
	IgG_{2a}	++++	++++
	IgG_{2b}	+++	+++
	IgG_3	++	+++
	IgM_1	variable	-
Pig	IgG	+++	+++
Rabbit	No distinction	++++	+++
Rat	IgG_1	-	+
	IgG_{2a}	-	++++
	IgG_{2b}	-	++
	IgG_3	+	++
Sheep	IgG	+/-	++

It is also well known that Protein A leaking from the column will interfere with analysis of the purified antibody (Godfrey MA et al., 1993). Secondly, if antibodies purified by bacterial F_c receptors are used as therapeutics, time-consuming analyses are required to ensure the absence of potentially hazardous contaminants putatively introduced via the affinity ligand. Pyrogens and viruses are possibilities that have to be taken into consideration in this context. Third, since these affinity ligand are limited in their selectivity to IgG, they are not useful for the purification of IgA, IgE, IgM and IgY, antibody types that are increasingly finding application in the cure and/or diagnosis of important diseases. Fourth, the typical conditions required for the elution of the antibody from such affinity columns, usually low pH, can alter the conformation of the immunoglobulins and thereby damage their biological activity (Vijayalakshimi MA 1998).

In order to overcome these drawbacks, attempts have been made to modify or mimic the structure of Protein A with the goal of obtaining affinity ligands that allow for milder elution conditions and/or selectivity for other subclasses of immunoglobulins. Gulich S et al. (2000) genetically engineered an IgG-binding domain of Protein A, creating the so-called Protein Z, which, e.g., allowed milder elution conditions.

2.1.2.3   Protein A mimetic ligands

The increasing number of monoclonals being developed for therapy, the role of the purification process in assuring the quality, consistency and safety of the products, and, finally, the emerging importance of other classes of immunoglobulines besides IgG as molecules of high medical interest, engendered considerable efforts towards the synthesis of low-molecular weight molecules able to bind antibodies, like Protein A but with improved properties. These synthetic ligands should have not only reduced production costs at large-scale, but also increased resistance to chemical and biological actions, reduced toxicity and less leakage from affinity sorbents, reduction in the amount of contaminants of biological nature, high capacity for large-scale purification, and extended selectivity for other classes of immunoglobulins not recognized by Protein A or G.

Recent investigations, based on the synthesis and screening of combinatorial peptide libraries or computer modeling, have provided several novel compounds with very promising characteristics.

- Tetramer of the IgG binding domains A and B of Protein A
  Artificial IgG-binding proteins ($pA(AB)_{1-6}$), have been expressed in *Escherichia coli* and immobilized on cyanogen bromide-Sepharose (Kihari Y and Aiba S, 1992). $PA(AB)_4$-Sepharose showed the highest IgG-binding capacity, about 30 % higher than Protein A.

- PAM (Protein A Mimetic, TG19318)

    A good example of the use of randomized synthetic peptide tetramers for affinity purification of antibodies has been reported by the group of Fassina G (Ruvo M et al., 1994). They performed a screening of a multimeric peptide library, composed of 5832 randomized tripeptide tetramers, by measuring the ability to interfere with the interaction between Protein A and biotinylated immunoglobulins. After several screening cycles, they identified the most active multimer as $(Arg-Thr-X)_4-K_2-K-G$ [PAM, Protein A Mimetic, TG19318]. The results obtained with PAM are very promising. The ligand seems to have a much broader specificity than Protein A. IgG has been successfully purified from different sources using this ligand (Fassina G et al., 1998, Guerrier L et al. 1998), as well as IgM from ascitic fluid, sera, or cell culture supernatants (Palombo et al.,1998a) and IgA (Palombo et al., 1998b) respectively IgE (Palombo et al., 1998c) from cell culture supernatants. Recent work has shown that IgY can be purified from egg yolk in a single step to more than 90% purity on a column of immobilized peptide TG19318 (Verdoliva et al., 2000).

- Peptide H

    Another ligand for mouse IgG purification has been identified by screening a dimeric tripeptide library, produced by starting from a bifunctional lysine residue at the C-terminus and structurally constrained by the presence of a disulfide bond formed by two cysteine residues at the N-terminus (Fassina G et al., 1994, Marino M et al., 1999). The screening of combinatorial libraries of cyclic peptides often gives excellent affinity ligand candidates, because cyclic peptides are more resistant to enzymatic degradation and less flexible compared to the linear form, which often does not display enough rigidity to provide a sufficiently selective recognition surface. This screening strategy led to the identification of Peptide H, a cyclic dimeric peptide of formula $(C-F-H-H)_2KG$, where the two cysteine residues at the N-terminus are covalently linked by a disulfide bridge. The capacity for mouse IgG was close to 1 mg IgG/ml of derivatized CH-Sepharose 4B support.

- 2-(3-aminophenol)-6-(4-amino-1-naphthol)-4-chloro-s-triazine (ApA- Artifical Protein A)

    The ability to combine knowledge of X-ray crystallography, NMR or homology structures with defined or combinatorial chemical synthesis and advanced computational tools has made the rational design of affinity ligands easier, more logical, and certainly faster. This approach has, e.g., been used by the group of Lowe and co-workers in order to find Protein A-mimetic ligands (Teng S.-F. et al., 1999). They designed a lead ligand for human IgG based on a key Phe-Tyr peptide, which was subsequently refined by screening a limited near neighbor library of mimetic ligands assembled on agarose by a modified mix-and-split procedure (Figure 5.2). Ligands displaying 3-aminophenol and 4-amino-1-naphthol moieties substituted on the triazine scaffold were found to bind human IgG. The resulting lead ligand, dubbed ApA (Artificial protein A), was found to bind to IgG in a competitive manner with an affinity constant of 1-10 µM, as deduced by competitive ELISA experiments

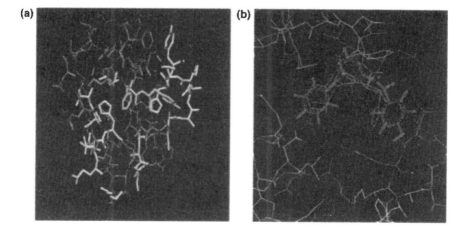

Figure 5-2. Design of a lead ligand for human IgG based on a Phe-Tyr dipeptide structure. (a) Structure of the complex between the F_b fragment of *Staphylococcus aureus* Protein A (SpA) and the F_c fragment of IgG. The residues in pink represent amino acids in SpA interacting with the residues in IgG (shown in yellow). The residues in green represent the key Phe-Tyr dipeptide motif of SpA in the complex. The dotted lines represent intermolecular and intramolecular hydrogen bonding. The interaction involves a total of 32 amino acids spanning an intersurface area corresponding to 400Å^2. (b) Molecular model of the complex between the F_c fragment of IgG and the synthetic ligand, artificial protein A (ApA). The ligand, in red, mimics the key dipeptide Phe-Tyr (shown in green) of SpA and contains anilino and tyramino moieties substituted on a triazinyl framework. ApA is located at the putative binding site among the amino acid residues involved in the interaction between the F_c part of IgG and the F_b fragment of SpA. (Reprinted from Current Opinion in Chemical Biology, 5, CR Lowe, *Combinatorial approaches to affinity chromatography.* 248-256, Copyright 2001, with permission from Elsevier Science)

(Li R et al. 1998). After immobilization on a solid support, such as agarose, ApA was used to purify IgG from human plasma and murine IgG from ascites fluid, and to remove bovine IgG from fetal calf serum with high yield (> 95%) and purity (> 99%). A follow-up study employing solution-synthesized ApA immobilized on beaded agarose indicated an affinity constant (K_a) for the immobilized ApA and human IgG of 1.4×10^5 M^{-1} and a theoretical maximum capacity of 152 mg IgG/g moist weight gel (Teng S.-F. et al., 2000). As in the case of PAM, ApA proved useful also for the purification of IgM and IgA. This study suggests that immobilized ApA, like the equivalent synthetic peptide PAM, may retain many of the advantages in regard to selectivity and capacity of immobilized Protein A, while being superior to the natural affinity ligand in terms of sterilisability, leakage resistance, and toxicity.

- FastMabs A® (UpFront Chromatography A/S)

    The group of Lihme and coworkers used a novel group of mixed mode adsorbents for the purification of monoclonal and polyclonal antibodies from a broad range of feeds including hybridoma cell culture supernatants, ascites fluid, animal sera, milk, whey, and egg yolk. These mixed mode adsorbents carry low molecular weight ligands that typically contain hydrophobic and hydrophilic functionalities within the same molecule (Hansen MB and Lihme A, 1996, Olander M Aa and Lihme A, 1998). In particular, these ligands consist of a hydrophobic core e.g. an aromatic or heteroaromatic ring structure, onto which hydrophilic or ionic substituents e.g. amino groups or carboxylic acid groups, were attached. The protein (antibody) binding mechanism seems to be rather complex, but mixed mode ligands generally show optimum binding under conditions where the substituents are in a non-charged form. The binding strength is therefore strongly pH dependent but in contrast to ion-exchangers, it is largely independent of the ionic strength of the feed. Binding will occur at pH values characteristic for a given mixed mode ligand / target protein-pair, and elution is most often performed by a simple pH-shift. The particular mixed mode ligands used for antibody purification consisted of an aromatic ring-system with a carboxylic acid substituent (Patent Application Lihme and Hansen). The ligand is bound covalently to 6% cross-linked agarose on a solid glass core to give the beads high density. The resulting mixed mode adsorbents showed selective binding of immunoglobulins from complex protein mixtures. IgGs bind to the adsorbent in the pH range of 4.0 to 6.0 and are typically eluted at pH 7.0 to 9.0. The high binding constant makes the adsorbent well suited for purification of monoclonal antibodies from dilute (< 100 µg Mab/ml) hybridoma cell culture supernatants (Lihme and

Hansen, 1997). The mixed mode ligand is furthermore stable to regeneration with 1M sodium hydroxide.

2.1.2.4 Anti-antibodies

Antibodies of the IgE class have also been developed for therapeutic applications. Purification of monoclonal and polyclonal IgE requires the use of convential, often complex and laborous fractionation procedures (Ikeyama S et al., 1986), since studies carried out with immobilized Protein A showed that this protein does not bind to monoclonal IgE, and binds only 12-14 % of the polyclonal IgE found in serum (Phillips TM et al., 1985). Therefore, polyclonal IgE are normally purified by a two-step procedure, using first Protein A to remove the IgG, followed by IgE adsorption to a conventional chromatographic support and elution of the target protein fraction (Zola H et al. 1978). For therapeutic applications, however, large amounts of highly purified material are required. In this case, monoclonal IgE are produced by hybridoma technology in media with low IgG and IgM content. These IgE antibodies are purified mainly by immunoaffinity chromatography using anti-IgE antibodies immobilized on solid supports (Lehrer SB, 1979).

2.1.2.5 Histidin

Antibodies from the sera of patients with autoimmune diseases are reported to have deviating catalytic functions. Their recovery by efficient purification methods is a crucial step in the study of the structural basis of these aberrations. The purification method of choice must not only assure good recovery, but also the conformational integrity of the immunoglobulins in question. Vijayalakshmi MA (1998) showed that in this regard adsorbents with immobilized histidin give excellent results both in yield and in purity, with the additional advantage of very gentle elution conditions. Catalytic autoimmune antibodies from sera of lupus patients were purified using histidyl-aminohexyl-Sepharose gel and compared with the antibodies purified by Protein A and Protein G affinity chromatography. The IgG preparations from the histidin affinity column had a much higher catalytic activity in hydrolyzing the peptide substrate Pro-Phe-Arg-methylcoumarinamide compared to the antibodies obtained by the conventional Protein A/G method (Nedonchelle E et al., 2000). This preservation of catalytic activity is attributed to the gentle conditions used in the histidin ligand method. Thus, histidin affinity offer a superior method for the isolation at least of autoimmune catalytic antibodies.

2.1.2.6 Metals

Immunoglobulins naturally present exposed histidin-rich sequences near to the carboxy terminus of the H-chain; this makes them suitable for purification by immobilized metal affinity chromatography (IMAC), introduced by Porath J and coworkers in 1975 (Boden V et al., 1995, Freyre FM et al., 2000). In addition, Hochuli E et al. (1987, 1988) showed that efficient purification of recombinant proteins with engineered histidin affinity sequences genetically attached to the N- or C-terminus is possible by IMAC, especially in combination with the Ni^{2+}-nitrilotriacetic acid matrices that recognize only adjacent histidins. Since such adjacent histidin residues are uncommon in native proteins, engineered oligo-histidin affinity tags form a unique basis for selectivity and efficiency in IMAC, often yielding proteins with more than 90% purity in a single isolation step. Today, IMAC is often the method of choice for the purification of recombinant single-chain antibodies or fusion proteins, which cannot be purified by Protein A / Protein G affinity chromatography since they lack the target of these F_c receptors, namely the F_c region. Commercial expression vectors, containing nucleotides coding for His6, His10, and some other fusions, are on the market since several years and a very large number of papers on the purification of recombinant antibodies by IMAC techniques has accumulated (some examples, Casey JL et al, 1995, Vaquero C et al., 1999, Yoshida S et al., 2001).

2.1.2.7   Thiophilic interactions

Thiophilic chromatography is another group-specific or pseudospecific affinity technique, which in general allows the retention of proteins that recognize a sulfone group in close proximity to a thioether. The possibility to use this approach for immunoglobulin separation was originally demonstrated by Porath and co-workers in 1985 (Porath J et al., 1985). They showed that it was possible to fractionate plasma proteins by chromatography on agarose-based beads activated by divinylsulfone and grafted with β-mercaptoethanol. Since then, this protein separation mode was mostly applied to antibody purification because the thiophilic gels (T-gels) are particular selective for immunoglobulins and may adsorb more than 20 mg of immunoglobulins per ml of gel (Hutchens TW and Porath J., 1986, Belew M et al., 1987, reviewed in Boschetti E et al., 2001). T-gels have a broad specificity towards immunoglobulins from various animal species, irrespective of the type or subclass. The thiophilic adsorption process can be controlled by varying either the pH or the salt concentration of the buffer (Hutchens TW and Porath J, 1986). Especially the salt concentration influences the adsorption of immunoglobulins on thiophilic gels. IgG are eluted from T-gels by an essentially salt free buffer at pH 7.0, thus reducing considerably the number of steps (such as neutralization) required before the purified protein solution can be used or stored. This one-step purification procedure also leads to a considerable concentration in the case of diluted feeds and can easily be adapted to large scale. A comparison between thiophilic chromatography and Protein A or Protein G based techniques shows that the main advantages of thiophilic chromatography are the mild elution conditions, the greater chemical stability of the affinity ligands (allowing even to autoclave the resin), the high binding capacity of the T-gels, the lack of ligand leakage, and the low cost of these adsorbents. However, the binding of antibodies to thiophilic adsorbents is less specific than the binding to bacterial F_c receptors. Thiophilic adsorption chromatography has also be used for the separation and purification of (recombinant) antibody fragments, lacking the F_c receptor (Lutomski D et al., 1995, Yurov GK et al., 1994). In addition, the method was optimized to separate monospecific forms from the bispecific species by salt-gradient elution (Kreutz FT et al., 1998).

2.1.2.8 Lectins

Immunoglobulins are glycoproteins, they may therefore be isolated by lectin affinity chromatography. Although different examples of such lectin based affinity chromatography purification of antibodies can be found in the literature (Peng Z et al., 1993, Roque-Barreira M et al., 1986), this purification procedure has mainly been used for the isolation of human IgA. The lectin Jacalin, isolated from jackfruit seeds (Roque-Barriera M and Campos-Neto A, 1985), binds to IgA and thus makes a most convenient affinity ligand for the purification of IgA from colostrum or serum (Kondoh H et al., 1987). Jacalin-adsorbents are available from different commercial suppliers. All steps in the Jacalin-affinity chromatography (adsorption-washing-elution) can be performed at neutral pH, and elution is done competitively with D-galactose or mellobiose. The major drawback of this type of lectin affinity chromatography is the high cost of D-galactose, which makes it almost impossible to use for large-scale purifications. Furthermore, it is known that Jalacin is a potent T cell mitogen and a strong B cell polyclonal activator (Bunn-Moreno MM et al., 1981). Therefore, the purified antibody preparation has to be checked carefully for the presence of residual ligand molecules.

2.1.3 Stationary phases for affinity chromatography of antibodies

The properties desired in a potential affinity chromatographic matrix are
o *Chemical resistance* under a wide range of experimental conditions such as high and low pH, presence of detergents as well as dissociating and sterilizing agents
o High density of *putative points of attachments*, which allow the easy covalent attachment of the affinity ligand. Examples from commercial matrices include primary hydroxyl groups that can be activated to form epoxides or tosyl groups to which NH_2-containing ligands can be linked in a straightforward manner.

o An appropriate *pore size* to allow free diffusion of the target molecules in and out of the bead.
o Finally, the support particles must be of sufficient *rigidity* to allow fast mobile phase flow for rapid separations.

In addition, it would seem vital that the separation occurs on the basis of the interactions of the antibody with the ligand alone, i.e. that the matrix should be nothing but an inert scaffold to present the ligand to the target protein. However, no matrix can be completely inert: hydrophobic sites can adsorb many proteins at high salt concentrations (conditions often used to elute protein from an affinity column) and ion-exchange sites occur on many materials. In all variants of affinity chromatography, the properties of the matrix thus influence and modify the process of adsorption and elution. As a consequence, the performance of one and the same ligand may differ considerably as a function of the support matrix used.

A bead-form of agarose, Sepharose, is the material of choice for many affinity applications as it comes close to the ideal properties mentioned above. It is highly hydrophilic with few non-specific, ion-exchange sites and possesses an abundance of immobilization sites for the affinity ligand. Originally, ligands were immobilized on Sepharose activated by cyanogen bromide (CN-Sepharose). However, ligands immobilized by the cyanogen bromide activation method were found to be prone to leaching, due to the rather instable nature of the linkage. In the recent years, more robust immobilization methods, e.g. based on the epoxide chemistry, have been established to alleviate this problem. In addition, several pre-activated Sepharose media that contain already the immobilized ligand (e.g. Protein A) have become commercially available. Their use saves time and avoids exposure to the potentially hazardous reagents that are required in some methods used to couple the ligand to the matrix.

A new and effective affinity chromatography matrix has been developed using doped sol-gel glass as a support system (Zusman R et al., 1990). With this method, large amounts of sheep immunoglobulin G have been isolated using Protein A trapped in such a sol-gel glass (Zusman R et al., 1992). More recently, the so-called gel fiberglass (GFG) matrix was invented as a further modification of the doped sol-gel glass one (Zusman R and Zusman I, 1995). This approach was, e.g., used to prepare a new class of affinity support for the purification of proteins (reviewed in Zusman R and Zusman I, 2001).

2.1.4 Developing an elution strategy for affinity chromatography

An important aspect of affinity chromatography is the ability to release and retrieve the isolated target molecule in *functional* form (reviewed in Firer MA, 2001). A list of all buffers and conditions suggested for the retrieval, or elution, of affinity-bound proteins would be almost as long as a list of successful applications of the technique. However, some general ideas will be given below.

2.1.4.1 Elution by bond-breaking buffers

Only a few studies have been made with the aim of a systematic investigation of the most appropriate elution conditions for a particular protein (for example, Tsang VCW and Wilkins PP, 1991, Kummer A and Li-Chan EC, 1998, Ben-David A and Firer MA, 1996). Tsang and Wilkins (1991) tested 13 buffers that differed in pH, salt concentration, chaotropicity or hydrophobicity. By comparing the specific activity and total recovery of the eluted goat anti-human IgG, they selected a buffer containing ethylene glycol as the most effective elution buffer for their system. The group of Ben-David and Firer (1996) extended the work of Tsang and Wilkins to the purification of monoclonal antibodies and showed that an ethylene glycol-containing buffer was also optimal for several monoclonals. Nahri LO et al. (1997) tested the structural and functional alterations in several monoclonal antibodies after treatment with three different buffers and used this information to optimize the elution buffer for a particular antibody population. The testing of many buffers on affinity columns is time and reagent consuming. To improve the efficiency of the selection process, buffers can initially be tested for their ability to elute target in immunoassays. This "ELISA-elution" assay has been used in several recent studies. For example, Kummer A and Li-Chan EC (1998) used the method to rapidly assay 54 buffers before selecting glycine-HCl, pH 2.8 to dissociate yolk antibody IgY from a bovine IgG-activated affinity column.

2.1.4.2 Competitive elution

An alternative is the use of competitive agents for elution, most simply by flushing the column with a mobile phase containing an excess of dissolved affinity ligand (or a derivative thereof). This strategy has several advantages but also some drawbacks.

Advantages are the preservation of the column's binding capacity due to the mild elution conditions and the specificity of the elution. Disadvantages are the necessity to have access to the free affinity ligand (it may not always be possible, practical, or economic to use the large molar excesses of ligand required for elution). In addition, competitive elution often takes longer than elution with bond-breaking buffers.

2.2 Ion-exchange chromatography

Ion-exchange chromatography is a rapid and inexpensive procedure that has been employed to purify antibodies from different sources and species (Sampson IA et al., 1984, Clezardin P et al., 1985). This type of chromatography is particularly useful for the isolation of antibodies that either do not bind or that bind only weakly to Protein A (e.g. mouse IgG1, Manil L et al., 1986). Contrary to affinity chromatography, ion exchange cannot be used as a single-step procedure to directly purify immunoglobulins from crude starting materials. It should either be preceded by an ammonium sulfate fractionation or by an affinity chromatography. It is also possible to use the sequence ion exchange chromatography – affinity chromatography with good results in terms of recovery and final purity.

In ion-exchange chromatography proteins – or indeed any other compound – are separated according to their surface (net) charge. As a consequence, this separation mechanism depends on the pI of the protein in question, the pH and salt concentration of the buffer, as well as on the charge of the ion-exchanger matrix. Matrices for protein ion exchange chromatography are typically made from beaded cellulose, agarose, dextran or polystyrene. Proteins of opposite charge are reversibly bound to the matrix under certain conditions. However, the interaction usually can easily be disrupted by increasing the ionic strength or changing the pH of the mobile phase.

Antibodies show most often a pI above 6, which renders them more basic than other serum proteins and the majority of the proteins described today (Table 5.2). In principle antibodies can therefore be purified be either cation- or anion-exchange chromatography (Graf H et al., 1994). In fact since they are more basic then most putative impurities, isolation by cation chromatography has some generic advantages. However, a study of the pertinent literature demonstrates that to date most antibodies isolated by ion-exchange chromatography were isolated using weak anion exchangers of the diethylaminoethyl (DEAE)-type. Two purification strategies can be perused. If the pH of the solution is maintained at pH 6.5 to 7.0, the antibodies will bear hardly any charge at all and therefore will not be retained on the column and elute first (Phillips TM, 1992). This approach is beset with the disadvantage that the trailing edge of the immunoglobulin peak is usually contaminated with other proteins. Alternatively, near pH 8, the immunoglobulins are bound to the stationary phase and may be eluted by a gradient of increasing ionic strength (Clezardin et al., 1985).

Monoclonal antibodies from ascites have also been successfully purified by ion-exchange chromatography on strong Mono Q anion exchangers (Pharmacia). The use of a strong ion exchanger allows the separations to be carried out in a pH-range of 3 – 11, which is particularly useful for those immunoglobulins that require a certain ionic strength for solubility (Burchiel SW et al., 1984, Tasaka K et al., 1984, Guse AH et al., 1994). At low buffer pH, antibodies will not bind to an anion exchanger. This may also be used for their purification. Jungbauer and co-workers (Necina R et al., 1998) described such a strategy using ion exchange media with high charge density. They showed that a combination of a negative purification (no binding of the target molecule, but binding of most impurities) with Q-Sepharose FF and a capturing with CM-HyperD (strong cation exchanger) gave sufficient yield and resolution for the capture of monoclonal antibodies from clarified hybridoma cell culture grown in media supplemented with fetal calf serum. When antibodies were captured from serum-free culture supernatant the antibody could be eluted in a single peak with substantial reduction of the contaminants.

However, it is clear that ion-exchange chromatography will typically be only one-step within a multi-step purification process in the case of an antibody intended for human therapy. The group of Guse (Guse A et al., 1994) gave one convincing example for the successful purification of a monoclonal antibody for therapeutic use using a series of different techniques, namely $(NH_4)_2SO_4$ precipitation, anion-exchange chromatography on MonoQ or Q-Sepharose, hydrophobic interaction chromatography on phenyl-Sepharose, and gel filtration chromatography on Superdex-20 as a final polishing step. It should be noted that affinity chromatography was not a necessity in this case.

2.3 Hydroxyapatite (pseudo) affinity chromatography

Hydroxyapatite (HA), a phosphate-based stationary phase, has interesting properties for both protein and DNA purification. In contrast to most other chromatographic phases, HA is an inorganic material, usually assumed to have the (idealized) formula $Ca_{10}(PO_4)_6(OH)_2$. In the case of biomacromolecules, HA shows some unique separation properties, together with high selectivity and resolution. However, the retention mechanisms for such molecules on HA are complex, since two types of interaction with the surface are possible (Deppert and Lukacin, 2000). Substances may, for example, interact with the phosphate moieties (P-sites) on the HA-surface.

This interaction requires either positive charges or groups with high phosphate affinity on the retained molecule. The interaction of negatively charged molecules, such as acidic proteins, is also possible on HA (Kawasaki T et al., 1990). In this case, an interaction of calcium-chelating or –binding groups on the retained molecule with the calcium-based C-sites on the HA-surface is assumed to be responsible for the retention. For large proteins, such as antibodies, complex mechanisms involving P- and C-site interaction have been observed, due to the inhomogeneity of their charge distribution (Gorbunoff M, 1985). Antibodies typically bind in a mixed mode manner to the HA-surface, which allows the fine-tuning of a separation strategy to a given purification problem, as illustrated for the purification of a recombinant antibody from cell culture supernatant by Giovannini and co-workers (Giovannini R and Freitag R, 2001a, Figure 5.3).

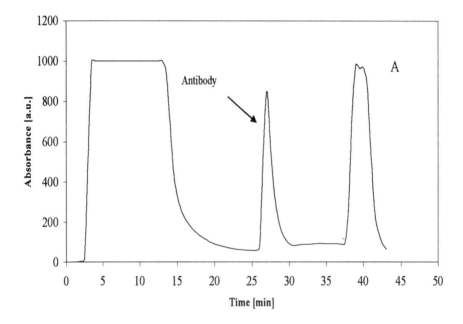

Figure 5.3. (a) Purification of a recombinant human antibody from CHO cell culture supernatants using a HA Macro-Prep R type I-column (Bio-Rad). Sample: cell culture supernatant diluted (1:3) with 1 mM phosphate buffer, pH 6, containing in addition 1 M NaCl. Sample volume 10 ml; gradient from 1 to 15 min, 100 % A ; from 15 to 35 min, from 100 to 85 % A; from 35 to 45 min, 0 % A. Buffer A: 1 mM phosphate, pH 6, containing in addition 1 M NaCl; buffer B: 400 mM phosphate, pH 6; flow rate 1 ml/min. (with kind permission of Kluwer Academic Publishers)

HA-chromatography has also been successfully applied for the purification of monoclonal antibodies from ascites (Juarez-Salinas H et al., 1986, Stanker LH et al., 1985, Pavlu B et al., 1986) and for the separation of different molecular forms of mouse IgA and IgM monoclonal antibodies (Aoyama K and Chiba J, 1993).

2.4 Hydrophobic interaction chromatography

Hydrophobic interaction chromatography (HIC) was developed in the 1970s especially for the preparative separation of proteins using predominately hydrophilic, agarose-based stationary phases into which some mildly hydrophobic ligands had been imbedded at fairly low density. The driving force for retention in HIC is a hydrophobic effect, i.e., less an attraction between the protein molecules and the stationary phase but rather the tendency of the surrounding water molecules to avoid contact with a hydrophobic surface and hence to bring such surfaces into direct contact with each other. At the same time, the environment of the target molecule (protein) remain sufficiently "hydrophilic" to avoid the denaturation that often occurs in reversed phase chromatography, hence the attractiveness of HIC for preparative applications.

HIC has been used for the purification of antibody subtypes and bispecific monoclonal antibodies. Abe N and Inouye K (1993) observed that monoclonal antibodies of the IgG_1 subclass produced by hybridomas raised with NS-1 myelomas, which were purified by anion-exchange chromatography, contained two types of immunoglobulin light (kappa) chain. Since the immunoreactivity of the hybrid monoclonal antibodies was different it was important to be able to separate the two. In their paper the authors showed that hydrophobic interaction HPLC was able to discriminate between antibodies based on very small difference in hydrophobicity, such as between kappa light chains from spleen and NS-1 cells and that the technique could therefore be used for the purification of the hybrid monoclonal antibodies.

It is known that the production and preparation of bispecific antibodies is very difficult since hybrid-hybridomas (tetradomas) secrete antibodies with a heterogeneous combination of heavy and light chains from both parental hybridoma cells, resulting theoretically in 10 different types of immunoglobulin. Among these only bispecific antibodies and bivalent parental antibodies represent correct associations of the related heavy and light chains. In order to meet the challenge of isolating the molecule of interest in the case of bispecific antibodies from a tetradoma supernatant it is therefore not only necessary to separate immunoglobulins from (proteineous) components of the cell culture media, but also to resolve the different types of antibody within the immunoglobulin fraction. Manzke and co-workers (Manzke O et al., 1997) showed that bispecific antibodies can be purified directly from culture supernatant by HIC, which resolves bispecific antibodies, monospecific immunoglobulins, and culture medium supplements in one single chromatographic step.

3. ALTERNATIVE SUGGESTIONS FOR ANTIBODY PURIFICATION

3.1 Continuous Annular Chromatography

The principle of continuous annular chromatography (CAC) has been known for several decades (Martin EJP, 1949). CAC is a continuous annular chromatographic mode, which lends itself to the separation of multi-component mixtures as well as of bi-component ones. In CAC, the mobile and stationary phases move in a crosscurrent fashion, which allows transforming the typical one-dimensional batch column separation into a continuous two-dimensional one. With the exception of linear gradient elution, all chromatographic modes have at present been applied in CAC (reviewed in Hilbrig F and Freitag R, 2003a). To our knowledge, Bayer AG is currently the only company developing CAC for a relevant bioseparation process, namely the concentration of a continuously produced recombinant factor VIII.

Recently, some groups optimized CAC for the purification of (recombinant) antibodies. Buchacher and co-workers (Buchacher A. et al., 2001, Iberer G et al., 2001) investigated the performance of protein (antibody) CAC in the size-exclusion mode. An IgG preparation rich in aggregates was used as an exemplary separation challenge. Under conditions, that maximized the throughput, the polymers could be separated from the monomers, but baseline separation could not be achieved. Baseline separation was, however, also not possible in the batch mode using equivalent conditions. For the separation of the aggregates from the monomeric product, the entire available separation space (360°) was used. The productivity of the annular chromatography was twice as high as that of the conventional batch chromatography, and the buffer consumption was halved. This was largely due to the fact that after steady state has been reached in the CAC no time is lost for column regeneration and that in CAC it is not necessary or customary to wait until all sample compounds have left the column before the new sample is applied.

Freitag and co-workers (Giovannini R and Freitag R, 2001) evaluated the possibilities of continuous annular affinity chromatography for antibody purification from a complex feed (cell culture supernatants) taken from an actual (bio)process. In particular, a commercially available preparative continuous annular chromatography (P-CAC) system was used to purify a recombinant antibody (human IgG$_1$-κ) from CHO cell culture supernatants by HA and rProtein A chromatography. Yields were between 87 % and 92 % in the case of HA and between 77 % and 82 % in the case of rProtein A chromatography. DNA removal was nearly quantitative in all cases. Concomitantly, the antibody fraction of the total protein content was raised by one order of magnitude in HA and by a factor of 50 by rProtein A chromatography.

3.2 High performance monolith affinity chromatography

Another recent development in (protein) chromatography concerns the morphology of the stationary phase. While conventionally the stationary phase is packed into the column in the form of small, usually porous beads, continuous bed-type stationary phases (sometimes called monoliths) constitute a block of porous polymer that fills the entire column space. Continuous bed columns are distributed under the trade name UNO™ by Bio-Rad. Especially for fast protein and antibody chromatography, another stationary phase geometry has been introduced for which the name High Performance Monolith Chromatography (HPMC) has been proposed (Tennikova TB and Freitag R, 1999). Typically, the stationary phases in HPMC are flat, monolithic and macroporous disks, which are now commercially available under the name of Convective Interaction Media (CIM™)-disks (BIA d.d.o.). The macroporous structure of the CIM™ material allows overcoming many of the disadvantages of conventional biochromatography. Most importantly, the mass transport is dramatically improved, since it occurs mainly by convection rather than by total or partial diffusion as in conventional chromatography. HPMC in general has been shown to be a useful technique for efficient and fast isolation of proteins from complex sources such as blood serum (Josic D et al., 1994, Platonova G et al., 1999) or cell culture supernatants (Kasper C et al., 1998). In general, HPMC combines high capacity and selectivity with low backpressure and short operation times.

Fast bioseparation of different IgGs, including recombinantly produced monoclonal antibodies, can be achieved by using CIM™ affinity disks (or columns) bearing different affinity ligands. Platonova and co-workers (1999) showed the potential for direct quantitative analysis of monospecific anti-peptide immunoglobulins and their semi-preparative isolation from precipitated blood fractions or crude blood serum of immunized animals. Synthetic peptides were immobilized as affinity ligands by a single-step reaction that involved the epoxy groups located on the pore surface of the porous polymer disc and the amino groups of the peptide molecules. Gel electrophoresis showed a high degree of purity of the anti-peptide antibody recovered after single step HPMC. Berruex and co-workers (Berruex L et al., 2000,2002) showed the direct quantitative isolation of antibodies from serum-free culture supernatants using immobilized group specific ligands (Protein A, G, and L) on CIM^{TM} disks. As shown in Figure 5.4 the HPCM separation took less then one minute to complete and presumably can be accelerated even more by further increasing the flow rate. Indeed, the chromatographic system rather than the binding kinetics pose the limits in HPCM. Furthermore, the combination of several disks with different affinity functionalities in the same cartridge allows the simultaneous separation of different antibodies (proteins) within a few minutes (Ostryanina ND et al., 2002). This makes HPMC an interesting tool for fast process monitoring or screening.

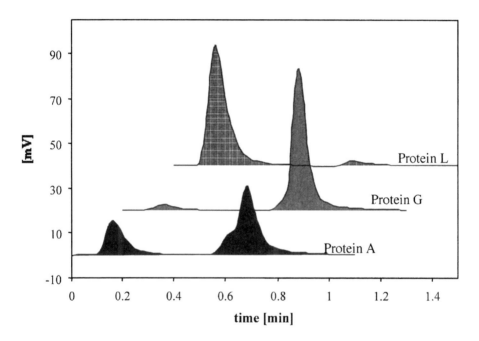

Figure 5.4. Comparison of the HPMA chromatograms of bovine IgG using disks with different affinity ligands. Conditions: CIM^{TM}-disks, 12x3 mm, flow rate 4 ml/min; UV detection at 280 nm; adsorption buffer was PBS pH 7.4 ; eluting buffer was 10 mM HCL pH 2.0 ; amounts loaded were 25 µg of bovine IgG in 100 µl buffer A. Chromatography : step gradient , 0-0.5 min 100 % A ; 0.5-0.51 min form 100 % A to 100 % B ; 0.51-1.1 min 100 % B ; 1.1-1.11 min from 100 % B to 100 % A and 1.11-1.3 min 100 % A. (Reprinted from J. Pharm Biomed Anal 24, Berruex LG, Freitag R and Tennikova TB, *Comparison of Antibody binding to immobilized group specific affinity ligands in high performance monolith affinity chromatography.* 95-104, Copyright 2000, with permission of Elsevier Science)

Purification of antibodies by chromatographic methods 157

3.3 Expended (Fluidized) Bed Chromatography

In an expanded or fluidized bed, the adsorbent particles are placed in a vessel with a porous bottom plate. A fluid flows upward through the porous plate at such a flow rate that the particles become "fluidized" within the confinements of the container, as illustrated in Figure 5.5. A major advantage of this approach is that particles in the feed (e.g. also residual cells) pose no problem. As long as they do not stick to the particles of the fluidized bed, solids move within the fluidizing liquid through the bed and are thus removed, while the product is bound to the adsorbent. The product is simultaneously concentrated and, to a certain extent, purified in a single-step operation. As a consequence, expended bed systems are very interesting for applications involving the direct processing of crude cell culture suspensions (e.g. hybridoma cell cultures), which can be passed directly into the system, thus bypassing the tedious step of cell and cell debris removal. First applications have been published, however the method still lacks wide acceptance.

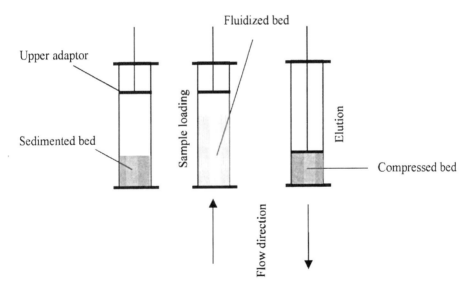

Figure 5.5. Schematic representation of a fluidized bed system. (Reprinted from Encyclopedia of Physical Science and Technology, Third Edition, Volume 14, LG Berruex and R Freitag, *Separation and Purification of Biochemicals*. 651-673, Copyright 2001, with permission from Elsevier Science)

Fluidized-bed receptor affinity chromatography for the purification of the humanized anti-Tac monoclonal antibodies has, e.g., been described by Spence and co-workers already in 1994 (Spence C et al., 1994). They used a soluble form of the interleukin-2 receptor chemically bound to an aldehyde derivative of controlled pore glass beads as affinity sorbent and successfully employed the corresponding fluidized bed in the purification of recombinant interleukin-2 and single chain anti-Tac (Fv)-Pseudomonas exotoxin immunotoxin from unclarified inclusion body extracts. Lütkemeyer and co-workers (Lütkemeyer D et al., 1999) investigated the extent of cell damage at the bench and pilot scale using a stabilized fluidized bed for direct recovery of IgG from cell culture broth. For this purpose, Streamline-25 and –200 columns containing 75 ml and 5 l of rProtein A matrix, respectively, were used. At the bench scale, 1 to 6 l of unclarified feed was applied directly to the Streamline-25 column. At the pilot scale, up to 95 l were processed using the Streamline-200 column. The authors observed that, despite the known sensitivity of hybridoma cells to shear forces, neither the high flow rate (300 to 450 cm/h) nor the passage of the cells through the expanded bed caused any relevant cell damage or clogging of the bed. An excellent DNA depletion was observed. These promising results indicate that expanded bed affinity chromatography can be used for cell removal and capture of antibodies. Subsequent processing of the eluate is possible after a simple filtration step.

3.4   Affinity precipitation for antibody purification

Affinity precipitation has been known for over 20 years (Larsson PO and Mosbach K, 1979, Schneider M et al., 1981, reviewed by Hilbrig F and Freitag R, 2003b), but has recently received more attention partially due to the development of new materials for its implementation, but also because it seems ideally suited to specific product capture at large scale.

Primary effect affinity precipitation was developed by Mosbach and co-workers in the late seventies based on the observation that the tetrameric enzyme lactate dehydrogenase (LDH) and bifunctional N_2,N_2'-adipodihydrazido-bis-(N^6-carbonylmethyl-NAD) (Bis-NAD) form at low temperature and in a certain concentration ratio a cross-linked, macromolecular network, which becomes insoluble and precipitates when the aggregates have grown sufficiently large. In primary effect affinity precipitation the formation of a precipitate is therefore the direct consequence of the affinity interaction between the multivalent enzyme and the bifunctional ligand. Bis-borate ligands have also been tested in this context. Borate was used as additive to induce the precipitation of polysaccharide protein A – IgG affinity complexes (Bradshaw AP and Sturgeon RJ, 1990). Biotinylated phospholipids can be strongly binding ligands for the tetrameric avidin. In aqueous solution such phospholipids form micelles by hydrophobic interaction, which can also be used for the separation of the captured target molecule from solution. Phospholipids have inter alia been successfully used for the isolation of antibodies (Powers DD et al., 1994).

In *secondary or indirect affinity precipitation* (Schneider M et al., 1981) the two aspects of the process – affinity and precipitation - can be performed and controlled independently. Instead of a precipitation caused by the affinity interaction, the two abilities are now combined in an especially designed agent called the affinity macroligand (AML). A typical AML consists of the actual affinity ligand (most affinity ligands known, e.g., from affinity chromatography may be used) and a stimulus-responsive polymer to which the affinity ligand is covalently linked. Stimulus-responsive polymers show abrupt changes in their water-solubility upon small changes in an environmental parameter such as the pH or the temperature. In particular, pH-responsive AML have been reported for the purification of monoclonal antibodies.

Eudragit S-100 is a commercially available high molar mass copolymer of methacrylic acid and methyl methacrylate (Mw 135'000 g/mol), which precipitates sharply below a pH of 4.5. The precipitation is fully reversible. Conjugation with affinity ligands shifts the transition to higher pH-values, because conjugation reduces the number of charged carboxylic acid groups in the Eudragit backbone (Taipa MA et al., 1998, 2000). In addition to Eudragit, several pH sensitive polymers known in nature have also been adapted to the affinity precipitation of proteins. These include alginate, chitosan, and derivatized cellulose (Hilbrig F and Freitag R, 2003). A general drawback of pH sensitive polymers like Eudragit S-100 or alginate is that they precipitate at a pH, which is outside the stability range of many proteins. Polyelectrolyte complex formation (PEC) was therefore proposed as a mean to shift the precipitation pH of such polymers into the physiological range. Dainiak and co-workers (Dainiak MB et al., 1999) used a nonstoichiometric polyelectrolyte complex (PEC) formed by poly(methacrylic acid) (PMAA) and poly(*N*-ethyl-4-vinyl-pyridinium bromide) (PEVP) to which inactivated glyceraldehyde-3-phosphate dehydrogenase (GAPDH) was covalently coupled to purify antibodies from hybridoma cell culture supernatants.

Crude antibody preparations were incubated with the GAPDH-containing PEC and the precipitation was carried out at 0.01 M NaCl and pH 4.5, 5.3, 6.0 and 6.5 using PECs with different PEVP/PMAA ratios. Purified antibodies were eluted at pH 4.0, where PECs of all compositions used were insoluble. PEC precipitation was accompanied only by small nonspecific coprecipitation of protein impurities. Precipitated PEC could be dissolved at pH 7.3 and used repeatedly. The same methodology was used to produce F_{ab} fragments of the same monoclonal antibody (Dainiak MB et al., 2000). These studies demonstrate that nonstoichiometric polyelectrolyte complexes can be successfully used as a carrier for the ligands in antibody affinity precipitation.

Thermoresponsive AML have also been evaluated for antibody purification. Chen and Hoffman (Chen JP and Hoffman AS, 1990) synthesized a copolymer of NIPAM (N-isopropylacrylamide) and N-acryloxysuccinimide having a molar mass of around 24'000 g/mol, an average of 5.5 activated ester groups per polymer chain, and a critical solution temperature (CST) of 32°C in pure water. Conjugation of protein A to this copolymer enabled the capture and recovery of IgG by thermoprecipitation of the formed AML-IgG complex. The dissociation constant of this affinity complex was $3 \cdot 10^{-6}$ M and the binding capacity of the AML was 25% of the theoretical one. The authors concluded that steric interference of the protein A binding sites with the polymer might be the reason for the low binding capability of the copolymer-AML, whereas they could exclude the occurrence of non-specific binding between IgG and the polymer backbone.

4. CONCLUSION AND PERSPECTIVES

Antibodies are fascinating molecules; because of their biology, their broad application spectrum in the life sciences, but because of their immense financial potential. Especially the latter aspect requires well-designed, economically feasible antibody production processes. The isolation of the functional antibody from its production source in such a process remains a challenge, which does not diminish as the molecules but also the production processes diversify. While Protein A was a safe solution only yesterday, many of today's most interesting "antibodies" don't even contain the Fc-part anymore. In this chapter we tried to give an overview over the chromatographic techniques used for antibody isolation. Both very "mainstream", but also less known approaches have been included. More than one process engineer has found a solution for a difficult antibody purification problem, e.g., in HA-chromatography, "after everything else failed". Chromatography and most certainly affinity chromatography remains an indispensable tool in the production of pure antibody preparations. At present there is no obvious alternative. However, conventional chromatography in the batch mode, employing columns packed with porous particles also has some drawbacks, e.g. in regard to speed, robustness, scalability. Towards the end of the chapter we therefore tried to point our some alternatives to conventional chromatography. Whether any of these do really constitute viable options remains to be seen.

ACKNOWLEDGEMENTS

We would like to thank all the colleagues who have helped in many invaluable ways in the production of this chapter, in particular, Rachel Flaction, Laure Berruex, Roberto Giovannini, Frank Hilbrig.

REFERENCES

Abe N., and Inouye K., 1993, Purification of monoclonal antibodies with light-chain heterogeneity produced by mouse hybridomas raised with NS-1 myelomas. *In application of hydrophobic interaction high-performance liquid chromatography. J Biochem Biophys Methods.* **27**: 215-227

Akerstrom B. and Bjorck L., 1989, Protein L: an immunoglobulin light chain-binding bacterial protein. Characterization of binding and physicochemical properties. *J. Biol. Chem.* **264**: 19740-19746

Aoyama K., and Chiba J., 1993, Separation of different molecular forms of mouse IgA and IgM monoclonal antibodies by high-performance liquid chromatography on spherical hydroxyapatite beads. *J Immunol Methods.* **162**: 201-210

Belew M., Juntti N., Larsson A., and Porath J., 1987, A one-step purification method for monoclonal antibodies based on salt-promoted adsorption chromatography on a "thiophilic" adsorbent. *J. Immunol. Methods* **102**: 173-182

Ben-David A., and Firer M.A., 1996, Immunoaffinity purification of monoclonal antibodies: in search of an elution buffer of general applicability. *Biotechnol. Tech.* **10**:799-802

Berger M., Shankar V., and Vafai A., 2002, Therapeutic applications of monoclonal antibodies. *Am J Med Sci* **324**: 14-30

Berruex LG., and Freitag R., 2002, Affinity-based interactions on disks for fast analysis, isolation and conversion of biomolecules. In: *Methods for affinity-based separations of enzymes and proteins.* Gupta MN. (Ed.), Birkhäuser Verlag, Basel, pp 82-114

Berruex LG., and Freitag R., 2002, Separation and purification of biochemicals. *In Encyclopedia of Physical Science and Technology. Third Edition, Academic Press.* **14**: 651-673

Berruex LG., Freitag R., and Tennikova TB., 2000, Comparison of antibody binding to immobilized group specific affinity ligands in high performance monolith affinity chromatography. *J Pharm Biomed Anal.* **24**: 95-104

Bjorck L., 1988, Protein L. A novel bacterial cell wand protein with affinity for IgL chains. *J. Immunol.* **140**: 1194-1197

Boden V., Winzerking JJ., Vijayalakshmi M., Porath J., 1995. Rapid one-step purification of goat immunoglobulins by immobilized metal ion affinity chromatography. *J. Immunol Methods.* **181**: 225-232

Boschetti E., 2001, The use of thiophilic chromatography for antibody purification: a review. *J. Biochem. Biophys. Methods* **49**: 361-389

Bradshaw AP., and Sturgeon RJ., 1990, The synthesis of soluble polymer-ligand complexes for affinity precipitation studies. *Biotechnol Tech.* **4**: 67

Bruck C., Portetelle D., Glineur C., and Bollen A., 1982, One-step purification of mouse monoclonal antibodies from ascitic fluid by DEAE Affi-Gel blue chromatography. *J. Immunol. Methods* **53**: 313-319

Buchacher A., Iberer G., Jungbauer A., Schwinn H., and Josic D., 2001, Continuous removal of protein aggregates by annular chromatography. *Biotechnol. Prog.* **17**:140-149

Bunn-Moreno M.M., and Campos-Neto A., 1981, Lectin(s) extracted from seeds of artocarpus integrifolia (jackfruit): potent and selective stimulator(s) of distinct human T and B cell functions. *J. Immunol.* **127**:427-430

Burchiel SW., Billman JR., and Alber TR., 1984, Rapid and efficient purification of mouse monoclonal antibodies form ascites fluid using high performance liquid chromatography. *J Immunol. Methods.* **69**: 33-42

Cao Y., Christian S., and Suresh M.R., 1998, Development of a bispecific monoclonal antibody as a universal immunoprobe for detecting biotinylated macromolecules. *J. Immunol. Methods* **220**:85-91

Casey JL., Keep PA., Chester KA., Robson L., Hawkins RE., Begent RH., 1995, Purification of bacterially expressed single chain Fv antibodies for clinical applications using metal chelate chromatography. *J. Immunol Methods.* **179**: 105-116

Chen JP., and Hoffman AS., 1990, Polymer-protein conjugates. II. Affinity precipitation separation of human immunogammaglobulin by a poly(N-isopropylacrylamide)-Protein A conjugate. *Biomaterials* **11**: 631

Cherednikova T.V., Muronetz V.I., and Nagradova N.K., 1980, Study of subunit interactions in immobilized D-glyceraldehyde-3-phosphate dehydrogenase. *Biochim. Biophys. Acta* **613**: 292-308

Cherednikova T.V., Muronetz V.I., and Nagradova N.K., 1981, Evidence for the stabilizing effect of antibodies on the subunit association of glyceraldehydes-3-phosphate dehydrogenase. *Mol. Immunol.* **18**: 1055-1064

Clezardin P., McGregor JL., Manach M., Boukercke H., and Dechavanne M., 1985, One-step procedure for the rapid isolation of mouse monoclonal antibodies and their antigen binding fragments by fast protein liquid chromatography on a mono Q anion-exchange column. *J Chromatogr.* **319**: 67-77

Dainiak M.B., Izumrodov V.A., Muronetz V.I., Galaev I. Yu., and Mattiasson B., 1999, Affinity precipitation of monoclonal antibodies by nonstoichiometric polyelectrolyte complexes. *Bioseparation* **7**: 231-240

Dainiak M.B., Muronetz V.I., Izumrudov V.A., Galaev I.Yu., and Mattiasson B., 2000, Production of Fab fragments of monoclonal antibodies using polyelectrolyte complexes. *Anal. Biochem.* **277**: 58-66

Deisenhofer J., 1981, Crystallographic refinement and atomic models of a human Fc fragment and its complex with fragment B of protein A from *Staphylococcus aureus* at 2.9- and 2.8-A resolution. *Biochemistry* **20**: 2361-2370

Deppert WR., and Lukacin R., 2000, *Hydroxyapatite chromatography.* In: Kastner M (ed), Protein Liquid Chromatography. Ch 5, pp 271-299, Elsevier, Amsterdam

Fassina G., Ruvo M., Palombo G., Verdoliva A., and Marino M., 2001, Novel ligands for the affinity-chromatographic purification of antibodies. *J. Biochem. Biophys. Methods* **49**:481-490

Fassina G., Scardino P., Ruvo M., Fucile P., Amodeo P., and Cassani G., 1994, Synthesis of conformationally constrained dimeric peptide libraries. In *Peptides* (H. Maia, ed.) ESCOM, Leiden, pp. 489-490

Fassina G., Verdoliva A., Odierna MR., Ruvo M., Cassini G., 1996, Protein A mimetic peptide ligand for affinity purification of antibodies. *J Mol Recognit.* **9**: 564-569

Fassina G., Verdoliva A., Palombo G., Ruvo M., and Cassani G., 1998, Immunoglobulin specificity of TG 19318 : a novel synthetic ligand for antibody purification. *J. Mol. Recognit.* **11**:128-133

Firer M.A., 2001, Efficient elution of functional proteins in affinity chromatography. *J. Biochem. Biophys. Methods* **49**: 433-442

Fleminger G., Wolf T., Hadas E., Solomon B., 1990, Eupergit C as a carrier for high-performance liquid chromatographic-based immuno-purification of antigens and antibodies. *J Chromatogr* **510**: 311-319

Forsgren A., and Sjoquist J., 1966, "Protein A" from *S. aureus*: I. Pseudo-immune reaction with human immunoglobulin. *J. Immunol.* **97**: 822-827

Freyre FM., Vasquez JE., Ayala M., Canaan-Haden L., Bell H., Rodriguez I., 2000, Very high expression of an anti-carcinoembryonic antigen single chain Fv antibody fragment in the yeast Pichia pastoris. *J. Biotechnol.* **76**: 157-163

Gaberc-Porekar V. and Menart v., 2001, Perspectives of immobilized-metal affinity chromatography. *J Biochem Biophys Methods.* **49**: 335-360

Giovannini R., and Freitag R., 2001a, Comparison of different types of ceramic hydroxyapatite for the chromatographic separation of plasmid DNA and recombinant anti-Rhesus D antibody. *Bioseparation 9*: 359-368

Giovannini R., and Freitag R., 2001b, Isolation of a Recombinant Antibody from Cell Culture Supernatant : Continuous Annular Versus Batch and Expanded-Bed Chromatography. *Biotechnol Bioeng.* **73**: 522-529

Godfrey M.A., Kwasowski P., Clift R., and Marks V., 1992, A sensitive enzyme-linked immunosorbent assay (ELISA) for the detection of staphylococcal protein A (SpA) present as a trace contaminant of murine immunoglobulins purified on immobilized protein A. *J. Immunol. Methods* **149**: 21-27

Godfrey M.A.J., Kwasowski P., Clift R., and Marks V., 1993, Assessment of the suitability of commercially available SpA affinity solid phases for the purification of murine monoclonal antibodies at process scale. *J. Immunol. Methods* **160**: 97-105

Gorbunoff M., 1985, Protein chromatography on hydroxyapatite columns. *Methods Enzymol.* **11**: 370-380

Goward C.R., 1995, Affinity chromatography and its application in large-scale separations. In *Process scale liquid chromatography* (G. Subramanian, ed.), Weinheim, Germany, pp-251-275

Graf H., Rabaud JN., Egly JM., 1994, Ion exchange resins for the purification of monoclonal antibodies from animal call culture. *Bioseparation.* **4**: 7-20

Grandics P.,1994, Monoclonal antibody purification guide: Part 1-3. *Am Biotechnol Lab.* **12** (6): 58-62, (7): 12-14, (8): 16-18

Guerrier L., Flayeuux I., Schwarz A., Fassina G., and Boschetti E., 1998, IRIS97: an innovative protein A-peptidomimetic solid phase media for antibody purification. *J. Mol. Recognit.* **11**:107-109

Gulich S., Uhlen M., and Hober S., 2000, Protein engineering of an IgG-binding domain allows milder elution conditions during affinity chromatography. *J. Biotechnol.* **76**: 233-244

Guse A.H., Milton A.D., Schulze-Koops H., Müller B., Roth E., and Simmer B., 1994, Purification and analytical characterization of an anti-CD4 monoclonal antibody for human therapy. *J. Chromatogr. A* **661**: 13-23

Hage D.S., 2002, High-performance affinity chromatography: a powerful tool for studying serum protein binding. *J. Chromatogr. B Analyt. Technol. Biomed. Life Sci.* **768**: 3-30

Hansen M.B.. and Lihme A., 1996, A new protein A mimicking affinity matrix for expanded bed purification of monoclonal antibodies. Poster at the First International Conference on Expanded Bed Adsorption, Queens'College Cambridge, UK 8-10 December 1996

Hilbrig F., and Freitag R., 2003a, Continuous Annular Chromatography. *J Chromatogr A.*: **790**: 1-15

Hilbrig F., and Freitag R., 2003b, Affinity precipitation for protein purification. *J Chromatogr A:* **790**: 79-90

Hochuli E., 1988, Large-scale chromatography of recombinant proteins. *J Chromatogr* **444**: 293-302

Hochuli E., Dobeli H., and Schacher A., 1987, New metal chelate adsorbent selective for proteins and peptides containing neighboring histidin residues. *J Chromatogr* **411**: 177-184

Huse K., Böhme H.-J., and Scholz G.H., 2002, Purification of antibodies by affinity chromatography. *J. Biochem. Biophys. Methods* **51**: 217-231

Hutchens T.W., and Porath J., 1986, Thiophilic adsorption of immunoglobulins – analysis of conditions optimal for selective immobilization and purification. *Anal. Biochem.* **159**: 217-226

Iberer G., Schwinn H., Josic D., Jungbauer A., and Buchacher A., 2001, Improved performance of protein separation by continuous annular chromatography in the size-exclusion mode. *J. Chromatogr. A.* **921**: 15-24

Ikeyama S., Nakagawa S., Arakawa M., Sugino H., and Kakinuma A., 1986, Purification and characterization of IgE produced by human myeloma cell line, U266. *Mol. Immunol.* **23**:159-167

Josic D., Lim YP., Strancar A., Reutter W., 1994a, Application of high-performance membrane chromatography for separation of annexins from the plasma membranes of liver and isolation of monospecific polyclonal antibodies. *J Chromatogr B Biomed.* **662**: 217-226

Josic D., Schwinn H., Stalder M., Strancar A., 1994, Purification of factor VIII von Willebrand factor from human plasma by anion-exchange chromatography. *J Chromatogr B Biomed.* **662**: 181-190

Juarez-Salinas H., Ott GS., Chen JC., Brooks TL., Stanker LH., 1986, Separation of IgG idiotypes by high-performance hydroxylapatite chromatography. *Methods Enzymol.* **121**: 615-622

Jungbauer A., Tauer C., Reiter M., Purtscher M., Wenisch E., Steindl F., Buchacher A., Katinger H., 1989, Comparison of protein A, protein G and copolymerized hydroxyapatite for the purification of human monoclonal antibodies. *J Chromatogr.* **476**: 257-268

Jungbauer A., Unterluggauer F., Steindl F., Ruker F., Katinger H., 1987, Combination of Zetaprep mass ion-exchange media and high-performance cation-exchange chromatography for the purification of high-purity monoclonal antibodies. *J Chromatogr.* **397**:313-320

Kasper C., Meringova L., Freitag R. and Tennikova T., 1998, Fast isolation of protein receptors from streptococci G by means of macroporous affinity discs. *J. Chromatogr. A* **798**: 65-72

Kawasaki T., Niikura M., and Kobayashi Y., 1990, Fundamental study of hydroxyapatite high-performance liquid chromatography. III. Direct experimental confirmation of the existence of two types of adsorbing surface on the hydroxyapatite crystal. *J Chromatogr.* **515**: 125-148

Kihira Y. and Aiba S., 1992, Artificial immunoglobulin G-binding protein mimetic to staphylococcal protein A. Its production and application to affinity purification of immunoglobulin G. *J Chromatogr* **597**: 277-283

Kondoh H., Kobayashi K., and Hagiwara K., 1987, A simple procedure for the isolation of human secretory IgA of IgA1 and IgA2 subclass by a jackfruit lectin, jacalin, affinity chromatography. *Mol. Immunol.* **24**:1219-122

Kreutz F.T., Wishart D.S., and Suresh M.R., 1998, Efficient bispecific monoclonal antibody purification using gradient thiophilic affinity chromatography. *J. Chromatogr.* **714**:161-170

Kristiansen T., 1978, Matrix-bound antigen and antibodies. Affinity chromatography. *Proc. Intern. Symp.*, Oxford, 191-206

Kummer A., and Li-Chan E.C., 1998, Application of an ELISA-elution assay as a screening tool for dissociation of yolk antibody-antigen complexes. *J. Immunol. Methods* **211**: 125-137

Langone J.J., 1982a, Applications of immobilized protein A in immunochemical techniques. *J. Immunol. Methods* **55**: 277-296

Langone J.J., 1982b, Protein A of *Staphylococcus aureus* and related immunoglobulin receptors produced by streptococci and pneumonococci. *Adv. Immunol.* **32**: 157-252

Larsson PO., and Mosbach K., 1979, Affinity precipitation of enzymes. *FEBS Lett.* **98**: 333
Lehrer S.B., 1979, Isolation of IgE from normal mouse serum. *Immunology* **36**: 103-109
Li R., Dowd V., Steward D.J., Burton S.j., and Lowe C.R., 1998, Design, synthesis, and application of a protein A mimetic. *Nat. Biotechnol.* **16**: 190-195
Lihme A., and Hansen M.B., 1997, Protein A mimetic for large-scale monoclonal antibody purification. American Biotechnology Laboratory, July
Lowe CR., Lowe AR., Gupta G., 2001, New developments in affinity chromatography with potential application in the production of biopharmaceuticals. *J Biochem Biophys.* **49**: 561-574
Lutkemeyer D., Ameskamp N., Tebbe IL., Wittler J., Lehmann J., 1999, Estimation of cell damage in bench-and pilot-scale affinity expanded-bed chromatography for the purification of monoclonal antibodies. *Biotechnol Bioeng.* **65(1)**: 114-119
Lutkemeyer D., Bretschneider M., Buntemeyer H., Lehmann J., 1993, Membrane chromatography for rapid purification of recombinant antithrombin III and monoclonal antibodies from cell culture supernatant. *J Chromatogr.* **639**: 57-66
Lutomski D., Joubert-Caron R., Bourin P., Baldier D., Caron M., 1995, Use of thiophilic adsorption in the purification of biotinylated Fab fragments. In *Journal of Chromatography B.* Biomed Sci Appl. **664**: 79-82
Manil L., Motte P., Pernas P., Troalen F., Bohuon C., and Bellet D., 1986, Evaluation of protocols for purification of mouse monoclonal antibodies. Yield and purity in two-dimensional gel electrophoresis. *J Immunol Methods.* **90**: 25-37
Manzke O., Tesch H., Diehl V., and Bohlen H., 1997, Single-step purification of bispecific monoclonal antibodies for immunotherapeutic use by hydrophobic interaction chromatography. *J Immunol Methods.* **208**: 65-73
Marino M., Campanile N., Ippolito A., Scarallo A., Ruvo M., and Fassina G., 1999, Structurally constrained selective ligands for mouse immunoglobulins. In *Peptides 98* (S. Bajusz, and F. Hudecz, eds.) Academia Kiado, Budapest, pp. 776-777
Martin AJP., 1949, Discussions faraday Soc. **7**: 332-336
Murray A., Sekowski M., Spencer DI., Denton G., and Price MR., 1997, Purification of monoclonal antibodies by epitope and minotope affinity chromatography. *J Chromatogr A* **782**: 49-54
Narhi L.O., Caughey D.J., Horan T., Kita Y., Chang D., and Arakawa T., 1997, Effect of three elution buffers on the recovery and structure of monoclonal antibodies. *Anal. Biochem.* **253**:236-245
Necina R., Amatschek A., and Jungbauer A., 1998, Capture of human monoclonal antibodies from cell culture supernatant by ion exchange media exhibiting high charge density. *Biotechn Bioengin.* **60**: 689-698
Nedonchelle E., Pitiot O., and Vijayalakshmi M.A., 2000, A preliminary study for isolation of catalytic antibodies by histidin ligand affinity chromatography as an alternative to conventional protein A/G methods. *Appl. Biochem. Biotechnol.* **83(1-3)**: 287-294
Ngo T.T., and Khatter N., 1990, Chemistry and preparation of affinity ligands useful in immunoglobulin isolation and serum-protein separation. *J. Chromatogr.* **510**:281-291
Nilson B.H., Logdberg L., Kastern W., Bjorck L., and Akerstrom B., 1993, Purification of antibodies using protein L-binding framework structures in the light chain variable domain. *J. Immunol. Methods.* **164**: 33-40
Nilson B.H., Solomon A., Bjorck L., and Akerstrom B., 1992, Protein L from Peptostreptococcus magnus binds to the kappa light chain variable domain. *J. Biol. Chem.* **267**: 2234-2239
Oleander M. Aa., and Lihme A., 1998, Mixed mode ligands – sophisticated "ion exchangers" for efficient capture of proteins from crude raw materials. Poster at the Second International Conference on Expanded Bed Adsorption. Napa Valley, CA, USA, 21-23 June 1998

Ostryania ND., Vlasov GP., Tennikova TB., 2002, Multifunctional fractionation of polyclonal antibodies by immunoaffinity high-performance monolithic disk chromatography. *J Chromatogr.* **949**: 163-171

Palombo G., Verdoliva A., and Fassina G., 1998a, Affinity purification of IgM using a novel synthetic ligand. *J. Chromatogr. Biomed. Appl.* **715**: 137-145

Palombo G., De Falco S., Tortora M., Cassani G., and Fassina G., 1998b, A synthetic ligand for IgA affinity purification. *J. Mol. Recognit.* **11**: 243-246

Palombo G., Rossi M., Cassani G., Fassina G., 1998c, Affinity purification of mouse monoclonal IgE using a protein A mimetic ligand immobilized on solid supports. *J Mol Recognit.* **11**: 247-249

Patent application: A. Lihme and M.B. Hansen, « Isolation of Immunoglobulins », PCT/DK97/00359

Pavlu B., Joansson U., Nyhlen C., Wichman A., 1986, Rapid purification of monoclonal antibodies by high-performance liquid chromatography. *J Chromatogr.* **359**: 449-460

Peng Z., Arthur G., Simons FE., Becker AB., 1993, Binding of dog immunoglobulins G, A, M, and E to concanavalin. *A. Vet Immunol Immunolpathol.* **36**: 83-88

Philips T.M., More N.S., Queen W.D., and Thompson A.M., 1985, Isolation and quantitation of serum IgE levels by high-performance immunoaffinity chromatography. *J. Chromatogr.* **327**: 205-211

Phillips TM., 1992, *Analytical Techniques in Immunochemistry.* Marcel Dekker, New York, pp. 22-39

Pimm M.V., Robins R.A., Embelton M.J., Jacobs E., Markham A.J., Charleston A., et al., 1990, A bispecific monoclonal antibody against methotrexate and a human tumor associated antigen augments cytotoxicity of methotrexate-carrier conjugate. *British J. Cancer* **61**:508-513

Platonova G.A., Pankova G.A., Il'omp I.Y., Vlasov G.P., and Tennikova T.B., 1999, Quantitative fast fractionation of a pool of polyclonal antibodies by immunoaffinity membrane chromatography. *J. Chromatogr A* **852**: 129-140

Porath J., Carlsson J., Olsson I., Belfrage G., 1975, Metal chelate affinity chromatography, a new approach to protein fractionation. *Nature.* **258**: 598-599

Porath J., Maisano F., and Belew M., 1985, Thiophilic adsorption – a new method for protein fractionation. *FEBS Lett.* **185**: 306-310

Powers DD., Carbonell RG., and Kilpatrick PK., 1994, Affinity precipitation of an antibody by ligand-modified phospholipids. *Biotechnol Bioeng.* **44**: 509

Raeder R., and Boyle M.D., 1995, Analysis of immunoglobulin G-binding-protein expression by invasive isolates *of Streptococcus pyogenes. Clin. Diagn. Lab. Immunol.* **2**: 484-486

Rapoport EM., Zhigis LS., Vlasova EV., Piskarev VE., Bovin NV., Zubov VP., 1995, Purification of monoclonal antibodies to Le(y) and Le(d) carbohydrate by ion-exchange and thiophilic-adsorption chromatography. *Bioseparatio.* **5**: 141-146

Roque-Barreira M.R., and Campos-Nieto A., 1985, Jacalin : an IgA-binding lectin. *J. Biol. Chem.* **134**:1740-1743

Roque-Barreira MC., Praz F., Halbwachs-Mercarelli L., Greene LJ., Campos-Neto A., 1986, IgA-affinity purification and characterization of the lectin jacalin. *Braz J. Med Biol Res.* **19**: 149-157

Ruvo M., Scardino P., Cassani G., and Fassina G., 1994, Facile manual synthesis of peptide libraries. *Protein Pept. Lett.* **1** :187-192

Sampson IA., Hodgen AN., and Arthur IH., 1984, The separation of immunoglobulin M from human serum by fast protein liquid chromatography. *J Immunol Methods.* **69**: 9-15

Santucci A., Soldani P., Lozzi L., Rustici M., Bracci L., Petreni S., and Neri P., 1988, High performance liquid chromatography immunoaffinity purification of antibodies and antibody fragments. *J. Immunol Methods* **114**: 181-185

Schneider M., Guillot C., and Lamy B., 1981, The affinity precipitation technique. Application to the isolation and purification of trypsin from bovine pancreas. *Ann NY Acad Sci.* **369**: 257

Siegel DL., 2002, Recombinant monoclonal antibody technology. *Transfus Clin Biol.* **9**: 15-22

Spence C., Schaffer CA., Kessler S., Ballon P., 1994, Fluidized-bed receptor-affinity chromatography. *Biomed Chromatogr.* **8(5)**: 236-241

Stanker LH., Vanderlaan M., Juarez-Salinas H., 1985, One-step purification of mouse monoclonal antibodies from ascites fluid by hydroxylapatite chromatography. *J Immunol Methods.* **76**: 157-169

Taipa MA., Kaul R., Mattiasson B., and Cabral JMS., 1998, Preliminary studies on the purification of a monoclonal antibody by affinity precipitation with Eudragit S-100. *J Mol Recognit.* **11**, 240

Taipa MA., Kaul RH., Mattiasson B., and Cabral JMS., 2000, Recovery of a monoclonal antibody from hybridoma culture supernatant by affinity precipitation with Eudragit S-100. *Bioseparation* **9**: 291

Tasaka K., Kobayashi M., Tanaka T., and Inagaki C., 1984, Rapid purification of monoclonal antibody in ascites by high performance ion exchange column chromatography for diminishing non-specific staining. *Acta Histochem Cytochem.* **17**: 283-286

Teng S.F., Sproule K., Husain A., and Lowe C.R., 2000, Affinity chromatography on immobilized "biomimetic" ligands. Synthesis, immobilization and chromatographic assessment of an immunoglobulin G-binding ligand. *J. Chromatogr. B: Biomed. Sci. Appl.* **740**: 1-15

Teng S-F., Sproule K., Hussain A., Lowe CR., 1999, A strategy for the generation of biomimetic ligands for affinity chromatography-Combinatorial synthesis and biological evaluation of an IgG binding ligand. *J Mol Recognit.* **12**: 67-75

Tennikova TB., and Freitag R., 1999, Analytical and preparative separation methods of biomolecules. Aboul-Ehnen HY: (Ed.), Marcel Dekker, New York, Basel, pp 255-300

Tsang V.C.W., and Wilkins P.P., 1991, Optimum dissociating condition for immunoaffinity and preferential isolation of antibodies with high specific activity. *J. Immunol. Methods* **138**: 291-299

Uretschläger A., and Jungbauer A., 2000, Scale-down of continuous protein purification by annular chromatography. Design parameters for the smallest unit. *J. Chromatogr. A.* **890**: 53-59

Uretschläger A., Einhauer A., and Jungbauer A., 2001, Continuous separation of green fluorescent protein by annular chromatography. *J. Chromatogr. A* **908**: 243-250

Vaquero C., Sack M., Chandler J., Drossard J., Schuster F., Monecke M., et al., 1999, Transient expression of a tumor-specific single-chain fragment and a chimeric antibody in tobacco leaves. *Proc. Natl. Acad. Sci. USA* **96**: 11128-11133

Verdoliva A., Basile G., and Fassina G., 2000, Affinity purification of immunoglobulins from chicken egg yolk using a new synthetic ligand. *J. Chromatogr. Biomed. Appl.* **749**: 233-242

Vijayalakshimi M.A., 1998, Antibody purification methods. *Appl. Biochem. Biotechnol.* **75(1)**: 93-102

Vola R., Lombardi A., Tarditi L., Bjorck L., and Mariani M., 1995, Recombinant protein L and LG : efficient tools for purification of murine immunoglobulin G fragments. *J. Chromatogr. B. Biomed. Appl.* **668**: 209-218

Wheatly J.B., 1992, Multiple ligand applications in high-performance immunoaffinity chromatography. *J. Chromatogr.* **603**:273-278

Yoshida S., Ioka D., Matsuoka H., Endo H., and Ishii A., 2001, Bacteria expressing single-chain immunotoxin inhibit malaria parasite development in mosquitoes. *Mol. Biochem. Parasitol.* **113**: 89-96

Yurov GK., Neugodova GL., Verkhovsky OA., Naroditsky BS., 1994, Thiophilic adsorption rapid purification of F(ab)$_2$ and Fc fragment of IgG1 antibodies from murine ascitic fluid. *J. Immunol Methods.* **177**: 29-33

Zola H., Garland L.G., Cox H.C., and Adcock J.J., 1978, Separation of IgE from IgG subclasses using staphylococcal protein A. *Int. Arch. Allergy Appl. Immunol.* **56**: 123-127

Zola H., Neoh SH., 1989, Monoclonal antibody purification. In choice of method and assessment of purity and yield. *Biotechniques.* **7**: 802, 804-808

Zusman R., and Zusman I., 2001, Glass fibers covered with sol-gel glass as a new support for affinity chromatography columns: a review. *J Biochem Biophys Methods* **49**: 175-187

Zusman R., Beckman D., Zusman I., and Brent B., 1992, Purification of sheep immunoglobulin G using protein A trapped in sol-gel glass. *Anal Biochem.* **201**: 103-106

Zusman R., Rottman C., Ottoenghi M., Avnir D., 1990, Doped sol-gel glasses as chemical sensors. *J Non-Cryst Solids.* **122** : 107-109

Zusman R., Zusman I., 1995, Gel fiberglass as a new support for affinity chromatography. *Biotechnol Appl Biochem.* **21**: 161-172

Chapter 6

QUALITY CONTROL OF ANTIBODIES FOR HUMAN USE

Andreas Richter[*], Mark Jostameling[*], Kerstin Müller[*], Andreas Herrmann[#] and Martin Pitschke[##]
[*]NewLab BioQuality AG, Erkrath, Germany, [#]Cardion AG, Erkrath, Germany, [##]Evotec Technologies GmbH, Erkrath, Germany

1. INTRODUCTION

The quality control of biopharmaceutical antibodies intended for human use are required to follow guidelines and regulations set down by national and international regulatory authorities. The US Food and Drug Administration (FDA) issued a guidance in 1997 specifically for antibody products in its „Points to consider in the manufacture and testing of monoclonal antibody products for human use". This guideline describes the quality control for the entire production process from cell line characterisation through to clinical considerations. In this chapter we will focus on analytical techniques for controlling the downstream processing and the release of the bulk material as well as finished product. For additional information on cell line characterisation refer to the relevant guidelines ICH Q5B and ICH Q5D or Fels, 2001.

Antibody production is generally shifting from murine hybridoma cells as production system to recombinant Chinese Hamster Ovary (CHO) cells. There is no major difference in the quality control between a hybridoma or a recombinant CHO cell-derived antibody product. Basically the regulations demand that the biopharmaceutical antibodies are safe and are characterised in accordance with the specified properties. To demonstrate this, a panel of analytical methods must not only be developed but also validated according to the relevant guidelines (FDA, 2001). Quality control testing accompanies drug development starting at the research stage through to process development and scale-up stages and continues to the production itself for market supply. There are, however, differences in the number of tests and the extent of validation which is required for the various stages of drug development. For example, it is normally not necessary to have fully validated analytical test procedures in place for the preclinical testing.

Normally a comprehensive set of data is collected during the initial phase of drug development using a broad variety of methods which results in the full characterisation of the antibody. In the later phases of development a subset of these methods is defined as lot-release testing methods and specifications will be set for this purpose. The specifications can be re-defined following further development and scale-up of the manufacturing process. Another subset of methods must be defined for studies demonstrating the stability of the antibody product during storage (according to relevant guidelines for stability testing, (ICH, 1996)).

In this chapter analytical methods normally employed for antibody quality control will be presented. In the first part, methods for controlling the purity of the antibody are discussed with a special focus on DNA and protein impurities as well as antibody aggregates. In the second part analytical procedures for the testing of in-process samples, bulk product and finished product will be discussed including antibody glycosylation and SDS-Page.

2. BIOANALYTICAL METHODS FOR IMPURITY CONTROL

2.1 Overview

During the downstream processing, the antibody molecules are purified from all the ingredients of the fermentation medium including host cell material such as DNA and cellular proteins as well as media components such as albumin, insulin or transferrin. As for all biologics special care must be taken to minimise bioburden and endotoxin levels.

The downstream processing itself can also be a source of impurities, for example by the introduction of enzymes such as proteases for the processing of the product or due to the leakage of materials such as Protein A during affinity chromatography purification steps. Product-related impurities such as cleaved or aggregated antibodies, deamidated or oxidised forms of the antibodies or incorrectly assembled antibody molecules should be controlled as well. Table 6.1 provides an overview of the different safety relevant impurities and the assays used in controlling them.

Quality control of biopharmaceutical antibodies 171

Table 6.1. Summary of quality assays for impurity control of biopharmaceutical antibodies

Analytical task	Test Method
Bioburden	Microbiological tests according to Pharmacopoeia
Endotoxins	LAL-testing according to Pharmacopoeia
Host Cell DNA	DNA Hybridisation, Threshold-System, qPCR
Host Cell Proteins	ELISA, Immunoligand Assay*
Media components such as insulin or transferrin	ELISA, Immunoligand Assay
Leachables such as Protein A	ELISA, Immunoligand Assay, HPLC
Aggregated Antibodies	SEC, Light scattering, Correlation spectroscopy**
Deamidated or oxidised antibody forms	Peptide Mapping ideally coupled with mass spectrometry, MALDI-TOF
Incorrectly assembled or disassembled chains	SDS-PAGE, SEC, Peptide Mapping

*for further details see chapter 2.1.2 ** for further details see chapter 2.1.4

Impurity control for residual DNA and Host Cell Protein (HCP) should follow a double safety strategy: the manufacturing process itself should be validated for its ability to consistently eliminate impurities and, in addition, the final bulk material must be tested to demonstrate that the required specifications have been met. If sufficient validation data are available concerning the process' robustness in DNA and HCP removal, it may be possible to omit these testing requirements for the lot-release testing (EMEA, position statement on residual DNA and HCP, 1997).

In the following subchapters we provide further information on quality control assays for residual host cell DNA, residual host cell proteins and residual Protein A as well as antibody aggregates.

2.1.1 Testing for Host Cell DNA

Depending on the fermentation system used and the method of cell harvest, the purification process normally starts with material containing significant amounts of host cell DNA. Although there are references suggesting that higher levels of DNA (World Health Organisation, 1996) may be allowed, the amount of residual DNA in the final bulk should be generally lower than 100 pg per therapeutic dose („Points to consider in the manufacture and testing of monoclonal antibody products for human use", FDA 1997). Keeping in mind that the DNA from one diploid CHO cell alone weights about 6 pg, this limit of 100 pg necessitates a purification process that is very effective and robust in removing DNA as well as requiring analytical methods which are extremely sensitive and reliable. High sensitive quantitation of trace amounts of DNA is performed by either hybridisation methods, by immunological methods such as the "Threshold™ System" (Molecular Devices Corp., Sunnyvale CA, USA)(Kung et al., 1989), or by quantitative PCR (q-PCR) methods (Lovatt, 2002). Table 6.2 presents selected validation data from residual DNA assays.

Table 6.2. Validation data of residual CHO cell DNA assays

Parameters	Hybridisation Assay	Threshold Assay
Precision		
Repeatability	4 %	2 %
Intermediate precision	10 %	14 %
Quantitation limit	10 pg	6.3 pg
Quantitation range	10 - 800 pg	6.3 - 200 pg

There are a few differences between the DNA testing procedures which should be taken into account when interpreting quantitative data. The hybridisation assay randomly measures total DNA from a few base pairs (bp) up to kilo base pairs in length. This assay is specific for the source DNA. The Threshold^{tm} assay requires that the DNA is longer than approximately 600 bp and it is not specific for the source DNA. PCR-based assays are specific for their target sequence and the amount of total DNA must be derived from the measured target copy numbers. A very important prerequisite for all of the assays is the availability of well-purified DNA. All assays differ in their sensitivity to residuals such as organic solvents, detergents, high salt concentrations, ethanol or residual protein. These can originate from the sample itself or from the DNA purification procedure. For these reasons the assays must always be designed as spike recovery assays in order to control the loss of material during sample preparation. Figure 6.1 illustrates the strategy of spike recovery controls for a hybridisation assay.

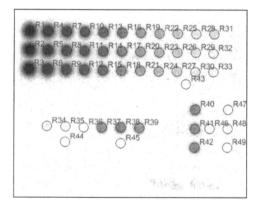

Figure 6.1. Dot blot hybridisation assay for the quantification of residual DNA. A calibration curve is applied from 1600 pg to 3 pg (no. R1 to R33). Samples are applied threefold (R34 - R36) as well as spiked samples (R36 to R39) spike controls (R40 to R42) and buffer controls (R47 to R49), R44 to R46 are background controls.

Quality control of biopharmaceutical antibodies 173

2.1.2 Testing for Host Cell Proteins

The purification process must be able to remove any residual Host Cell Protein (HCP) in order to minimize that risk of adverse immune reactions to impurities in the antibody. HCP represents a variety of different proteins which cannot be analysed by classical protein methods. This is because HCP exists only as trace amounts in the final material having large excesses of product antibody. Therefore, immunological methods are the only methods which can be applied to determine the levels of possible HCP contamination. Great care must be taken to ensure there is no unspecific binding to the product itself. Product and process specific assays must normally be used in determining HCP levels. The development of these specific assays are very time consuming. Mock fermentation and mock purification runs are performed to obtain a suitable antigen. Various samples along the purification process must be analysed using, for example, Western blotting and PAGE to determine which appears to be the most likely candidate for immunization. Once this has been determined, the antigen is immunised into animals such as rabbits or goats. The resulting antiserum is the basis for the development and validation of a quantitative assay which should have a sensitivity in the range of 10 - 100 parts per million (ppm). Frequently, ELISA (Immuno-linked) or ILA (Immunoligand) assays are used.

Recently the possible use of generic host cell protein assays for comparable processes instead of product-specific assays has been in discussion (Hoffman, 2000). In these generic assays the antiserum which is used has been raised against the host cell protein preparation representing the most probable residual proteins in the first downstream processing steps. The advantage of a generic assay is that the time consuming antigen production, the immunisation procedure and assay development and validation are not necessary. A generic anti-CHO HCP serum is shown in Figure 6.2 by gel electrophoresis and Western blotting. During early phases of clinical testing, generic assays can be very useful not only for process development but also for lot-release or the final process validation. For the later phases of clinical studies or for marketing of product, product-specific HCP assays, however, are normally required by the regulatory authorities.

Both specific and generic host cell protein assays have some limitations: The ELISA or ILA signal used for quantitation of HCP represents an average signal from hundreds of different antibody-antigen bindings. Not every single HCP-antigen is detected with the same sensitivity. Therefore, it is possible that due to a strong binding detection antibody a certain host cell protein is over-estimated in the HCP measurement or vice versa. As shown in Figure 6.2 low molecular weight antigens often result in a lower immune response compared to higher molecular weight proteins. This would lead to an underestimation of those proteins in HCP assays.

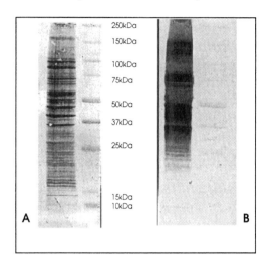

Figure 6.2. Western Blot analysis of a generic CHO cell protein assay. Proteins secreted from CHO cells have been prepared and used as antigen for immunisation of goats. A: silver stained SDS-PAGE of antigen proteins. B: Western blot analysis. The antiserum was developed at NewLab BioQuality AG.

As presented in Table 6.3 commonly used host cell protein assays are sensitive up to a few ppm. With the antibody preparations, it must be carefully checked to ensure that there is no cross reaction of the HCP detection system. The ILA system has proven to be relatively insensitive against cross reaction because it is based on fluorescein-recognising secondary antibodies and not on IgG-recognising antibodies as usually used in sandwich ELISA.

Table 6.3. Validation data from a generic CHO-HCP assay (Immunoligand Assay)

Parameters	Validation data
Precision	
Repeatability	11 % CV
Intermediate precision	18 % CV
Quantitation limit	5 ppm
Quantitation range	5 - 500 ng/ml

2.1.3 Testing residual Protein A

Purification of antibodies commonly employs an affinity chromatography step using Protein A as the antibody-binding ligand. After consecutive purification runs with the same chromatographic medium, the risk of ligand leakage increases and consequently, a Protein A contamination of the antibody product is possible (Iyer *et al.*, 2002). Regulatory authorities advise that it must be demonstrated that Protein A is eliminated during purification and that the final bulk product is free of any Protein A contamination. As in the case of HCP assays, due to their sensitivity and specificity, immunological assays are normally employed. Recently a technology has been introduced for Protein A detection using an immunological detection principle combined with a fluorescence-based single molecule detection system referred to as fluorescence intensity distribution assay (FIDA) (Richter *et al.*, 2001). This assay has the advantage of a short measurement time compared to classical ELISA and possibly demonstrates an upcoming technology when fast in-process controls are required. In Table 6.4 key parameters of Protein A assays which are in use for biopharmaceutical quality control have been summarized.

Table 6.4. Comparison of different assays for Protein A detection

Parameters	ELISA	ILA	FIDA
Precision			
Repeatability	5.1 % CV	7.0 % CV	4.9 % CV
Intermediate precision	9.1 % CV	9.0 % CV	8.8 % CV
Quantitation limit	2 ppm	0.025 ppm	1.4 ppm
Quantitation range	2 - 100 ng/ml	0.025 - 2 ng/ml	1 - 18 ng/ml

2.1.4 Antibody aggregates as product-related impurities

Impurities originating from aggregated monomers may result in lot-to-lot variability (May *et al.*, 1992) and may result in reduced bioactivity, immunogenic reactions, or unacceptable physical appearance (Kataham *et al.*, 1995). *In vivo* applications of therapeutics containing aggregated material may have a dramatic effect on the bioavailability and pharmacokinetics and can preclude its absorption all together. Present techniques available for the evaluation of the aggregate ratio are size exclusion chromatography (SEC-HPLC) (Goetz, 2001) and gel electrophoresis with silver staining. These methods normally have a sensitivity with detection limits of 1% protein content. Using dynamic light scattering in a dust-free environment, this sensitivity can be increased to 0.1%. (Moradian-Oldak, 1995). In this chapter an alternative technology, **NIPP**, nucleation-induced-protein-polymerisation in combination with a technology called **FIDA**, fluorescence-intensity-distribution analysis is described. These methods offer significantly improved sensitivity for the detection of even single aggregates with a concurrent high specificity for the detectable aggregates.

The *de novo* formation of aggregates can be described as a two-step process (Fig. 6.3). During the initial nucleation reaction, oligomers (seeds) are formed transiently from monomers in a concentration and microenvironmental dependent manner. Once a seed is formed, the subsequent addition of further sub-units results in the kinetic fast growth reaction (nucleation induced polymerisation) (Harper *et al.*, 1997).

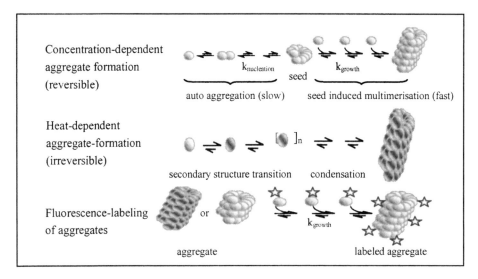

Figure 6.3. Mechanism of protein aggregation fluorescence detection technology: Formation of multiple labelled aggregates resulting from the addition of fluorescence labelled monomers to the sample solution. Evotec Technologies-GmbH and Evotec OAI AG, Hamburg, Germany, patents pending for NIPP and FIDA technology.

Aggregation under denaturing conditions is initiated by loss the secondary structure which is subsequently followed by irreversible condensation of the unstructured monomers. Both types of aggregates can be detected using a fluorescence-based homogenous assay. Therefore, single fluorescence labelled monomers are added to the sample of interest. Subsequently, multiple fluorescence-labelled aggregates are formed in those samples containing intrinsic seeds due to the NIPP mechanism (Pitschke *et al.*, 1998). The assay system has been further developed for antibody testing as reported by Storm *et al.*, 2002 and Clemens *et al.*, 2003.

The combination of the NIPP technology and FIDA provides a detection tool which allows to detect and quantify aggregates down to the single aggregate level. It is especially suited to control and optimise the production process of antibodies in a early phases which are not accessible by other analytic aggregation techniques. The combination of NIPP and FIDA offers a very sensitive and specific test for the valuation of biopharmaceutical products and in the optimisation of antibody formulations.

3. BIOANALYTICAL METHODS FOR ANTIBODY CHARACTERISATION

3.1 Overview

There are 5 classes of human antibodies (IgA, IgD, IgE, IgG, IgM) but in the biopharamceutical industry IgG antibodies and their derivatives play by far the most predominant role. Due to the complex rearrangement processes of antibody gene elements, different IgG subclasses exist with different light and heavy chains and differences in the inter-chain disulphide bonds. For example, human IgG can have a λ or a κ-light chain and four different types of heavy chains: IgG1 to IgG4 (Overview: e.g. Roitt and Rabson, 2000, King 1998).

IgG represents a class of protein molecules with a complex structure. Two units of two different protein chains (heavy and light chain) are connected via disulphide bonds to form a four peptide unit. In addition intra-molecular disulphide bonds stabilise the structure of the chains. The molecules are usually glycosylated at each heavy chain. The glycosylation pattern depends on their host cells and the conditions during the fermentation procedure (Ip *et al.* 1994). There are different "recognition" regions on an IgG molecule, the hyper-variable antigen binding regions and the highly conserved regions which are the contact sites for effector function (fc-receptors, complement system). Both the formation of the correct antigen binding site as well as the correct formation of the sites for interaction with other molecules in the patient contribute to the efficacy of the drug. In addition, glycosylation plays an essential role in determining the lifetime of an antibody drug product in the patient. Consequently, alterations not only in the binding region but also in the heavy chain fine structure could lead to an altered performance of the drug in the patient.

A consistent micro-heterogeneity pattern is one of the most important indicator for the consistency of the batches and, therefore, for the consistency of the production process.

In addition to the original immunoglobulin-modified biopharmaceutical antibodies, defined antibody fragments, chimeric antibodies and antibody fusion proteins have also been developed. For quality control of such products additional individual assays have to be employed.

Due to the structural specialities, a panel of analytical methods should be available to demonstrate that the products are in accordance with the expectations. As it is recommended by authorities, state-of-the-art methods should be applied but not before having shown that the assays can be validated and are reliable. Table 6.5 presents a summary of analytical methods commonly used today for biopharmaceutical antibody characterisation. In the following chapter the relevant test methods are briefly described and some more details are provided for glycosylation analysis and quantitative SDS-PAGE.

Table 6.5. Summary of commonly used assays for characterisation of biopharmaceutical antibodies

Analytical task	Test Method
Identity: Subclass determination	Immunological methods
Identity	Peptide Mapping, N- and C-terminal sequencing, ELISA
Identity and Isoform analysis	Isoelectric focussing, Ion exchange HPLC, Capillary electrophoresis
Protein concentration	UV-Absorbance, Colorimetric assays
Protein concentration for determination of the extinction coefficient	Amino acid analysis, Nitrogen determination
Primary structure of antibody chains	N-Terminal Sequencing, C-Terminal Sequencing, Mass spectrometry
Secondary structure	Circular Dichroism*
Molecular Weight	SDS-PAGE, MALDI-TOF, Size Exclusion HPLC
Disulfid bond structure	Reducing and non reducing SDS-PAGE, Analysis of free SH-Groups
Carbohydrate structure	HPAEC-PAD, Differential Deglycosylation and SDS-PAGE, Mass Spectrometry, Isoform analysis

For further reading: Cantor and Schimmel, 1980

3.2 Identity

The demonstration of the identity is usually performed by comparison to a reference standard. Data are generated which should be in accordance with the reference standard within set limits. The allowed range is a case by case decision but should be very well justified by the manufacturer. The justification of acceptance criteria and specification is usually based upon the set of data which has been collected.

For evaluating the identity of biopharmaceutical antibodies, the following methods are applicable: SDS-PAGE in a reducing and non-reducing mode (chapter 3.7); N-terminal and C-terminal amino acid sequencing of the heavy and light chain; peptide mapping; MALDI-TOF; and isoelectric focussing (IEF).

IEF is an iso-protein analytical method and, therefore, very useful in demonstrating the antibody identity and micro-heterogeneities. Typically an IEF pattern is generated which should resemble the standard pattern within set limits. The acceptance limits should be carefully worked out on the basis of an adequate number of experiments. It is important to be able to

Quality control of biopharmaceutical antibodies 179

differentiate between the normal error of the assays and the acceptable or unacceptable variations of the product.

3.3 Protein concentration

One of the most important analytical tasks is the determination of the protein concentration. Once defined the protein concentration is the basis for the application of the correct protein amount in further analyses and finally for the formulation.

In principle there are four different methods available: colorimetric methods such as Bradford or BCA, UV-absorbency, amino acid analysis and nitrogen determination. All of these assays have their advantages and drawbacks and therefore are utilised for different analytical purposes (Ritter and McEntire, 2002).

Colorimetric assays are easy to use and also applicable with in-process samples since they do not need an optically clear solution as is the case with the UV-absorbency. It is important to have a reference standard calibration curve from comparable or identical proteins. UV-absorbency is very easy to perform because there is no staining required. The calculation of the protein concentration is according to the Lambert-Beer equation. Therefore, the molar extinction coefficient must be available which is dependent upon UV-absorbing residues of certain amino acids, predominantly tyrosine and tryptophane. For both the colorimetric assays and the UV-absorbency the most important prerequisite is a representative calibration curve with a well-known linear range.

The amino acid analysis provides information on protein concentration and amino acid composition (Anders, 2002). It is a powerful method for determining the molar extinction coefficient. Due to the different principle of measurement, the amino acid analysis is often used as an additional method to colorimetric assays or UV absorbency. Amino acid analysis of glycoproteins such as antibodies may lead to imprecise results due to incomplete hydrolysation or incomplete solubilisation following hydrolysation. Therefore, great care has to be taken for method optimisation and validation of the procedure.

3.4 HPLC-Methods: isoforms and purity

Separation by HPLC methods can lead to information on antibody identity, concentration, purity, molecular weight and structure. For antibody quality control a separation on the basis of charges (Cation exchange chromatography (CIEX)) and molecular weight (Size Exclusion Chromatography (SEC)) is commonly used.

For antibody products show micro-heterogeneity the isoprotein pattern can be observed by CIEX, IEF or related methods (Kaltenbrunner *et al.*, 1993, Hamilton *et al*, 1987). The assays are usually evaluated by qualitatively comparing the resulting peak pattern and the retention times with the reference standard pattern.

HPLC-methods for determination of concentration, purity and molecular weight needs to be designed and validated as quantitative assays. Usually "purity " is defined as the absence of impurities below a set limit. The limit can be defined as the portion of the areas of impurity peaks and the area of the peak(s) that can clearly be related to the active pharmaceutical antibody. As mentioned in Chapter 2.1 antibody related impurities may occur due to imprecise processing, cleavage of the disulphide bonds, protease cleavage or aggregation of the antibodies. SDS page as an alternative purity determining method will be presented in more detail in chapter 3.7.

3.5 Peptide Mapping

For peptide mapping the antibodies are cleaved by a proteolytic enzyme and the resulting fragments are separated by HPLC. Further analysis of the fragments can be performed using mass spectrometry or N-terminal sequencing. The resulting fragment pattern is used for identity confirmation by comparison to the reference standard. But beyond that peptide mapping is a very powerful method for the analysis of chemical and structural changes. Incorrect or missing disulphide bond are clearly detected. Even small changes in the antibody molecule as for example deamidation or oxidation of methionine usually leads to a well detectable shift in the peptide pattern. Especially for the further analysis of small structural changes mass spectrometry is the most appropriate method (Nguyen *et al.*, 1995, Greer, 2001).

3.6 Antibody Glycosylation

Since the glycosylation plays an important role in pharmacokinetic (clearance), bioactive (carbohydrate ligand, protein conformation) and immunogenetic characteristics the glycosylation of biopharmaceutical antibodies becomes more and more interesting during the recent years. Apart from these pharmacological relevants glycosylation also affects biochemical properties such as solubility, aggregation and stability against protease degradation (Jenkins *et al.*, 1996).

In order to guarantee the production of a comparably glycosylated antibody with regards to biological safety and Batch-to-Batch consistency the regulatory authorities are increasingly asking for carbohydrate analyses as final product or process control. Therefore the comparability of the glycosylation pattern has to be shown. In addition special attention should be drawn to the occurrence of non-human and thereby potentially antigenic structures like NGNA and terminal Galactose(α1-3)Galactose as well as to the degree of sialylation which has a direct impact on in-vivo half life.

A

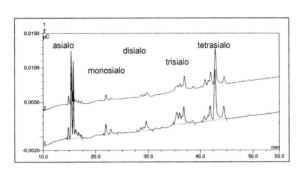

B

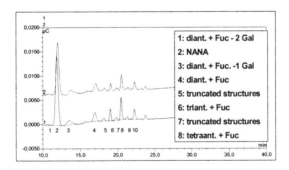

Figure 6.4. Chromatograms obtained by HPAEC-PAD analysis of the native (A) and asialo N-glycans (B) of an antibody-fusion protein derived from a CHO cell line which was purified from harvests.

For this reason the attempt of a routinely used, quick, robust and cost-effective chromatographic or electrophoretical method is existing which can replace the complex methods such as GC-MS, FAB-MS or ^{1}H-NMR-spectroscopy (Lottspeich and Zorbas, 1998). A simple and reliable carbohydrate analysis method which is used for process and quality control is the FACE (Fluorophore associated carbohydrate electrophoresis) technology where oligosaccharides or monosaccharides are labelled with a fluorescent tag, electrophoretical separated and detected by UV imagining. A more comprehensive technology is known as HPAEC-PAD (high pH anion exchange chromatography using pulsed amperiometric detector) which separates oligosaccharides or monosaccharides on an anion matrix at high pH and detects them by an amperiometric detector as they can be oxidized on the surface of a gold electrode. The oligosaccharide analysis by HPAEC-PAD includes two kind of assays: a "native" and an "asialo" N-glycan analysis. In case of native N-glycan analysis the allocation of different sialylated N-glycans are determined whereas asialo N-glycan analysis detects the proportion of asialo N-glycans and splitted sialic acid (Figure 6.4).

The glycosylation pattern of an antibody depends on different factors: First the glycosylation structure applicable depends on the expression system (mammalian or non-mammalian expression system). Furthermore, in case of a mammalian cell culture it could be shown that protein expressed by different host cells (Grabenhorst et al., 1999), even different clones made from the identical host cell, reveal a different glycosylation pattern (Gawlitzek et al., 2000). In addition, during the process development many factors such as type of fermentation, media, supplements, pH or the carbohydrate source have severe influence on the glycosylation pattern (Gawlitzek et al., 2000, Gawlitzek et al., 1998). Therefore, for a recombinant antibody production the comparability of glycosylation has to be shown along the fermentation (Table 6.6 shows a native N-glycan analysis of a fermentation in-process control by HPAEC-PAD) and purification process, for final Batch-to-Batch consistency, and after storage.

Table 6.6. Area allocation of different sialylated native N-glycans of an antibody-fusion protein by HPAEC-PAD: All samples which were purified from harvests are derived from a 100L- continuous flow CHO fermentation

Area-%	100L-CFF-day 3	100L-CFF-day 9	100L-CFF-day 15	100L-CFF-day 21	100L-CFF-day 27	100L-CFF-day 33
Asialo	32 %	27 %	30 %	31 %	27 %	29 %
Monosialo	5 %	7 %	6 %	5 %	6 %	6 %
Disialo	11 %	14 %	10 %	11 %	14 %	15 %
trisialo	25 %	28 %	24 %	27 %	27 %	27 %
tetrasialo	26 %	24 %	30 %	26 %	26 %	23 %
Mean sialylation per native N-glycan	2,08	2,14	2,19	2,13	2,19	2,08

3.7 SDS-Polyacrylamid Gel Electrophoresis (SDS-PAGE)

As mentioned above antibodies consist of heavy and light chains which are combined via disulfid bonds. Therefore SDS-PAGE under nonreducing conditions will lead to a single band with an apparent molecular weight of about 150 kDa. Under reducing conditions heavy and light chains will be separated and generate bands at approximately 52 and 26 kDa. SDS-PAGE gels can be stained using a protocol on the basis of Coomassie stain. This staining procedure leads to band intensities which are proportional to the amount of protein on the gel within the working range. The Coomassie staining is not depending on the individual protein sequence. Alternatively SDS-PAGE gels can be evaluated by silver-staining which is more sensitive.

Table 6.7. Validation data of the SDS-PAGE analysis

Parameters	Validation data molecular weight determination	Validation data impurity control
Accuracy	Not determined	> 94 %
Precision		
Repeatability	1 %	7 %
Intermediate precision	2 %	9 %
Quantitation limit	Not tested	0.1 µg
Quantitation range	Precision data verified for 25 and 50 kDa proteins	Precision data verified for 10% to 35% impurities

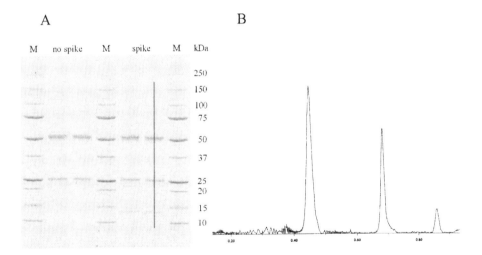

Figure 6.5. SDS Polyacrylamid gel, coomassie stained and spiked with an "impurity control". A 8 – 18% gradient gel under reducing conditions was used to separate 1 µg of a recombinant IgG antibody (lanes: "no spike") and 1 µg antibody and 0,1µg lactalbumin as impurity control (lanes "spike"). Figure B shows the scanning data evaluated with a scan analysis software ("Quantity One, BioRad, USA). For quantitative analysis the peak areas have been determined and the relation between "impurity"- and "antibody"-related signals was calculated.

For evaluation of SDS-PAGE gels electronic scanning systems with quantitation software are available from different manufacturers. Having qualified and validated such a systems a quantitative analysis of SDS-PAGE becomes fast and accurate. In principle two kind of information can be drawn from that analysis: apparent molecular weight and purity. As mentioned above, purity is defined as the absence of impurities. Impurities would occur as additional bands. In Figure 6.5 an example of SDS-PAGE evaluation is demonstrated leading to information on molecular weight and purity. As it represents a quantitative method the SDS-PAGE should be validated according to the appropriate guidelines. Typical validation data are shown in Table 6.7.

3.8 Testing the potency of a biopharmaceutical antibody

Potency of an antibody is defined by its ability to bind specifically to its antigen. Binding studies are performed to evaluate apparent binding affinity constants. Routine testing is performed by comparing the binding activity of the test item with the reference material.

When possible a bioassay is used for demonstrating the biologic activity. Cell-based bioassays often demonstrate an influence of the antibody on the proliferation of indicator cells. Those bioassays are very product specific and, therefore, individually designed and developed. Nevertheless there are regulations and guidelines concerning the statistical evaluation of bioassays which must be followed (e.g.: European Pharmacopoeia, 2002 or United States Pharmacopoeia 2002).

The specificity of the antibody is also tested *in situ* by staining assays where labelled antibodies are applied to various tissues in human tissue cross reactivity assays. This is performed, however, more under the aspect of product safety and not as a part of characterisation itself.

4. QUALITY CONTROL FOR THE FILLED AND FINISHED ANTIBODY PRODUCT

Special quality control assays should be applied especially for the filled and finished product in the final container. Sterility testing under the rules of the appropriate guidelines and pharmacopoeia methods is an important product safety issue. Product characterisation tests as mentioned above do not necessarily have to be repeated with the filled and finished product. This depends on the fill finish procedure whether an alteration of the bulk product properties could happen or not. In addition to the antibody itself other ingredients like buffers, stabilisers or bulking agents are added during filling and finishing. Examples of such substances are: L-histidine-HCL, PBS-buffer, sodium citrate, glycine, histidine, mannitol, sucrose, trehalose or polysorbate 80. Appropriate quantitative assays for these substances have to be established. If possible pharmacopoeia methods should be used.

In addition to the quantitative determination of the ingredients in the final container, pH, appearance and the uniformity of mass should be specified and tested. If a lyophilisation procedure is performed issues such as reconstitution time and residual moisture must be tested as well.

5. CONCLUSIONS

Antibodies are some of the most promising biopharmaceutical proteins. The cost effective manufacturing of these products which are of high quality is a challenging task. The rapidly growing experience and the establishing of standardised production and analytical processes will support both economic effectiveness and ensure a high level of product quality and safety. Nevertheless, the introduction of new analytical techniques should be supported in order to gain new insights into the product characteristics. Especially the further investigation into the micro-heterogeneities will lead to a better understanding of the relationships between the fine structure and the functionality of antibodies and their potential effects in patients. This can be the basis for the further improvement of these biopharmaceuticals.

ACKNOWLEDGEMENTS

We would like to thank our collegues at NewLab BioQuality AG, Cardion AG and Evotec Technologies GmbH for supporting us with data and discussions. A special thank to Dr. Helga Siakkou and Dr. Guy Berg for critical reading the manuscript.

REFERENCES

Anders, J.C. 2002, Advances in amino acid analysis, *Biopharm*, April 2002

Cantor, C.R. and Schimmel, P.R. 1980, Biophysical Chemistry, W.H. Freeman and Company, 409-433

Clemens, C:, Hecks, B., Langer, J., Pitschke, M. 2003, Quantification of Aggregate contamination in antibodies; ; *paper presented on the IBC conference „Scaling up of Biopharmaceutical Proteins" 22.-24. January 2003 Basel Switzerland*

European Agency for the Evaluation of Medicinal Products, EMEA, 1997, CPMP position statement on DNA and Host Cell Proteins (HCP) impurities, routine testing versus validation studies

European Pharmacopoeia 2002, Statistical analysis of biological assays and tests, 4th edition, section 5.3, pp 429-456

Fels, A., 2001, Cell Banking A critical starting point for GMP-compliant manufacturing of biopharmaceuticals, Bioforum International, **5** (1): 29-31

Food and Drug Administration, USA, 1997, Points to consider in the manufacture and testing of monoclonal antibody products for human use

Food and Drug Administration, USA, 2001, Guidance for Industry, Bioanalytical Method Validation

Gawlitzek, M., Ryll, T., Lofgren, J. and Sliwkowsi, M.B. 2000, Ammonium alters N-glycan structures of recombinant TNFR-IgG: Degradative versus biosynthetic mechanisms. *Biotechnology and Bioengineering* **68** (6):637- 646.

Gawlitzek, M., Valley, U. and Wagner, R., 1998, Ammonium ion and glucosamine dependent increases of oligosaccharide complexity in recombinant glycoproteins secreted from cultivated BHK-21 cells. *Biotechnology and Bioengineering* **57**:(5), 518- 528.

Goetz, H. 2001, Protein analysis by aqueous size exclusion chromatography (SEC), Application note 5988-4266 EN, Agilent Technologies, Palo Alto, USA

Grabenhorst, E., Schlenke, P., Pohl, S., Nimtz, M. and Conradt, H.S. 1999, Genetic engineering of recombinant glycoproteins and glycosylation pathway in mammalian host cells. *Glycoconjugate Journal* **16**: 81- 97.

Greer, F. M. 2001, MS analysis of biopharmaceutical products, *Innovations in Pharmaceutical Technology*

Hamilton, R.G., Roebber, M., Reimer, C.B. and Rodkey, L.S. 1987, Quality control of murine monoclonal antibodies using isoelectric focusiung affinity immunoblot analysis, *Hybridoma* **6**: 206

Harper, J.D. & Lansbury, P.T.Jr. 1997, Models of amyloid seeding in Alzheimer's disease and scrapie: mechanistic truths and physiological consequences of the time-dependent solubility of amyloid proteins, *Annu. Rev. Biochem.* **66**: 385-407

Hoffman, K. 2000, Strategies for host cell protein analysis, *BioPharm* **13** (6): 38-45

International Conference on Harmonization, ICH, 1996, Guideline on stability testing of biotechnological/biological products (Q5B)

International Conference on Harmonization, ICH, Tripartite Guideline (Q5D), 1997, Derivation and characterisation of cell substrates used for production of biotechnological/biological products

International Conference on Harmonization, ICH, Tripartite Guideline (Q5B), 1995, Quality of biotechnological products: Analysis of the expression constructs in cells used for production of r-DNA derived protein products

Ip, C.C., Miller, W.J., Silberklang, M., Mark, G.E., Ellis, R.W., Huang, L., Glushka, J., van Halbreek, H., Zhu, J. and Alhadeff, J.A. 1994, Structural characterisation of the N-glycans of a humanised anti-CD18 murine immunoglobuline G. *Arch. Biochem. Biophys.*, **308**: 748-752

Iyer, H., Henderson, F., Cunningham, E., Webb, J., Hanson, J., Bork, C. and Conley, L. 2002, Considerations during development of a protein A-based antibody purification process, *BioPharm* January 2002, 14-20

Jenkins, N., Parekh, R.B. and James, D.C.,1996 Getting the glycosylation right: Implications for the biotechnology industry. *Nature Biotechnology* **14**: 975- 981.

Kaltenbrunner, O., Tauer, C., Brunner, J., Jungbauer, A. 1993, Isoprotein analysis by ion exchange chromatography using a linear pH gradient combined with a salt gradient.. *J. Chromatogr.*, **639**: 41-49.

Katakam M., Banba A.K., 1995, Aggregation of insulin and its prevention by carbohydrate excipients, *J Pharm Sci Technol*, **49(4)**: 160-165

King, D.J. 1998, Application and engineering of monoclonal antibodies, Taylor and Francis, London, UK

Kung, T.V., Panfili, P.R., Sheldon, E.L., King, R.S., Nagainis, P.A., Gomez, B., Ross, D.A., Briggs, J. and Zuk, R.F. 1989, Picogram quantitation of total DNA using DNA-binding proteins in silicon sensor-based system, *Analytical Biochemistry* **187**: 220-227

Lottspeich, F. and Zorbas, H., 1998, Bioanalytik, Spektrum Akademischer Verlag, 504- 531.

Lovatt, A., 2002, Applications of quantitative PCR in the biosafety and genetic stability assessment of biotechnology products, *Reviews in Molecular Biotechnology* **82**: 279-300

May P.C., Gitter BD, Waters DC, Simmons LK, Becker GW, Small JS, Robinson PM 1992, Beta-Amyloid peptide in vitro toxicity: lot-to-lot variability. *Neurobiol Aging* **3**: 605-607

Moradian-Oldak J, Simmer JP, Lau EC, Diekwisch T, Slavkin HC, Fincham AG, 1995, A review of the aggregation properties of a recombinant amelogenin. *Connect Tissue Res.* **32(1-4)**:125-30

Nguyen DN, Becker GW, Riggin RM, 1995, Protein mass spectrometry: applications to analytical biotechnology, *J Chromatogr* **705**(1):21-45

Pitschke, M., Haupt, M., Prior, R., Riesner, D. 1998, Detection of single amyloid beta-protein aggregates in the cerebrospinal fluid of Alzheimer's patients by fluorescence correlation spectroscopy, *Nature Med.* **4**:832-834

Richter, A., Wolter, T., Matika, A., Christoph, S. und Meyer-Almes, F.J., 2001 Novel assay for protein impurities in biopharmaceuticals based on Fluorescence Intensity Distribution Assay (FIDA), in Animal cell technology: From target to market, (E. Lindner-Olsson *et al.*, eds.) Kluwer Academic Publishers, The Netherlands, 488-490

Ritter, N., and McEntire, J. 2002, Determining protein concentration, *Biopharm*, April 2002

Roitt, I., Rabson, A. 2000, Essential Immunology, Blackwell Publishing, UK

Storm, S:, Hecks, B., Langer, J., Pitschke, M., 2002, Quantification of Rare Peptide & Protein Aggregates; *paper presented on the IBC conference: Formulation strategies for Biopharmaceuticals, 4th to 6th febuary. 2002, Miami, FL, USA*

United States Pharmacopoeia 2002, Design and analysis of biological analysis, 25th edition, section 111

World Health Organisation, 1996, Technical Report Series **878**: 25*ff*

Chapter 7

EXPRESSION OF HUMAN ANTI-Rh (D) MONOCLONAL ANTIBODIES INTO DIFFERENT CELL LINES: INFLUENCE ON THEIR FUNCTIONAL PROPERTIES

Christophe de Romeuf*, Christine Gaucher*, Arnaud Glacet*, Sylvie Jorieux*, Philippe Klein*, and Dominique Bourel*
* Département Recherche & Développement, Laboratoire Français du Fractionnement et des Biotechnologies, 3 avenue des Tropiques, B.P. 305, Les Ulis, 91958 Courtabœuf cedex, France.

1. INTRODUCTION

Human polyclonal antibodies have been used for many years in infectious diseases, auto-immune diseases. Polyclonal antibodies that recognise and bind specifically Rhesus positive red blood cells (RBC) prevent the allo-immunisation against RBC and, hence, the hæmolytic disease of the new-born (HDN). These anti-Rhesus D antibodies (anti-D) are also used in cases of the following cases, abortion, extra-uterine pregnancies, amniocentesis, fetal transplacental hemorrhage, uncompatible Rhesus blood transfusion and ITP (Ware et al., 1998).

Polyclonal anti-D antibodies are isolated from the plasma of hyper-immunised Rh-negative volunteers. The mechanisms by which these anti-D antibodies prevent immunisation are not fully understood. It is unlikely that the absence of immunisation is due to the masking of Rhesus molecules present on red cells by the anti-D antibodies for two reasons. First, it has been shown that Fab' fragments, by contrast to the intact IgG, are not effective in preventing the immunisation (Nicholas et al., 1969). Second, the amount of polyclonal antibodies that is infused is not always sufficient enough to saturate all the Rhesus molecules. Thus, the precise mechanisms involved in the tolerance induced by the infusion of polyclonal anti-D antibodies are still a matter of controversy. On the one hand, polyclonal anti-D antibodies may induce a rapid clearance of red cells from peripheral blood through phagocytosis and/or antibody-dependent cell cytotoxicity (ADCC). These two mechanisms involve the high affinity receptor for IgG (FcγRI/CD64), present on monocytes, activated macrophages and neutrophils, and two low affinity Fcγ receptors present on monocytes, macrophages and dendritic cells (FcγRIIa/CD32) and on NK cells (FcγRIIIa/CD16) (Hulett and Hogarth, 1994). On the other hand, the prevention of allo-immunisation could be due to an inhibition triggered by the presence of RBC and anti-D antibodies, involving the low affinity Fcγ receptor FcγRIIb that has been shown to inhibit B cell activation (Amigorena et al., 1992).

The immunisation of male volunteers has sharply decreased in Europe, due to the possible, although extremely low, hazards linked to RBC infusion. This decrease may lead to a shortage in polyclonal antibody supply in the coming years. Thus, human monoclonal antibodies (mAbs) against RhD have been produced by several groups in order to propose an alternative for HDN prevention (Kumpel et al., 2002). Clinical trials performed with some of these mAbs have shown that only a few of them (Kumpel et al., 1995, Miescher et al., 2000) are able to suppress the anti-RBC immune response. BRAD-5, a mAb developed by Bio Products Laboratory (BPL) (Kumpel et al., 1995) was the first antibody capable to eliminate Rhesus positive red blood cells from the circulation in Rh (D) negative volunteers and to prevent the appearance of an immune response. This activity did not appear related to the affinity of the antibody, but rather to its ability to interact with FcγRIIIa (CD16), the low affinity receptor involved in ADCC. In vitro, BRAD5 could trigger an efficient red blood cell lysis by FcγRIII positive NK cells By contrast, mAbs that proved to be inefficient in clinical trials did not mediate ADCC in vitro through FcγRIIIa. Thus, all these data suggested that the ability of the mAbs to efficiently bind low affinity FcγR is critical for preventing allo-immunisation.

In this work we showed that depending on the cell expression system used, it is possible to modulate the Fc related functional properties of mAbs.

2. SCREENING OF ANTI-D HUMAN ANTIBODIES ACCORDING TO A FCγRIII-DEPENDENT ADCC ASSAY

First, an ADCC assay was set up to screen for anti-D mAbs capable of triggering ADCC through FcγRIII. In that assay, antibodies or antibody-containing culture supernatants are incubated overnight with papain-treated RBC and with Human Peripheral Blood Mononuclear Cells (PBMC), in the presence of various doses of polyclonal human IgG (IVIg, TEGELINE®) which spontaneously bind the high-affinity FcγRI (CD64) expressed on monocytes (Fig. 7.1). In these conditions, the ADCC is essentially due to the recruitment of the low affinity FcγRIII expressed on NK cells, as demonstrated by the complete inhibition of cytotoxicity obtained in presence of the anti-FcγRIII/CD16 mAb 3G8, an antibody that binds to the IgG-binding site of this receptor. The assay includes polyclonal anti-D antibodies (WinRho®) and DF5 or AD1 mAbs, as positive and negative controls, respectively. DF5 and AD1 mAbs have been shown to be unable to induce the disappearance of RhD$^+$ RBC from human peripheral blood in an earlier clinical trial. AD1 or DF5 mAbs do not mediate ADCC *in vitro* in presence of IVIg, by contrast to the WinRho® polyclonal anti-D antibodies. Thus, the experimental procedure allows the discrimination between mAbs with high and low FcγRIII reactivity.

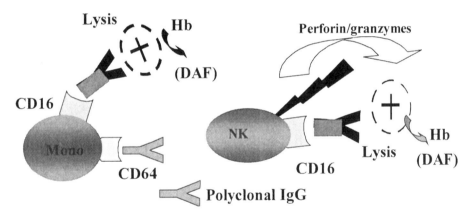

Figure 7.1. Principle of screening of cytotoxic mAbs by an ADCC assay performed in presence of polyclonal IgG.

Second, the sera of immune blood donors were then tested for their ability to induce a strong ADCC *in vitro* through FcγRIIIa. Two subjects among 38 donors were selected and their peripheral blood mononuclear cells (PBMC) were used as a source of B cells for EBV transformation (Boylston *et al.*, 1980; Kumpel *et al.*, 1989; Mc Cann-Carter *et al.*, 1993). A number of EBV-transformed B cell lines were obtained and cloned by limiting dilution. The ADCC screening assay allowed the selection of several clones exhibiting a strong FcγRIIIa-dependent ADCC. To confer more stability, the selected clones were fused with cells from the hetero-myeloma cell line K6H6 (Bron *et al.*, 1984; Foung *et al.*, 1987). One stable hetero-hybridoma cell line producing a human anti-D mAb (IgG1, κ) (termed T125-F60) exhibiting a strong ADCC activity was selected.

Third, the cDNAs encoding for the heavy and light chains of the T125-F60 antibody were cloned into an eukaryotic expression vector engineered for optimised Ig expression. Chinese Hamster Ovary (CHO) cells were then stably transfected and clones were selected and isolated, based on their ability to produce functional anti-D recombinant antibodies (Fig. 7.2).

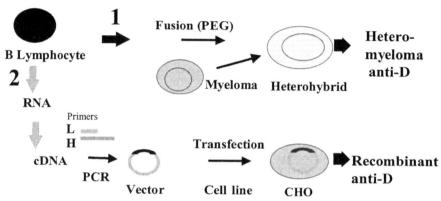

Figure 7.2. Generation of the heterohybridoma T125-F60 and the corresponding recombinant human monoclonal anti-D antibody.

3. MODULATION OF ANTIBODY EFFECTOR FUNCTIONS

Cells from different other cell lines [Baby Hamster Kidney (BHK), Cos7, Vero, U293, Jurkat, Wil-2, YB2/0, K6H6] were then transfected with the T125-F60 encoding expression vector (see above). As shown in Figure 7.3, the recombinant human IgG1 antibodies produced by cells from these different cells lines exhibited an heterogeneous pattern of cytotoxicity in the ADCC assay. Only two cell lines, YB2/0 and Vero, expressed anti-D antibodies with a Poly-D like ADCC activity.

Since the nine mAbs secreted by these different cell lines have the same primary sequence, these results suggested that post-translational modifications could account for the difference observed in ADCC. Notably, we hypothesised that these antibodies might exhibit different glycosylation patterns due to the use of cell lines derived from different species. Bi-antennary N-glycan with bissecting GlcNac are found in human IgG but not in their mouse counterparts. Similarly, both α2-3 et α2-6 sialic acids are

Expression of human anti-Rh (D) monoclonal antibodies

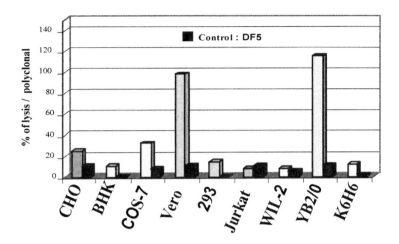

Figure 7.3. ADCC activity of the recombinant anti-D T125-F60 antibody produced by cells from different cell lines. The % of lysis/polyclonal (ordinate) represents the % of cytotoxicity of the T125-F60 mAb produced by a given cell line (abscissa) as compared to an arbitrary value of 100 attributed to the % of cytotoxicity obtained with the WinRho® polyclonal anti-D antibodies. The DF5 mAb was used as a negative control in these experiments.

found in mouse and human species, whereas they are exclusively α2-3 linked in carbohydrates synthesised by CHO cells (Yu *et al.*, 1994). In addition, it had been known for more than two decades that the glycosylation pattern of IgG has a profound impact on their ability to bind FcγR.

To confirm these results, the DF5 antibody, produced by a human EBV B cell line obtained from an immunised D-negative donor (DF5-EBV), and that neither induces the disappearance of RhD$^+$ RBC from human peripheral blood nor triggers a significant FcγRIII-dependent ADCC in *vitro* (see above), was cloned and expressed in the rat myeloma cell line YB2/0 (DF5-YB2/0). Interestingly, the DF5-YB2/0 mAb induced a strong RBC lysis, to the same extent as the anti-D polyclonal antibodies (WinRho®). By contrast, the DF5-EBV mAb was unable to provoke RBC lysis. The addition of the anti-FcγRIII/CD16 mouse 3G8 mAb totally abolished the RBC lysis induced by the DF5-YB2/0 mAb, showing the major contribution of FcγRIII in this ADCC assay (Fig. 7.4). Thus, as previously observed with the T125-F60 mAb (Fig. 7.3), the DF5-EBV mAb, although exhibiting the same primary sequence as the DF5-YB2/0 mAb, is not able to efficiently trigger ADCC through FcγRIII, confirming the importance of post-translational modifications in supporting biological activity or not.

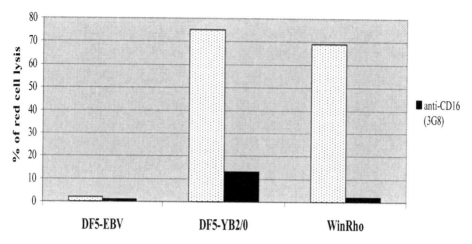

Figure 7.4. DF5 human mAb produced in YB2/0 cells (DF5-YB2/0) but not in EBV-transformed B cells (DF5-EBV) mediates a strong FcγRIII-dependent ADCC. The 3G8 mouse mAb inhibits both the DF5-YB2/0 and the WinRho® mediated ADCC.

4. ROLE OF CARBOHYDRATES IN EFFECTOR FUNCTION OF RECOMBINANT HUMAN ANTIBODIES

Structural analysis were then performed with these two antibodies (DF5-EBV and DF5-YB2/0) and revealed that they have different glycosylation patterns which could be responsible for their ability to mediate ADCC or not. Glycosylation can be modified by the addition of glycosidase inhibitors in culture medium, such as deoxymannojirimycin or castanospermin (Rothman et al., 1989). Thus, cells from a hetero-myeloma cell line producing an antibody with a low ADCC activity (AD1) was cultured in presence of DMM. After two weeks of culture, the lytic activity of the secreted antibody was dramatically increased (Fig. 7.5), indicating that changes in the carbohydrate content can induce a strong increase in ADCC. Since it is known that DMM induces high-mannose type oligosaccharide corresponding to immature complex carbohydrates, this result indicates that a glycan with a low content in sialic acid, galactose and fucose confers increased reactivity of IgG toward the FcγRIII.

The relationship between the biological activity of IgG and the carbohydrate moiety linked to the Asn 297 (CH2 domain) has been investigated in details. Twenty years ago, Leatherbarrow *et al.* (1985) demonstrated that the culture of antibody-producing cells in the presence of tunicamycin induces a tremendous decrease of the IgG binding to FcγRI

Expression of human anti-Rh (D) monoclonal antibodies

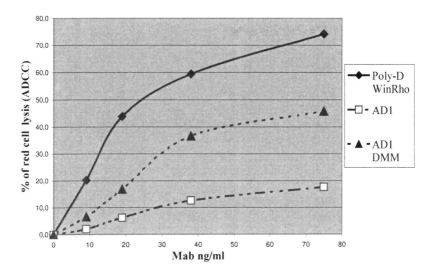

Figure 7.5. Modulation of ADCC by DMM. The AD1 mAb was produced in presence or in absence of the glycosidase inhibitor DMM. The presence of DMM in culture medium for two weeks allowed to produce antibody mediating a strong ADCC, by contrast to the antibody produced in culture medium lacking DMM.

expressed by monocytes or macrophages. It has been also reported that ADCC is dependent on the glycosylation of IgG. Removal of glycan from IgG by endoglycosidase H completely abolishes ADCC activity (Boyd et al. 1995). More recent studies have shown that the binding of fucose-deficient IgG1 to human FcγRIII is improved up to 50-fold. It parallels a strong increase in ADCC when purified peripheral blood monocytes or natural killer cells are used as effector cells, especially at lower antibody concentrations (Shields *et al.*, 2001; Shinkawa *et al.*, 2003). Thus, the low fucose content (Shields *et al.*, 2002; Shinkawa *et al.*, 2003), as well as the presence of bisecting GlcNAc (Umana *et al.*, 1999) have been shown to play a critical role in the enhancement of ADCC.

The modification of the primary sequence of the Fc region has also an impact on the biological activity of IgG. The presence of specific amino-acid residues at well-defined positions of human IgG enhances the binding to all FcγR or to some of them, or improves the binding to one type of receptor while reducing the binding to another type. Recent data indicated that some IgG1 variants with an improved binding to FcγRIIIA exhibits up to a 100% increase in ADCC (Shield *et al.*, 2001). These data are in agreement with a previous work showing that amino-acid residues (246 and 258) interact with the carboydrate moiety of IgG (Lund *et al.*, 1993).

5. CONCLUSION

The biological activity of monoclonal antibodies is highly dependent on the cell expression system. Monoclonal anti-D antibody expressed in YB2/0 supports ADCC to the same extent as polyclonal anti-D antibodies. The improvement of the FcγRIII binding and ADCC observed *in vitro* when the glycosylation pattern of mAbs is modified suggests that such optimised antibodies could be more efficient when used *in vivo*, especially in oncology. However, the clinical benefit achieved when using such optimised antibodies may be different depending on the FcγRIII phenotype of the patients. Recent data have shown that the clearance of RBC coated with an IgG3 anti-D monoclonal antibody (BRAD-3) is more rapid in five subjects homozygous for FcγRIIIa-F/F158 than in three subjects expressing the FcγRIIIa-V158 allele (Kumpel *et al.*, 2003). A clinical trial performed by the LFB should indicate whether the injection of an anti-D mAb, produced in YB2/0 cells and exhibiting a stronger interaction with FcγRIIIa, induces a better clearance of Rhesus positive red cells and can prevent an anti-RBC immune response in all treated patients. In another recent study, Cartron *et al.* (2002) also reported an association between the FCGR3A genotype and the clinical and molecular responses to Rituxan® (anti-CD20) in patients with non-Hodgkin lymphomas. However, in contrast to the Kumpel's study (2003), the clinical response was better in the 158V/V homozygous patients than in 158F/F carriers.

The production of monoclonal antibodies optimised for their ability to interact with FcγR, although being exciting as one can expect a better efficacy at least in some pathological conditions, should be nevertheless carefully evaluated. Potential side effects induced by stronger IgG/FcγR interactions, due to a massive release of cytokines such as TNFα, cannot be ruled out, as suggested by a recent clinical trial (Pangalis *et al.*, 2001). In any case, the engineering of optimised Fc region of therapeutic antibodies should allow to use antibodies more efficiently in carefully chosen pathologies.

ACKNOWLEDGEMENTS

We would like to thank all our colleagues who participated in our work on monoclonal antibodies and technicians from our group for their excellent technical assistance. We also specially thank Dr. J.L. Teillaud for its critical review of the manuscript

REFERENCES

Amigorena, S., Bonnerot, C., Drake, J., Choquet, D., Hunziker, W., Guillet, J.G., Webster, P., Sautès, C., Mellman, I., and Fridman, W.H., 1992, Cytoplasmic domain heterogeneity and functions of IgG Fc receptors in B-lymphocytes. *Science* **256**: 1808-1812

Boyd, P.N., Lines, A.C., and Patel, A.K., 1995, The effect of the removal of sialic acid, galactose and total carbohydrate on the functional activity of Campath-1H. *Mol Immunol* **32**: 1311-1318

Boylston, J.M., Gardner, B., Anderson, R.L., and Hughes-Jones, N.C., 1980, Production of human IgM anti-D in tissue culture by EB virus-transformed lymphocytes. *Scand. J. Immunol.* **12**: 355-358

Bron, D., Feinberg, M.B., Teng, N.N.H. and Kaplan, H.S., 1984, Production of Human Monoclonal IgG Antibodies against Rhesus (D) Antigen. *Proc. Nat. Acad. Sci. USA* **81**: 3214-3217.

Cartron, G., Dacheux, L., Salles, G., Solal-Celigny, P., Bardos, P., Colombat, P., and Watier H., 2002, Therapeutic activity of humanized anti-CD20 monoclonal antibody and polymorphism in IgG Fc receptor FcgammaRIIIa gene. *Blood* **99**: 754-758

Foung, S.K.H., Blunt, J.A., Wu, P.S., Ahearn, P., Winn, L.C., Engleman, E.G. and Grumet, F.C., 1987, Human monoclonal antibodies to Rho (D). *Vox. Sang.* **53**: 11-17

Hulett, M.D., and Hogarth, P.M., 1994, Molecular basis of Fc receptor function. *Adv. Immunol.* **57**: 1-127

Kumpel, B.M., Poole, G.D. and Bradley, B.A., 1989, Human Monoclonal Anti-D Antibodies.I. Their Production, Serology, Quantitation and Potential Use as Blood Grouping Reagents. *Brit. J. Haemat.* **71**: 125-129

Kumpel, BM., Goodrick, M.J., Pamphilon, D.H., Fraser, I.D., Poole, G.D., Morse, C., Standen, G.R., Chapman, G.E., Thomas, D.P., and Anstee, D.J., 1995, Human Rh D monoclonal antibodies (BRAD-3 and BRAD-5) cause accelerated clearance of Rh D+ red blood cells and suppression of Rh D immunization in Rh D- volunteers. Blood **86**: 1701-1709.

Kumpel, B.M., Beliard, R., Brossard, Y., Edelman, L., de Haas, M., Jackson, DJ., Kooyman. P., Ligthart. P.C., Monchatre, E., Overbeeke, M.A., Puillandre. P., de Romeuf, C., and Wilkes, A.M., 2002, Section 1C: Assessment of the functional activity and IgG Fc receptor utilisation of 64 IgG Rh monoclonal antibodies. *Transfus. Clin. Biol.* **9**: 45-53.

Kumpel, B.M., De Haas, M., Koene, H.R., Van De Winkel, J.G., and Goodrick, M.J, 2003, Clearance of red cells by monoclonal IgG3 anti-D in vivo is affected by the VF polymorphism of Fcgamma RIIIa (CD16). *Clin. Exp. Immunol.* **132**: 81-86

Leatherbarrow, R.J., Rademacher, T.W., Dwek, R.A., Woof, J.M., Clark, A., Burton, D.R., Richardson, N. , and Feinstein, A., 1985, Effector functions of monoclonal aglycosylated mouse IgG2a ; binding and activation of complement component C1 and interaction with human Fc receptor. *Molec. Immun.* **22**: 407-415

Lund, J., Takahaski, N., Nakagawa, H., Goodall, M., Bentley, T., Hindley, S.A., Tyler, R., and Jefferis, R., 1993, Control of IgG/Fc glycosylation : a comparison of oligosaccharides from chimeric human/mouse and mouse subclass immunoglobulin G5. *Molec. Immun.* **30**: 741-748

Mc Cann-Carter, M.C., Bruce, M., Shaw, E.M., Thorpe, S.J., Sweeney, G.M., Armstrong, S.S., and James, K., 1993, The production and evaluation of two human monoclonal anti-D antibodies. *Transf. Med.* **3**: 187-194

Miescher, S., Zahn-Zabal, M., De Jesus, M., Moudry, R., Fisch, I., Vogel, M., Kobr, M., Imboden, MA., Kragten, E., Bichler, J., Mermod, N., Stadler, BM., Amstutz, H., Wurm, F., 2000, CHO expression of a novel human recombinant IgG1 anti-RhD antibody isolated by phage display. *Br J Haematol.* **111**:157-66.

Nicholas, R., and Sinclair, SC., 1969, Regulation of the immune response. I. Reduction in ability of specific antibody to inhibit long-lasting IgG immunological priming after removal of the Fc fragment. *J. Exp. Med.* **129**: 1183-1201.

Pangalis, GA., Dimopoulou, MN., Angelopoulou, MK., Tsekouras, C., Vassilakopoulos, TP., Vaiopoulos, G., and Siakantaris, MP., 2001, Campath-1H (anti-CD52) monoclonal antibody therapy in lymphoproliferative disorders. *Med Oncol.* **18**: 99-107.

Rothman, R.J., Perussia, B., Herlyn, D., and Warren, L., 1989, Antibody-dependent cytotoxicity mediated by natural killer cells is enhanced by castanospermine-induced alterations of IgG glycosylation. *Mol. Immunol.* **26**: 1113-1123

Shields, RL., Lai, J., Keck, R., O'Connell, L.Y., Hong, K., Meng, Y.G., Weikert, S.H., Presta, L.G., 2002, Lack of fucose on human IgG1 N-linked oligosaccharide improves binding to human Fcgamma RIII and antibody-dependent cellular toxicity. *J Biol Chem* **277**: 26733-26740.

Shields, RL., Namenuk, AK., Hong, K., Meng, Y.G., Rae, J., Briggs, J., Xie, D., Lai, J., Stadlen, A., Li, B., Fox, J.A., and Presta, L.G., 2001, High resolution mapping of the binding site on human IgG1 for Fc gamma RI, Fc gamma RII, Fc gamma RIII, and FcRn and design of IgG1 variants with improved binding to the Fc gamma R. *J Biol Chem* **276**: 6591-6604.

Shinkawa, T., Nakamura, K., Yamane, N., Shoji-Hosaka, E., Kanda, Y., Sakurada, M., Uchida, K., Anazawa, H., Satoh, M., Yamasaki, M., Hanai, N., and Shitara, K., 2003, The absence of fucose but not the presence of galactose or bisecting N-acetylglucosamine of human IgG1 complex-type oligosaccharides shows the critical role of enhancing antibody-dependent cellular cytotoxicity. *J Biol Chem* **278**: 3466-3473.

Umana, P., Jean-Mairet, J., Moudry, R., Amstutz, H., Bailey, J.E., 1999, Engineered glycoforms of an antineuroblastoma IgG1 with optimized antibody-dependent cellular cytotoxic activity. *Nat. Biotechnol.* **17**: 176-180

Ware, RE., and Zimmerman, S.A., 1998, Anti-D: mechanisms of action. *Semin Hematol.* **35**: 14-22.

Yu, I.P.C., Miller, W.J., Silberklang, M., Mark, G.E., Ellis, R.W., Huang, L., Glushka, J., Van Halbeek, H., Zhu, J., and Alhadeff, J.A., 1994, Structural characterization of the N-Glycans of a humanized anti-CD18 murine immunoglobulin G. *Arch. Biochem. Biophys.* **308**: 387-399

Chapter 8

MONOCLONAL ANTIBODY PRODUCTION: MINIMISING VIRUS SAFETY ISSUES

John Bray* and Malcolm K. Brattle[#]
*Business Development Manager, Validation Services [#] Director, Q-One Biotech, Todd Campus, West of Scotland Science Park, Glasgow, G20 0XA

1. INTRODUCTION

1.1 Viral safety issues for monoclonal antibodies

Therapeutic compounds derived from biological fluids or tissues, or biopharmaceutical products, pose a number of problems for manufacturers and regulatory authorities when considering virus safety. Previous experience has demonstrated the potential for transmission of infectious viruses from a small number of biopharmaceutical products. Examples include the transmission of *Human immunodeficiency virus* (HIV) and *hepatitis C virus* (HCV) in blood products, and the transmission of *Simian virus 40* (SV40) in vaccines. Monoclonal antibodies intended for therapeutic use pose similar virus safety concerns since the cell culture process used for production of such products can support the growth of adventitious virus particles. These virus contaminants may be inadvertently introduced into the final formulation via raw materials or personnel. For these reasons it has been a regulatory requirement for several decades now that any manufacturer of biopharmaceuticals of human or animal origin assess the safety of the product for use in humans. Although there are several types of potential microbial contaminants of concern, the majority can be removed by standard sterile filtration. Such filtration treatment would have little, or no, effect on the level of virus particles within a product. Therefore, a major element in the safety assessment of biopharmaceuticals is ensuring, as far as possible, the product's freedom from contaminating viruses. There are three principle complimentary approaches used to control for potential viral contamination of biologicals:

- Selection of the source material
- Testing of source materials and products from various stages of the manufacturing process for the absence of detectable virus
- Testing the capacity of the manufacturing process to remove or inactivate viruses

The latter is referred to as a virus clearance study, or a virus validation study, and plays an important role in establishing the safety of biopharmaceuticals. The regulatory definition of validation of this type is:

"A documented programme, which provides a high degree of assurance that a specific process will consistently manufacture a product, meeting predetermined specifications" (CPMP/ICH/295/95, 1997)

There are inherent limitations in testing both starting materials and bulk product; the sample size sets a statistical lower limit on the level of contamination that can be detected and the assay methods determine the range of viruses that may be revealed. With increasing sophistication of techniques new viruses are being uncovered in biological materials, for instance circoviruses have recently been found as significant contaminants of both human and animal biological materials. The limitations on testing, indicated above, underscore the importance of choosing optimal virus clearance technologies and conducting appropriate virus clearance studies.

Since virus clearance study data would represent a significant part of a submission to a regulatory body for a biopharmaceutical product, an in-depth understanding of the regulatory requirements for virus clearance in different countries, for different product types, and at different phases of development would be required.

To address the virus safety concerns for biopharmaceutical products, and to help manufacturers understand the level of clearance study required for their particular product, world-wide regulatory agencies have prepared guidelines detailing the testing and safety evaluation that should be performed prior to any submission. A number of guidelines from individual regulatory bodies are available which cover specific topics or products. The most relevant guidelines for virus safety assessment of an antibody product are listed in Table 8.1 below:

Table 8.1. Regulatory Guidelines

ICH Topic Q5A. 4th March 1997	Note for Guidance on Quality of Biotechnology Products: Viral Safety Evaluation of Biotechnology Products Derived from Cell Lines of Human or Animal Origin
FDA CBER Points to Consider (1993)	Points to Consider in the Characterisation of Cell Lines used to Produce Biologicals
EMEA/410/01 rev 1. May 2001	Note for Guidance on Minimising the Risk of Transmitting Animal Spongiform Encephalopathy Agents via Human and Veterinary Medicinal Products
FDA CBER Points to Consider (1997)	Points to Consider in the Manufacture and Testing of Monoclonal Antibodies for Human Use.
CPMP/BWP/268/95. 14th Feb 1996	Note for Guidance on Viral Validation Studies:The Design, Contribution and Interpretation of Studies Validating the Inactivation and Removal of Viruses

2. VIRUS CLEARANCE STUDIES AND MONOCLONAL ANTIBODIES

The aim of a virus clearance study is to assess the effectiveness of individual steps in the manufacturing process at removing or inactivating viruses (CPMP/ICH/295/95, 1997: CPMP/BWP/268/95, 1996; FDA points to consider on Monoclonal Antibodies, 1997; CPMP/BWP/95 rev 3, 2001). These data are used to give a quantitative estimate of the overall level of virus clearance obtained by the manufacturing process. A similar approach can be used to demonstrate the removal of other potential contaminants, *e.g.* DNA, mycoplasma and prions.

A virus clearance study should reflect the virus risks associated with the product, and include a selection of viruses that vary in size, shape, genome type, structure and resistance to various methods of physico-chemical inactivation.

The ICH Q5A regulatory guideline (CPMP/ICH/295/95, 1997) indicates that a manufacturer of biological products for human use should demonstrate the capability of the manufacturing process to remove or inactivate known contaminants.

To determine the effectiveness of a process step in removing and/or inactivating infectious agents, the preferred method when considering viruses is an infectivity assay. Alternative assays may be used to provide useful information in certain circumstances. For example, valuable additional data on the partitioning of viruses can be obtained by the use of a quantitative polymerase chain reaction (Q-PCR) assay (Lovatt, 2002).

2.1 Viruses of concern

When considering monoclonal antibody or recombinant proteins products derived from animal cell culture, the cells themselves may harbour endogenous viruses (*e.g.* rodent cell lines may harbour endogenous retrovirus particles). Bovine serum or porcine trypsin, commonly used in the culture of animal cells, may be contaminated with several viruses. *Bovine viral diarrhoea virus* (BVD) and *Bovine polyomavirus* (BPyV), a potentially zoonotic virus, are the most commonly encountered agents in bovine serum. A major concern for other products of bovine origin is the agent responsible for bovine spongiform encephalopathy (BSE). *Porcine parvovirus* (PPV) and *porcine circovirus* (PCV) are prevalent infections of pigs and are often found to be contaminants of porcine trypsin. Moreover, circoviruses may resist inactivation by the levels of irradiation commonly used to treat trypsin (Plavsic & Bolin, 2001). Other viruses have been identified as contaminants of rodent cell lines during production, including *Murine minute virus* (MMV) and *Cache valley virus* (CVV).

Finally, in any manufacturing process contaminants may be introduced via operators during manufacture, although this is a rare occurrence. Viruses of particular concern include those transmitted by aerosol or contact, such as paramyxoviruses, adenoviruses and enteroviruses. More detail on factors to consider when selecting a panel of viruses for a virus clearance study is given in section 3.

2.2 Design of a virus clearance study

Virus clearance studies are a costly and time-consuming component of the bio-safety portfolio of any biopharmaceutical product. Increasing emphasis is being placed by the regulatory authorities on the correct implementation of these studies, in order to ensure that the data generated is an accurate representation of the ability of the manufacturing process to remove or inactivate viruses. Consequently, it is extremely important to ensure that the design, planning and implementation of the virus clearance study are discussed well in advance, to ensure compliance with the various regulatory guidelines.

Because there are many factors to be considered when planning a virus clearance study, and no two products or processes are identical, the approach taken should be to view each study as an individual project. The aim should be to identify the most cost-effective method to generate the necessary data to ensure safe passage of the product through to licensure. To achieve this, it is important to design the study well in advance of any submission date. Without good planning it is possible that one small oversight with regard to, for example, sample collection, could cause a long and costly delay to a submission.

It is also extremely important that the manufacturing process be designed with virus safety in mind. It is much easier to alter the manufacturing process during development than to try to introduce changes to a process once it is established. Ideally, you should include at least one, and preferably two, robust virus clearance steps with different modes of action, within a manufacturing process. Examples of different types of manufacturing process steps often assessed in virus clearance studies are shown in Table 8.2.

2.2.1 Process steps

Table 8.2. Manufacturing processes studied for virus removal/inactivation.

Inactivation	Partitioning
Heat Treatment	Precipitation
Pasteurisation	Ethanol
Lyophilisation/dry heat	Polyethylene Glycol
Solvent Detergent	Chromatography
	Ion Exchange
pH Treatment	Affinity
Low pH (column elution)	Hydrophobic Interaction
High pH (sanitisation)	Reverse Phase
	Nanofiltration

Many different types of process steps may be effective for virus removal/inactivation, as indicated in Table 8.2. Robust steps are those steps considered to be effective under a wide range of conditions (*e.g.* different buffers, pH conditions, protein concentrations, temperatures etc.), and include steps such as heat treatment, and for enveloped viruses, low pH and solvent/detergent treatments. Partitioning steps, such as chromatographic steps and precipitation are generally considered to be less robust. Chromatographic partitioning steps can, however, be effective for virus removal *i.e.* reproducibly allow the removal of a high level (> 4 logs) of virus, within the range of the manufacturer's process conditions. Nanofiltration processes, where separation is considered to be predominantly on the basis of size, are generally considered robust, for viruses significantly larger than the nominal pore size of the filter. Nanofiltration would, therefore, be an obvious method of choice to remove virus particles from a biological product. Unfortunately, for large protein products, such as certain monoclonal antibodies, nanofiltration is not always a viable option as the antibody product may not easily pass through the nanofilter. Therefore, those nanofilters of a small enough average pore size capable of removing the more robust virus contaminants, such as parvoviruses and picornaviruses, may have a negative impact on yield of high molecular weight protein products.

Many monoclonal antibody products cannot tolerate the harsh conditions that are required to inactivate some viruses (or other contaminants). When considering heat treatment (*e.g.* 60°C for 10 hours) the antibody product may not be stable for the length of time necessary to inactivate most viruses. Solvent/detergent treatment may affect the efficacy of the antibody. Whether a low pH treatment can be included in a manufacturing process is influenced by whether the product can withstand being held at a pH below 3.8 for approximately 30-60 mins. In such cases, some other means of virus reduction will need to be considered. Therefore, other potential virus reduction processes, such as chromatography, are often required to contribute to virus removal during the manufacture of a product. The study of a chromatography step does, however, create further issues, which are discussed in more detail in section 2.2.2.2

With any virus clearance study, the objective is to look at the total manufacturing process. Each process step to be studied is spiked (or challenged) with an appropriate preparation of high titre test virus. The data for each individual process step can then be combined, to give a reduction value for the chosen virus over the total manufacturing process. This is outlined in Figure 8.1 which shows a typical manufacturing process for a monoclonal antibody, indicating the potential virus log reduction values for each individual step, for a retrovirus model (*e.g. Murine leukaemia virus* (MLV)).

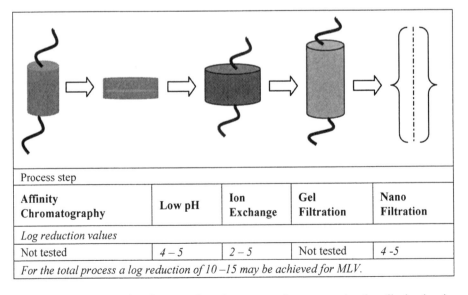

Process step				
Affinity Chromatography	Low pH	Ion Exchange	Gel Filtration	Nano Filtration
Log reduction values				
Not tested	4 – 5	2 – 5	Not tested	4 -5
For the total process a log reduction of 10 –15 may be achieved for MLV.				

Figure 8.1. An example of a manufacturing process for a monoclonal antibody showing possible values for virus* removal at each step. (*virus example: MLV)

2.2.2 Established removal and inactivation steps

The removal from and inactivation of viruses within a biopharmaceutical product has been accomplished to date using those methods indicated in Table 8.2. A more detailed description of each method is given below.

2.2.2.1 High temperature

Heat inactivation of viruses is a classic and attractive non-invasive physical treatment for high value pharmaceutical proteins. Pasteurisation is a method that has been used for albumin products since 1948, and involves heating of the end product to +60°C for at least 10 hours. However, a practical problem in biotechnology is the inefficient heat transfer associated with processing large volumes. A further drawback is the limited resistance of proteins to elevated temperatures for long periods of time. In order to maintain the biological function of more heat labile proteins, stabilisers such as amino acids, citrate or sugars may be added. This may be counter productive, however, as the stabilisers may protect certain viruses from inactivation by heat. Moreover, when sugars are employed as stabilisers they may result in aberrant glycosylation of the proteins.

2.2.2.2 Chromatography

In some chromatography processes, for example, the buffers used may result in virus inactivation. Although the inactivation kinetics of the buffer may be studied as an independent step, it may not be possible to demonstrate how the virus partitions during the chromatography process using infectivity assays. In other words, any physical removal of virus due to the chromatography process itself could not be studied. However, with the introduction of Quantitative Polymerase Chain Reaction (Q-PCR) assays, many chromatography processes may now also be studied, at least with respect to removal or partitioning of virus genomes. Such studies would be performed in parallel with infectivity studies.

Most purification processes for biopharmaceutical products include chromatographic steps. Although such steps are not generally considered robust for virus removal, certain chromatographic steps can be considered effective under specific conditions. The effectiveness of a chromatographic step depends on many factors including the type of chromatography resin, the type of ligand, the types and concentration of buffers, the temperature and pH conditions, protein concentration, and column flow rates. Several chromatographic processes may result in partitioning of viruses, although some methods also include specific buffers which may inactivate enveloped viruses. Where this is the case, the effect of the inactivating buffer should be demonstrated. This can be achieved either by studying the inactivating buffer alone in batch mode, or by the incorporation of an assay to determine the number of virus genomes passing through the column, such as Q-PCR. Q-PCR data can be used to determine the level of removal and/or inactivation occurring on the column itself, in conjunction with an infectivity assay (Lovatt, 2002). A major disadvantage of chromatography steps is that they may not be predictable or reproducible. It is possible, however, that a manufacturing process does not contain enough robust steps to obtain the level of virus clearance required, and so chromatography steps can be useful to demonstrate an increase in the level of clearance obtained for a particular virus. However, regulatory authorities have expressed concern over the potential build up of viruses on re-used resins. To address this issue, sanitisation of the column is necessary. A common sanitisation procedure involves cleaning the column with sodium hydroxide (NaOH). Q-One Biotech has investigated the ability of NaOH treatment to inactivate several viruses and have demonstrated that a concentration of 0.5M is effective against many enveloped and non-enveloped viruses (Amersham Biosciences Application Note 18-1124-57).

Regulatory authorities have also expressed concerns regarding the ability of re-used column resins to clear viruses to the same extent as new resin. The latest ICH guideline does indicate that "over time and after repeated use, the ability of chromatography columns and other devices used in the purification scheme to clear virus may vary. Some estimate of the stability of the virus clearance after several uses may provide support for the repeated use of such columns" CPMP/ICH/295/95 (1997). To address this issue, a study of re-used resin may be performed in conjunction with a study of new resin.

Regulatory authorities are now also asking to see data on the robustness of a process, looking at extremes of conditions such as pH, temperature, and protein concentration. These data give an indication of the virus reduction capabilities of a manufacturing process under worst case conditions.

2.2.2.3 Nanofiltration

Filtration is a robust virus removal process with little detrimental effect on the structure or activity of biological materials. It is therefore an ideal step to include in a manufacturing process to remove contaminating virus particles. Since other robust virus inactivation steps may have limited or no effect on non-enveloped viruses, nanofiltration systems have recently been developed specifically aimed at increasing the safety of biopharmaceuticals by removing viruses, such as picornaviruses and parvoviruses. One advantage of filtration is that virus particles are physically removed from the product of interest, the efficiency of virus removal being a function of size and shape of the virus. One of the drawbacks with nanofiltration, however, is that a small number of biopharmaceutical products are larger than the average pore size of nanofilters capable of removing the smaller, more robust viruses. As indicated in section 2.2.1, this can be a significant issue for monoclonal antibody products, and particular care should be taken when selecting a suitable nanofilter. Several factors should be considered, including efficiency of the filter and yield of the product. Nanofiltration (Johnston *et al.*, 2000) has been demonstrated to be useful second robust step. A variety of different nanofilters are now available, with the range of average pore size from 70nm – 15 nm. However, parvoviruses are not totally removed by nanofiltration, even through the smaller 15 nm filter.

2.2.2.4   Precipitation

Several precipitation methods have been used for virus removal for many years. Ethanol fractionation, for example, has been used for more than 50 years to prepare therapeutic proteins from human plasma. Ethanol is known to be both bactericidal and virucidal and is the principal agent in Cohn fractionation used in the manufacture of blood products. The highest concentration of ethanol used during Cohn fractionation is 40% and in some steps is as low as 8-25%. The most efficient disinfectant concentrations of ethanol are, however, in the order of 70% (Bailey and Suomela, 1998).

As an alternative to cold ethanol fractionation, precipitation using polyethylene glycol (PEG) has been investigated. An advantage of using PEG precipitation over the use of ethanol is that less foaming occurs. PEG is non-flammable and also can be used above 0°C, with little risk of denaturation of the protein products. PEG has been widely used as a means of precipitating viable viruses under low gravitational force. It can only be considered a partitioning method and the efficiency with which different viruses are precipitated is influenced by the molecular weight of the PEG polymer, the gravitational force applied and the sedimentation constant of the virus.

2.2.2.5   Solvent/Detergent

To address the concern of contamination of pooled plasma products with enveloped viruses including HIV, *Hepatitis B virus* (HBV) and HCV, the New York Blood Center investigated the use of different solvent/detergent (S/D) combinations to establish which was most effective. Organic solvent/detergent mixtures are known to disrupt the lipid envelopes of viruses such as retroviruses. The result is either complete structural disruption, or destruction of the viral cell receptor. In either case the virus is rendered non-infectious. The treatment of plasma with organic S/D mixtures has been shown to enhance the virus safety of final products.

Since the advent of S/D treatment for blood and blood products, there has been no reported transmission of HIV, HBV or HCV by treated products (Robertson and Erdmann, 2000). This safety record for S/D treated blood products regarding enveloped virus contamination, has encouraged the adoption of S/D for the treatment of non-blood products such as monoclonal antibodies and recombinant proteins. Although solvent/detergent has been used in the blood industry for more than 15 years, this treatment generally has no effect on unenveloped viruses. Consequently, biopharmaceutical manufacturers are paying particular attention to systems capable of removing unenveloped viruses such as parvoviruses and picornaviruses from bulk products.

2.2.2.6   Low/High pH

The manufacturing process for monoclonal antibodies often includes an affinity chromatography step as a capture process. In many cases the ligand on the affinity resin for a monoclonal antibody product is protein A. Elution of the product from such resin generally occurs in a low pH buffer. Where it is possible to hold the product in such an elution buffer for 30 mins after elution, the step can be studied as a kinetic step for its ability to inactivate enveloped viruses. For a low pH treatment to be effective against enveloped viruses, a pH of less than 3.8 is useful, and a pH of 3.5 is desirable for the step to be effective (unpublished data, Q-One Biotech). Such a low pH range, however, has no effect against non-enveloped viruses. As previously discussed, high pH buffers (such as NaOH) are often used for sanitisation of manufacturing instruments because of their virucidal activity.

2.2.3   Virus clearance methods in development

Historically, purification processes have depended on chromatographic partitioning steps for virus removal, with inactivation being dependent on inherent steps in the process, such as low pH. As indicated above, chromatographic steps are not considered robust, and there has been a recent move to implement two robust orthogonal steps within a downstream process to provide virus reduction, with at least one of these being an inactivation process. Many protein products may not, however, be stable under conditions of extreme heat, high or low pH or solvent/detergent conditions. Therefore, there has been a drive to develop new technologies to inactivate viruses in biopharmaceutical products. Many studies have demonstrated that, for the more robust non-enveloped viruses in particular, the introduction of a second virus reduction step may significantly increase the total reduction level for a particular virus type. Nanofiltration is an example of a second step now being used widely in the manufacture of biologicals.

A number of new, proprietary technologies for virus inactivation that could be applied to standard downstream processes are being developed. Such processes should display high effectiveness for a broad range of viruses (enveloped and non-enveloped) and pose no enhanced risk (for toxicity, mutagenicity and carcinogenicity) to the recipients of products treated with these new processes. When introducing a second robust step to a manufacturing process, it is important to establish that the introduction of this second step does not, however, compromise the stability of the end product. Physical systems in general, cause less regulatory concern because there are generally no toxicology issues. Nevertheless, physical systems can lead to product degradation whilst newer chemical systems may prove to be very safe, and generally have little impact upon the stability of the product.

It is not only the collateral effects on the product and virus clearance capabilities of these newer technologies that will determine their suitability for inclusion in a manufacturing process, but also their scalability. Downscaling of a manufacturing process for a validation study is an essential part of the design and planning of the study. Process steps chosen to be studied must have operating parameters and physical characteristics that can be scaled down, and the downscaled process must be validated to demonstrate it does mimic as closely as possible the full scale manufacturing process. The validity of any virus clearance data is dependent on the accuracy with which the downscaled process mimics the full-scale process.

Table 8.3 lists technologies in development for virus inactivation.

Table 8.3. Emerging methods of virus inactivation.

Physical Inactivation Methods	Chemical Inactivation Methods
Microwave	Phenothiazine Dyes
Gamma Irradiation	Psoralens
Broad Spectrum Pulsed Light	Imines
High Pressure	Haloacetaldehydes
	Hypericin
	Beta Propiolactone
	Riboflavin
	Caprylate

The introduction of any of these systems requires a number of factors to be considered:
- *Cost*
- *Scalability*

- *Product quality and functionality*
- *Product safety*
    - toxicology of compounds used
    - ease of removal
    - neoantigen formation
- *Virus reduction capabilities*

As an alternative to heating, a number of companies are investigating the use of microwave technology for in-process virus inactivation. Microwaves have been demonstrated to have biocidal effects due to the heating they induce. In addition, there exists a phenomenon called the microwave effect which appears to destroy viruses for reasons other than heating (Kakita 1995). A more specific High Temperature Short Time (HTST) microwave treatment has been developed to overcome the traditional problem of heat treatment for long periods of time denaturing the therapeutic protein of interest. Temperature gradients are also less of a concern using this system. The basis of the system is to expose the product of interest to a continuous flow of microwave radiation whilst using a specially designed heat exchanger to heat and cool fluids in milliseconds rather than minutes. This process may be appropriate for certain proteins like immunoglobulins that resist such treatment. Smaller proteins, like tissue plasminogen activator, were shown to be resistant to the higher temperatures ($97^\circ C$) required to inactivate small unenveloped viruses such as PPV, whereas, under these conditions significant loss of clotting factors is observed (Walter, 1998). While microwave technology is promising, its use may well be dependent on the thermostability of the product and the expected contaminants. It may not yet offer a commercially acceptable trade-off of virus inactivation versus product loss for coagulation factors, but may be acceptable for products like monoclonal antibodies. Microwave HTST, however, has a lot to offer as it can be incorporated into a continuous flow downstream process. Nevertheless the thermostability of the product and the rapid cooling needed are issues to consider. In addition, the effects of individual buffers will require optimisation and validation for each new product.

Gamma irradiation has a long history of use in the sterilisation of products including food. A limiting factor in its application to biological products has been the heat generated during the process. Gamma irradiation is, however, capable of inactivating a wide range of pathogens, can be used as a terminal or intermediate step in a process, and is well understood. This technology has the added advantage that it can avoid using exogenous chemicals, but cost and complexity may make it prohibitive to implement for biotechnology products. It may have a role in the batch treatment of plasma pools as this process can be centralised. In addition much more extensive validation of virus inactivation should be undertaken before these processes can be regarded as acceptable. The disadvantages of using gamma irradiation include the introduction of protein modifications, and the difficulties of using the technology at small scale.

Intense pulses of light applied in short duration flashes (Broad Spectrum White Light) are known to have a biocidal effect on many micro-organisms, including viruses. For most applications, a few pulses of light applied in a fraction of a second are enough to provide an effective inactivation treatment.

There are some disadvantages to broad spectrum pulsed light technology. Obtaining good virus kill without affecting proteins may not always be possible. The technology may also require customised equipment, since not all materials transmit broad spectrum light effectively. Many materials such as polystyrene, polyethylene terephthalate (PET), and glass absorb light in the ultraviolet region. Since all wavelengths used in the pulsed light technology emission spectrum must contact the product to be sterilized, sterilization through these materials is not possible, and applications using these materials are limited to surface sterilization.

Inactivation of viruses by hydrostatic pressure, is a novel approach to the inactivation of pathogens in biopharmaceuticals that retains the therapeutic properties of the products being treated. Bradley *et al.* (2000) indicate that high-pressure procedures may be useful for the inactivation of viruses in blood and other protein-containing components. Whilst high-pressure technology has shown some promise, it is not at the stage of development where it can be realistically considered for biotechnology products.

The virus safety of protein solutions can be enhanced by treatment with short wavelength ultra violet (UV) irradiation. For example, UVC treatment of foetal calf serum was demonstrated to consistently give high clearance rates for a selection of enveloped and unenveloped viruses including *Picornavirus* and *Parvovirus* examples (Kurth *et al.*, 1999). The addition of such a step to existing processes may provide an added margin of safety for non-enveloped or heat stable viruses.

Although UV light alone can have an inactivating effect on viruses, recently, there has been a high degree of interest expressed in photochemical methods (methods involving the addition of a photoreactive chemical agent and specific wavelengths of light). The use of photoreactive chemical agents and long wave UV light is proving particularly suitable for virus inactivation and several classes of photoreactive chemicals are being investigated. There are several important properties that photoreactive compounds must possess to be suitable for inactivation of viruses in biopharmaceuticals. They must be

- soluble in water
- non toxic/pathogenic/mutagenic or carcinogenic

- highly effective against a broad range of viruses
- able to maintain biological activity of labile products
- effective at low photochemical energy levels

Phenothiazine dyes produce singlet oxygen after photoactivation. This feature coupled with their affinity for nucleic acid suggests that part of the virucidal effect of these compounds may be associated with free radical damage to DNA. Methylene blue (MB) and its derivatives are photoactive and in principle are suitable for photodynamic virus inactivation of biopharmaceutical products. MB induces singlet oxygen formation, which acts on the viral genome (Mohr, 1998). Much experience has been gained in the use of methylene blue to treat red blood cells although more recently 1,9-dimethylmethylene blue has been shown to be more effective (Wagner et al., 1998). The reason for its greater virucidal specificity is believed to be its higher affinity for DNA and the level of singlet oxygen production from 1,9, dimethylene blue is 50% greater than that for methylene blue. While methylene blue appears to be a promising technology, there are some reservations over the available genotoxicological data. A major weakness of MB systems is their comparative inefficiency in inactivating unenveloped viruses, although some inactivation of Adenovirus, Calicivirus and Papovavirus (SV40) was observed (Mohr et al., 1995).

Psoralens are a class of ultraviolet-activated DNA intercalating compounds which form covalent mono and di-adducts with thymine bases. Psoralens, in the presence of UVA light, are effective at inactivating a wide range of enveloped viruses and are capable of penetrating cells to inactivate the proviruses of HIV and *Human T-cell lymphotrophic virus* (HTLV). The introduction of psoralen technology will be dependent on the production of sound genotoxicological data.

The major failing of psoralen systems is their poor capacity to inactivate non-enveloped viruses. It remains to be fully determined if a new range of derivatives can overcome this problem.

Of most concern is the direct mutagenic activity of photoactive compounds. The required safety evaluation of these compounds involves both *in vitro* and *in vivo* genotoxicological assays. It is necessary to evaluate the photo-products as well as the primary material. There are some concerns over the ability of the standard genotoxicological assays to reveal critical mutagenic events; the use of systems like the $p53^{-/-}$ mouse may be needed to fully evaluate the oncogenicity of some of these compounds or their adducts.

Recent studies of virus inactivation agents have focused on the naturally occurring chemical, vitamin B2, or riboflavin. Riboflavin, being water soluble, is able to penetrate a wide variety of targeted viruses and cells. Therefore, it is likely to penetrate traditionally hard to kill non-enveloped viruses and intracellular viruses. Goodrich (2000) reported on the use of riboflavin and its ability to inactivate viruses. Riboflavin intercalates with the pathogen nucleic acid. The photochemical reaction that ensues breaks bonds in the viral DNA or RNA. Riboflavin has a well known clinical history, and so the ability of this compound to inactivate a wide range of viruses should be viewed by the biopharmaceuical industry with great interest.

Hypericin is a naturally occurring polycyclic quinone which has been investigated as a potential virucidal agent with activity against a broad range of enveloped viruses. The effective virucidal activity emanated from a combination of photodynamic and lipophilic properties. Hypericin binds cell membranes (and, by inference, virus membranes) and crosslinks virus capsid proteins. This action results in the loss of infectivity and reverse transcriptase activity, (Lavie, 1995). The fact that hypericin does not have an effect on non enveloped viruses is, however, a severe disadvantage to this product. The same can also be said of caprylate. Caprylate is a fatty acid that is used as a stabiliser during pasteurisation and subsequent formulation of albumin. Under certain conditions of pH and caprylate concentration, the non-ionised form of caprylic acid is maximised. The non-ionised form demonstrates virucidal properties against enveloped viruses by a mechanism believed to be an interaction with the lipid envelope of the virus. The activation is enhanced at elevated temperatures.

There is a large body of experience in the vaccine industry of using electrophilic agents like acetylethyleneimine (AEI) and ethyleneimine monomer for the inactivation of viruses. Ethyleneimine monomer is prepared from β-bromoethylamine by treatment with alkali and is often referred to as binary ethyleneimine or BEI. These products have not been used to inactivate human viral vaccines but billions of doses of vaccine for *Foot and Mouth disease virus* (FMDV) have been produced using these agents. Of the chemical systems, imines have the advantage of inactivating certain non-enveloped viruses like parvoviruses and, provided detailed toxicological studies confirm their safety, they are likely to play an important role in the treatment of biological products.

Significant data on the effect of haloacetaldehydes on viruses was discovered in collaboration between American Red Cross and Amersham Biosciences. Virus spiked protein solution was run in a column process consisting of a column packed with iodinated DEAE (di-ethylaminoethyl) Sephadex® resin in sequence with a DEAE-Sephadex capture column for removal of excess released coloured substances (different forms of hydrated iodide and tri-iodide ions). Extensive studies of the column effluent with different analytical methods (nuclear magnetic resonance, gas chromatography and mass spectroscopy) later showed that the active ingredient released from the Iodine resin was a low molecular weight non-charged compound, Iodoacetaldehyde (IAA). This compound was probably formed by Iodine's oxidative action on the ionic ligand bound to the resin, the DEAE (di-ethylaminoethyl) group. Whilst haloacetaldehydes do show promise as an inactivation technology, the toxicity of these reagents has still to be evaluated.

The efficacy of combined beta-propiolactone /UV radiation for inactivation of HBV in labile blood derivatives has been reviewed. (Prince et al. 1983)

It remains to be seen which of these new technologies will be adopted by the different biopharmaceutical manufacturers, but we are already seeing some encouraging data for several of the different techniques. In addition to this data, the opinion of the regulatory authorities regarding these different techniques will also have an impact on their inclusion in any manufacturing process.

3. VIRUS CHOICE FOR A MONOCLONAL ANTIBODY CLEARANCE STUDY

The virus choice will depend on a number of factors including the cell substrate and the manufacturing process. The virus panel chosen should include selected model viruses that differ in their sensitivity to physical and chemical agents. These models should be representative of all possible virus contaminants for a product. It is not possible to predict all potential contaminants, and it is possible that the product (or starting materials) could contain as yet unknown contaminants. Using a large panel of viruses with varying size, genome type, and resistance to physico-chemical inactivation, will help to address unknown, as well as predicted, virus contaminants.

In selecting a virus panel, it is important to consider the origin of reagents used in the manufacturing process, as well as the starting material. For example, affinity chromatography columns often contain monoclonal antibodies; cell culture medium may contain bovine serum. Operating personnel may also contribute to the contamination of a product and so the virus panel chosen should include examples of virus families that would cover potential contaminants from an operator. Other considerations include the indication for the product, the health status of the patients, the route of administration of the product, and the number of patient doses. An additional practical consideration in choosing a virus panel is that there should be a reliable assay with a defined end-point available for the viruses chosen. There should also be no undue risk to the operator(s) performing the virus clearance study.

Monoclonal antibody production: minimising virus safety issues 215

For a virus clearance study on a product entering phase I/II clinical trials, a minimum of a single study should be performed using a single virus. For biopharmaceuticals derived from rodent cell lines, a retrovirus such as MLV would be the virus chosen. Increasingly, regulatory authorities have been asking for a second robust virus (e.g. parvovirus) to be included in such early phase studies to show, at an early stage, the overall robustness of the process.

Where a product is due to enter phase III clinical trials virus clearance study data should demonstrate the capacity of a process to reproducibly remove a range of viruses with different physico-chemical properties. Thus a study should be performed at least in duplicate, and would generally include a panel of 4 (for recombinant proteins and monoclonal antibodies) or 5 (for human blood products) viruses.

When studying the manufacturing process for a monoclonal antibody, a typical virus panel might include MLV, *Porcine pseudorabies virus* (PRV), *Reovirus Type 3* (Reo 3), and MMV. For a CHO cell derived recombinant product, *Parainfluenza virus type 3* (PI3) is generally used instead of a herpesvirus since incidences of paramyxovirus contamination have been observed in CHO derived cell lines. Examples of virus panels that might be used in studying a monoclonal antibody product are shown in Table 8.4.

Further details of model viruses can be found in Table 8.5.

Table 8.4. Virus selection for a mammalian cell derived product validation study

Model	Contaminant	Properties
MLV	Retroviruses	Enveloped, ss RNA, 80-130 nm Low resistance to physico-chemical inactivation
HSV-1 PRV BHV-1	Herpesviruses	Enveloped, ds DNA, 150-200 nm Low-medium resistanceto physico-chemical inactivation
PI3	Paramyxoviruses	Enveloped, ss RNA, 150-300 nm Low-medium resistance to physico-chemical inactivation
BVD	Flaviviruses	Enveloped, ss RNA, 40-50 nm Low-medium resistance to physico-chemical inactivation
Reo 3	Reoviruses *Bluetongue virus*	Non-enveloped, ds RNA, 60-80 nm Medium resistance to physico-chemical inactivation
MMV CPV PPV	Parvoviruses	Non-enveloped, ss DNA, 18-26 nm High resistance to physico-chemical inactivation

Validation studies should be discussed at the earliest possible occasion with the relevant regulatory authorities. This would usually be done at a pre IND or NDA meeting, and then again prior to phase III clinical studies to make sure that no outstanding issues remain prior to licensing application.

4. STUDY DESIGN

There are several stages in the design and performance of a virus clearance study (TSE studies also follow a similar design):

Since it is necessary to deliberately spike virus into the manufacturing process to perform a virus clearance study, it is essential that such a study be performed in laboratories designed for this purpose and operated fully in compliance with the principles of Good Laboratory Practice (GLP). The chosen lab should be separate from the manufacturing facility, and the study performed by personnel experienced in performing virus clearance studies. It is, therefore, common for virus clearance studies to be out-sourced to dedicated contract labs.

Under these circumstances, it is essential that, at the earliest stage in study design, to enter into detailed technical discussions to allow the most appropriate design to be agreed.

Viral clearance study reports for submission to regulatory authorities should be very extensive and include all of the raw data from the titrations, interference and cytotoxicity studies, and all of the calculations used in preparing the results. All correction factors for changes in volume resulting from pH neutralisation or processing should be clearly indicated in the report, in addition to any other controls (*e.g.* ultracentrifugation control).

Because of the complexity of a virus clearance study, the time taken from agreeing on the study design to putting together the report for submission to the regulatory authorities could be several months.

4.1 Preliminary studies

The initial lab work should consist of extensive preliminary studies. Preliminary studies are performed to demonstrate whether samples to be tested in the virus clearance study may interfere with the assay systems used. Control samples, representative of all the process samples to be tested, should be used. It is advisable to test up-front the effect of the process samples on the cells and viruses used in any particular assay. The regulatory authorities throughout Europe, the US and Japan have raised the issue of addressing potential cytotoxicity and interference effects, and require that such preliminary studies be performed in a virus clearance study (CPMP/ICH/295/95, 1997).

4.1.1 Cytotoxicity

Cytotoxicity assays are performed to demonstrate whether process buffers and/or samples are toxic to the indicator cells used in the virus titration assays. Samples representative of all the process samples and intermediates should be tested for cytotoxicity, on each of the cell lines to be used.

4.1.2 Interference

Interference assays are performed to determine whether samples interfere with the ability of the relevant virus to infect the indicator cell lines or prevent detection of the appropriate virus-induced cytopathic effect (cpe). Interference assays are performed on samples representative of the product fractions, as this is the sample used for assessing the level of virus reduction achieved. It is important to allow the interference assays to run for the full length of the assay. Since a low dilution of virus would be used for these assays, the interference effect may not necessarily be observed until the last few days of the assay.

4.1.3 Load controls

A number of additional preliminary studies, termed load controls, may be performed, depending on the nature of the study. Load control assays are performed to determine whether the starting materials (and in some cases other buffers or samples) could have an effect on the viruses used, during the process step. These assays would typically involve spiking selected samples with a high level of virus, and incubating for a given period prior to titration.

For example, virus may be spiked into starting material, or relevant process buffers, to determine whether these may inactivate virus during the course of the clearance study. For inactivation studies, selected samples may be spiked with virus after dilution or quenching of the inactivant, to ensure that the inactivant under study has been effectively quenched, and does not continue to inactivate virus following sample collection.

All the preliminary studies must be performed and completed before commencing with the spiked process runs. This requires close coordination regarding the timing of the study and the availability of materials necessary to complete these preliminary tests.

4.2 Spiked process runs

Once the preliminary studies are complete, the spiked process runs can be performed.

For each individual step to be studied, starting material from the full scale manufacturing process should ideally be used. This material is then spiked with a high titre of virus, and then taken through the individual downscaled process step. Relevant process samples are collected, diluted to the appropriate non-cytotoxic and non-interfering dilution, and then assayed. The total virus load in the start material can then be compared with the total virus recovered in the relevant product fraction (this is illustrated in Figure 8.2).

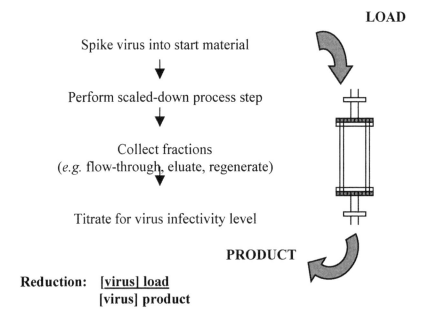

Figure 8.2. Example of the spiking process for a chromatography step.

4.3 Titrations

After performing the spiked process runs, the collected samples are assayed as described below. For viruses used routinely in virus clearance studies, a 50% tissue culture infectious dose ($TCID_{50}$) assay is often used. Serial dilutions of sample are inoculated onto the appropriate cell line. Assays are incubated for the appropriate time, and each well is scored as either positive or negative, and the proportion of positive wells then determined.

Samples generated during a spiked process run should generally be assayed directly (*i.e.* without freezing). The length of the titration assays will vary, depending on the virus used, and range from around 1 week to 4 weeks.

With any biological assay, however, it is possible that repeat assays may be required. For this reason, excess samples should also be frozen and stored as a precaution.

Appropriate controls must also be incorporated for any sample manipulations that do not form part of the process step (for example, if a sample is ultracentrifuged to remove toxicity, or if a sample is frozen prior to titration).

Once the data is available on the number of wells scored positive for each dilution the virus titre is then calculated, using the method of Karber (Karber, 1931).

4.4 Calculation of virus clearance

Once the virus titrations have been performed then the next stage is to calculate the virus reduction factors for each step tested in the clearance study. The virus reduction factor for an individual purification or inactivation step is defined as the $\log_{10}$ of the ratio of the virus load in the pre-purification material (Spiked starting material - SSM) divided by the virus load in the post purification material (Output Material). The formula takes into account both the titres and volumes of the materials before and after the purification step.

$$10^{R'} = \frac{v' \cdot 10^{a'}}{v'' \cdot 10^{a'}}$$

Where: R' = reduction factor for a given stage

v' = volume of the input material
a' = titre of the virus in the input material

v'' = volume of the retained output material

a'' = titre of the virus in the output material

The virus clearance factor is calculated similarly by substituting the theoretical total virus spiked into the SSM by the total virus input.

The 95% confidence limits for the calculation of virus clearance and reduction factors are calculated as follows:-

$$= \sqrt{(a^2 + b^2)}$$

where a = Standard error from total virus spiked/recovered in starting material
b = Standard error from total virus recovered in sample

For example, if a column purification step was spiked with 10ml of virus at a titre of 5.0×10^7 pfu ml^{-1} and the eluate volume was 50ml which contained virus at a titre of 1.5×10^1. The reduction factor for this step would be:

$$10^{RI} = \frac{10 \times 5.0 \times 10^7}{50 \times 1.5 \times 10^1}$$

$$= 6.7 \times 10^5$$

$$= 10^{5.8}$$

Therefore the above step of the process can remove 5.8 logs$_{10}$ of virus under the conditions used in the purification step. Because of the inherent imprecision of some virus titrations, an individual reduction factor should be greater than 1 log$_{10}$ to be significant. A clearance factor of greater than 4 logs$_{10}$ represents an effective virus clearance step.

4.5 Interpretation and limitations of viral clearance studies

Interpretation of the effectiveness of a virus clearance step is not a simple procedure. A combination of factors must be considered, and assessment of a step based solely on the quantity of virus inactivated/removed can lead to the conclusion that a process meeting specified levels of virus reduction will produce a safe product. This is not necessarily the case. Many factors contribute in defining the effectiveness of a step, and the data must be carefully evaluated in each case. The factors to consider include:

- suitability of the test viruses used
- design of the clearance study
- log$_{10}$ reduction achieved
- rate of inactivation kinetics

- nature of removal/inactivation
- variability in the virus clearance step
- limit of sensitivity of the assay

It is the combined evaluation of the above factors that will lead to a decision on whether a process step can be regarded as effective or not. If a low level of virus reduction is obtained using a particular process, the introduction of a specific removal/inactivation step may be required.

Whenever significant changes in the production or purification process are made, the effect of that change, both direct and indirect, on viral clearance should be considered, and the system re-evaluated as needed. Such changes can affect the level of virus clearance obtained.

Validation studies are useful in contributing to the assurance that an acceptable level of safety in the final product is established but do not categorically establish safety. A number of limitations in the design and execution of virus validation experiments may lead to an incorrect estimate of the ability of the process to remove virus infectivity. One of these limitations is the use of model viruses or viruses that have been adapted for growth in tissue culture. Such model virus stocks may not behave in the same way as the actual wild type virus contaminants. In particular, virus stocks may differ markedly in their degree of purity and aggregation. Virus in the centre of an aggregate can, for example, be protected from inactivation. There also can exist resistant sub-populations of virus which are extremely difficult to remove or inactivate. Therefore a virus resisting a first inactivation step may be more resistant to subsequent steps and as a consequence the overall reduction factor is not necessarily the sum of the reduction factors calculated from individual steps each time with a fresh virus spike-suspension. Virus clearance may have also been over-estimated by summing the logarithmic clearance factors for steps where the virus reduction occurred by a similar mechanism i.e. adsorption onto the column matrix. It is very difficult to reproduce exactly the full-scale manufacturing process at a smaller scale and maintain exactly the equipment and conditions found in the full manufacturing scale. For these reasons it is generally recommended that at least one individual stage of the validation process can remove or inactivate virus by a significant number (e.g. at least 4 $\log_{10}$). This provides an extra degree of assurance that the virus validation results are meaningful and contribute to the safety of the final product.

There are many variable parameters within a monoclonal antibody manufacturing process and some of these could impact on the results of a viral clearance study. There is increasing interest from the regulatory authorities, prior to product approval, for the impact of some of these variables on viral clearance studies to be examined. Such variables include,

Table 8.5. Typical virus models used for clearance studies

Virus	Family	Structure Size / Physico-chemical resistance	Model/host
Human immunodeficiency virus	Retroviridae	Enveloped ss RNA 70-100nm Low	Model for HIV 1, HIV 2, HTLV-1 and HTLV-2. Mandatory for products derived from human plasma/blood.
Murine leukaemia virus (Ecotropic and Xenotropic)			Represents a non-defective C type retrovirus. Mandatory for biological products derived from CHO cell lines and monoclonal antibody products.
Maedi visna virus			Model for lentiviruses. May be used as a model for HIV, and/or a model for potential contaminants of ovine derived material, particularly ovine blood products.
Herpes simplex virus type 1	Herpesviridae	Enveloped ds DNA 120-200nm Low to medium	Models for human or animal herpesviruses, e.g. Human herpes virus 1- 8 which may be transmitted in blood and plasma products; bovine or equine herpesviruses present in animal blood products. Models for Epstein Barr virus used in hybridoma generation.
Infectious bovine rhinotracheitis virus (Bovine herpes virus type I)			
Porcine pseudorabies virus			
Parainfluenza virus type 3	Paramyxoviridae	Enveloped ss RNA 150-200nm Low to medium	Potential contaminant of bovine serum. Incidences of contamination of CHO derived recombinants with this virus family observed.
Vesicular stomatitis virus	Rhabdoviridae	Enveloped ss RNA 50 x 200nm Low to medium	Model for rhabdoviruses such as Rabies virus.
Bovine viral diarrhoea virus	Flaviviridae	Enveloped ss RNA 40-60nm Low to medium	Models for potential togavirus or flavivirus contaminants. BVD is the preferred model for Hepatitis C virus in human blood and plasma derivatives. Alternatively Sindbis virus may be used.
Sindbis virus	Togaviridae	Enveloped ss RNA 60-70nm	
Contagious pustular dermatitis virus (ORF)	Poxviridae	Enveloped ds DNA 220-400nm Low to Medium	Model for potential pox virus contaminants, model for potential contaminants of ovine derived material.

Monoclonal antibody production: minimising virus safety issues 223

Adenovirus type 2 and 5	*Adenoviridae*	Non-enveloped ds DNA 70-90nm Medium	Model for human and animal adenoviruses
Reovirus type 3	*Reoviridae*	Non-enveloped ds RNA 60-80nm Medium to high	Infects human and animal cells, potential contaminant of hybridoma and recombinant cell lines. Model for orbiviruses and rotaviruses, model for Bovine blue tongue virus.
Encephalomyocarditis virus Human hepatitis A virus Human poliovirus Theiler's mouse encephalomyelitis virus	*Picornaviridae*	Non-enveloped ss RNA 25-30nm Medium to high	Model for Hepatitis A virus contamination of human blood/plasma, or picornavirus contamination of other products.
Feline calicivirus	*Caliciviridae*	Non-enveloped ss RNA ~40nm Medium to high	Model for Hepatitis E virus, a Calici-like virus. It is also a model for Rabbit haemorrhagic disease virus, a Calicivirus family member.
Simian virus 40	*Papovaviridae*	Non-enveloped ss DNA ~45nm High	Model for polyomaviruses including Bovine polyomavirus, and JCV and BKV (both human polyomaviruses)
Bovine parvovirus Canine parvovirus Murine minute virus Porcine parvovirus	*Parvoviridae*	Non-enveloped ss DNA 18-25nm High	Model for Human parvovirus B19, representing a severe test of the downstream process. Parvoviruses are known contaminants of CHO cell fermenters, and are also potential contaminants of rodent derived biopharmaceuticals

*ss = single stranded
ds = double stranded

buffer concentration, temperature, pH, protein concentration and chromatography column flow rates. Such studies are extensive and involve looking at the upper and lower ranges of these key parameters for the key relevant viruses Biopharma and biotech companies with a pipeline of monoclonals often use a generic approach as a solution to this issue. They study all these parameters in their standardised manufacturing process and use this data to support early clinical trials. The acceptability of such generic data to the regulatory authorities is viewed on a case by case basis. Issues such as generic data and looking at old and new resins for their ability to remove viruses is just part of the evolving regulatory experience to continue to ensure the safety of biologicals.

In summary, viral clearance studies are complex but, coupled with the cell bank characterisation and quality control testing of each unprocessed bulk harvest and final purified product, provide the virus safety assessment for a monoclonal antibody. It is essential that all these studies are performed in a manner acceptable to the regulatory authorities and according to the latest guidelines and experience. It is advisable to discuss the complete safety strategy in advance with the regulatory authorities, before embarking on what are time consuming and expensive safety studies. It is the experience of the author that most questions regarding viral safety of a biological arise from an incomplete or poorly performed viral clearance study.

REFERENCES

Amersham Biosciences Process Chromatography Application Note 18-1124-57. Use of sodium hydroxide for cleaning and sanitizing chromatography media and systems.

Bailey, A., Suomela, H., (1998). Process validation for the inactivation or removal of viruses in blood and plasma products. Q-One Biotech technical bulletin 13.

Bradley, D.W., Hess, R.A., Tao, F., Sciaba-Lentz, L., Remaley, A.T., Laugharn, J.A. Jr, Manak, M., (2000) Pressure cycling technology: a novel approach to virus inactivation in plasma. *Transfusion* **40** (2): 193-200

Committee for Proprietary Medicinal Products (CPMP), (1997). ICH Topic Q5A, step 4 Consensus Guideline. Note for Guidance on Quality of Biotechnology Products: Viral Safety Evaluation of Biotechnology Products Derived from Cell Lines of Human or Animal Origin, Publisher; The European Agency for the Evaluation of Medicinal Products: Human Medicines Evaluation Unit. (CPMP/ICH/295/95).

Committee for Proprietary Medicinal Products (CPMP), (1996). Note for Guidance on Virus Validation Studies: The Design, Contribution and Interpretation of Studies Validating the Inactivation and Removal of Viruses (CPMP/BWP/268/95). Publisher: The European Agency for the Evaluation of Medicinal Products: Human Medicines Evaluation Unit.

Committee for Proprietary Medicinal Products (CPMP). (2001) Note for guidance on Plasma Derived Medicinal Products: (CPMP/BWP/269/95 rev 3). Publisher; The European Agency for the Evaluation of Medicinal Products: Human Medicines Evaluation Unit.

Committee for Proprietary Medicinal Products (CPMP) and Committee for Veterinary Medicinal Products (CVMP), (2001). Note for guidance on Minimising the Risk of Transmitting Animal Spongiform Encephalopathy Agents via Human and Veterinary Medicinal Products: (EMEA 410/01 rev 1). Publisher; The European Agency for the Evaluation of Medicinal Products:

Food and Drug Administration, Center for Biologics Evaluation and Research. (1997) Points to Consider in the Manufacture and Testing of Monoclonal Antibody Products for Human Use.

Goodrich, R.P. (2000) The use of riboflavin for the inactivation of pathogens in blood products. *Vox Sang*; **78** Suppl 2:211-5

Johnston, A., MacGregor, A., Borovec, S., Hattariki, M., Stuckley, K., Anderson, D., Goss, NH., Oates, A., Uren, E. (2000) Inactivation and clearance of viruses during the manufacture of high purity factor IX. *Biologicals*, **28**(3):129-36

Kakita, Y., Kashige, N., Murata, K., Kuroiwa, A., Funatsu, M. and Watanabe, K., (1995) Inactivation of Lactobacillus bacteriophage PL-1 by microwave irradiation. *Microbiol. Immunol.* **39**: 571-576

Karber, J. Beitrag zur kollectiven Behandlung Pharmakologische Reihenversuche. (1931). *Arch Exp. Path. Pharmak.*, **162**, 480-483

Kurth, J., Waldmann, R., Heith, J., Mausbach, K., Burian, R. (1999). Efficient inactivation of viruses and mycoplasma in animal sera using UVC irradiation. *Dev. Biol. Stand.* **99**:111-8

Lavie, G., Mazur, Y., Lavie, D., Prince, AM., Pascual, D., Liebesd, L., Levin, B., Meruelo, D. (1995). Hypericin as an inactivator of infectious viruses in blood components. *Transfusion*, **35** (5): 392-400

Lovatt, A. (2002). Applications of quantitative PCR in the biosafety and genetic stability assessment of biotechnology products. *Rev. Mol. Biotechnol.* **82**. 3. 279-300

Mohr, H, (1998). Virus inactivation of fresh plasma. *Vox Sang* **74** pp171-172

Mohr, H., Lambrecht, B. and Selz, A. (1995) Photodynamic virus inactivation of blood components. *Immunological Investigations*, **24**: 73-85.

Plavsic, M., Bolin, S., (2001) Resistance of Porcine Circovirus to Gamma Irradiation, *BioPharm*, **14** (4) pp: 32-36.

Prince, A.M., Stephan, W., Brotman, B. (1983). Beta propiolactone/ ultraviolet irradiation: a review of its effectiveness for inactivation of viruses in blood derivatives. *Rev. Infect. Dis.* **5** (1): 92-107

Robertson, B.H., Erdmann, D.D., (2000). Non-enveloped viruses transmitted by blood and blood products. *Dev. Biol. Stand.* **102**: 29-35.

Walter, J.K., Nothelfer, F., Werz, W. (1998) Validation of Viral Safety for Pharmaceutical Proteins. In: *Bioseparation and Bioprocessing, Vol 1*, Subramanian G, Wiley-VCH Weinheim: 465-496

Wagner, S.J., Skirpchenko, J., Robinette, J.W.F.D., Cincotta, L., (1998) Factors affecting virus photoinactivation by a series of phenothiazine dyes. *Photochem. Photobiol.* **67**: 343

Chapter 9

CONTRACT MANUFACTURING OF BIOPHARMACEUTICAL GRADE ANTIBODIES

Leo A. van der Pol and Douwe F. Westra
DSM Biologics Company BV, PO Box 454, 9700 AL Groningen, The Netherlands

1. INTRODUCTION

The success of over a dozen approved human antibodies on the therapeutic market supports the mature status of pharma-grade antibodies as group of biopharmaceuticals. With a significant higher number in clinical trials and the search for new recombinant proteins as a result of the human genome sequencing program it is expected that many more human antibodies will enter the market in years to come (Gura, 2002, Walsh, 2000).

That a group of products become successful is an attractive observation for a CMO (Contract Manufacturing Organization) because such a company can offer a targeted program for development, validation, and cGMP production based upon the performance of a number of similar projects. The availability of blueprints for the production of pharmaceutical-grade antibody that have demonstrated their feasibility is beneficial for both the CMO and the customer because time and money are saved.

A targeted approach will only work well if a target production process has the required status with respect to quality and robustness and a competitive efficiency. Meanwhile, such a process must possess sufficient flexibility to incorporate the relevant trends, such as the implementation of animal-source-free (ASF) or mammalian-source-free (MSF) culture medium. This is illustrated in this chapter.

2. TRENDS IN THE ANTIBODY PRODUCTION PROCESS

2.1 Cells

Antibodies became an important group of biopharmaceutical products since humanized antibodies were more effective in patients than their respective murine type counter parts. With the change to humanized antibody the cell lines changed from murine hybridomas to recombinant myeloma (NS0 and SP2/0) and CHO cells. The hybridomas are expected to re-enter the stage as fusion cells from transgenic mice producing 100% human type antibody. In addition human cell lines, such as PER.C6 and HEK293, are candidate antibody production cell lines if they can demonstrate an accepted safety status and a high specific production rate for correctly modified and secreted product.

2.2 Culture media

An important regulatory-driven trend for the upstream process is the use of serum-free and mammalian-source-free (MSF) or Animal-Source-Free (ASF) medium to minimize the risk of transfer of viruses such as human immunodeficiency virus (HIV) and prions (Bovine Spongiform Encephalopathy, Creutzfeld Jacob Disease). The larger-scale production of antibody in serum-containing medium and later in serum-free reached a mature status in the 1980's and 1990's. Since many serum-free media contained different components from various mammalian sources (especially human and bovine) the serum-free status was not always a great leap in process safety. Therefore, the target medium became Protein-Free medium but because this could still include 10 kD filtered plasma fractions from animals a better target medium was described as ASF or MSF culture medium.

For ASF/MSF medium the whole cycle of development for the upstream production process had to be completed, including adaptation procedure, freeze/thaw procedure, pre-culture and fermentation until a robust process at scale has demonstrated its feasibility. It is expected that a mature status will be reached for ASF/MSF medium in this decennium and that animal cell culture will eventually greatly benefit from the knowledge that is obtained in chemically defined - and to a lesser extend undefined - MSF media.

2.3 Bioreactors

The bioreactor used for the production of the harvest containing the crude antibody for therapeutic applications is exclusively a stirred tank reactor.

The stirred tank reactor creating a homogeneous cell suspension allows better process development and supports superior process control compared to gradient systems used for cell culture, especially because representative samples of the culture can be evaluated. For large-scale culture in stirred tanks no special mild impeller type seems required (Reichert, 2000) and direct sparging of gas can be applied for aeration provided that the culture medium contains protective components such, as Pluronic F68 (Clayton et al., 1999, Chisti, 2000).

Until some years ago there was discussion whether for a fermentation process in a homogeneous stirred tank reactor a batch/fed-batch process or a continuous perfusion process was more efficient or preferred for a cGMP process. The finding that the quality of an antibody product may vary dependent on the phase of a batch culture (growth, stationary, decline) has disturbed the idea of simple batch definition. The choice to use a homogeneous stirred tank reactor in either batch or continuous perfusion mode will depend more and more on cell and product features rather than on historical sentiments.

With respect to cell features the correlation between growth rate and specific production rate will determine whether it is worthwhile to develop a production process using stationary cells at low growth rate (fed-batch and continuous perfusion) or using cells at high growth rate (repeated batch, fill and draw). Product properties such as the stability in harvest will determine whether a prolonged residence time in harvest is feasible (fed-batch) or that a short residence time is required (short batch, continuous perfusion at high medium flow rate).

For antibody producing suspension cells there is usually a favorable specific production rate at low growth rates while antibody product is quite stable in fermenter harvest. Resulting best options for the upstream fermentation process are fed-batch and continuous perfusion at moderate medium flow rate.

2.4 IgG purification

The purification of an antibody to biopharmaceutical grade requires a downstream process that consists of a combination of individual operation units. The key technologies that are used for the purification of biopharmaceutical grade antibodies are liquid chromatography and filtration. A critical step in the purification scheme of an antibody is the capture of the antibody from the fermentation harvest. The initial capture of antibodies from the fermentation harvest is in most cases performed with the use of protein A-based chromatography purifications (Fahrner et al., 1999, Hahn et al., 2003, Iyer et al., 2002,). Protein A binds strongly and selectively to human antibodies without the need of adjusting the fermentation harvest before application to the column. The characteristics enable protein A-based purification schemes to render antibodies with already a relatively high purity early in the downstream process. A drawback of the use of protein A resins lies in its limited stability at high pH, thereby limiting the lifetime of such resins. Furthermore, protein A leachables have to be removed below certain limits in the further downstream process because protein A leachables can cause unwanted immunogenic reactions. Finally, the costs of the resins are high because of the complexity in the resin manufacturing.

In the current development of resins, resins are developed which reduce the costs associated with the capture of antibodies. In typical protein A-based purification processes, the fermentation harvest is clarified from the cells and other particles either by filtration or centrifugation and is subsequently concentrated to reduce the volume that has to be applied to the column. Resins are developed that allow high flow rates to limit the need for reducing the volume of the fermentation harvest before it is applied to the column. Fermentation harvest can be applied to the column directly after clarification at a high flow rate (up to 1500 cm h^{-1}) and saving the costs for the concentration operation unit. Other protein A resins are developed for expanded bed adsorption and fluidized bed adsorption techniques. These techniques allow cells that are present in the start material to flow through the column, thereby eliminating the need for the clarification of the fermentation harvest before application. These techniques combine the clarification, concentration and capture of antibodies.

Another trend that is seen is the development of synthetic ligands that can compete with the selectivity of protein A. It is expected that synthetic ligands are cheaper to manufacture, thereby reducing the resin costs. In addition, resins using such synthetic non-protein ligands could have a higher stability at high pH. This stability allows a cleaning cycle with the use of high concentration of sodium hydroxide and thereby potentially increasing the column lifetime. Examples for these ligands are the thiophilic ligands and the ligand used for hydrophobic charge induction chromatography resins.

Another relatively new technology is the use of membranes with ligands bound to it, i.e. membrane-based chromatography. An attractive application of this technology is the use of membranes with an anion exchange ligand for the removal of residual DNA. Disposable capsules are available that can be used in stead of packed anion exchange columns. Careful thoughts have to be given on the process economics when evaluating using disposable capsules (Warner and Nochumson, 2003). In addition to this application, membrane-based chromatography offers potential improvements for the purification of large molecules like IgM or plasmid DNA. The membranes have a more open structure than resin beads and the ligands are therefore more readily available for binding these large molecules resulting in higher binding capacities.

2.5 Regulatory affairs

A trend ongoing for several years in regulatory affairs is the harmonization of regulations by the International Conference on Harmonization (Hesse and Wagner, 2002). For a CMO active in the production of biopharmaceuticals for different customers spread around the world it is beneficial that a universal quality policy is provided instead of having to deal with different national guidelines per project.

3. CONTRACT MANUFACTURING OF BIOPHARMACEUTICALS

Besides the given trends in the previous section lots of new additional developments could be presented for the dynamic field of manufacturing of biopharmaceuticals. However, for a CMO to operate successful and to provide optimal service for customers a focus on potential standardization is required.

The advantages of working with a target process for the production of a group of products such as antibodies with mammalian suspension cells include:

1. the (larger) equipment is present in the facility, therefore
2. no project specific (large) investments are required,
3. the blueprints for the bulk of the required documentation is available;
4. the targeted approach for the development phase results in time benefit for the majority of the projects
5. a reduction of risk: if a target process has demonstrated its feasibility for a number of cell lines it is likely to succeed for the next similar cell line.

Potential disadvantages include:

1. that the production process is not fully "tailor made", not all areas that might give a better performance for the particular cell line and product have been explored and
2. if the target process is not adapted to the relevant trends the resulting production process becomes no longer "state of the art".

Overall it is considered that for the majority of Antibody projects the benefits of a targeted approach outweigh by far potential benefit of the "tailor made" approach, certainly for projects with great priority for time to market.

DSM Biologics has chosen a targeted approach for two product groups: plasmid DNA produced by *E.coli* and antibodies produced by mammalian suspension cells. The approach aiming at the implementation of a target IgG process is presented in the next sections.

4. ANTIBODY PROJECT APPROACH

A project starts with information transfer from customer on the specific items of an antibody project, such as specific assays to support product quantity and quality. For a targeted antibody program actually little information is required to get started beyond a tests showing that the cell line that produces the antibody is free of mycoplasma. A project plan describes the activities to be performed from process development to a certain cGMP manufacturing phase. In a Process Development Plan and a Master Validation Plan it can be described what studies are planned as part of a certain phase of a project and which activities such as cGMP production and validation studies can be combined.

A project usually starts at a CMO in a development phase to prepare for clinical phase I production or alternatively is transferred before phase III. In the first case the emphasis is on the fast evaluation of a small-scale production process to demonstrate feasibility for further scale-up towards a pilot process before the transfer of the scaled production process to the production department. In the second case the emphasis is on evaluation if the existing production process can be performed at the site, whether it is reproducible and robust enough to "freeze" the process, and whether the level of validation is sufficient to support this status.

Ideally for a project the different phases R&D to Development to Validation to cGMP production phase I, II, III and the manufacturing of licensed product would follow as sequential blocks. Given the importance on time to market while meeting regulatory requirements, in reality development, validation and cGMP activities will exist in parallel phases and it has to be evaluated what process changes will require a certain study to demonstrate that the change has no impact on the safety and quality of the product.

5. TARGET MANUFACTURING PROCESS

5.1 Upstream: expansion preculture

The standard DSM IgG production process according to cGMP guidelines starts with the thawing of a single vial of the (M)WCB (see schematic in figure 9.1). Standard criteria for the thawing include a minimum viability of 50% and an increase in viable cell numbers at day 3 after thawing. The thawing of the antibody producing cells is the start of an expansion preculture to generate a sufficient amount of suspension cells to inoculate a stirred bioreactor. The expansion preculture starts in T-flasks of increasing size and ends with a number of roller bottles (10-20) containing a minimum of 5 x10^9 viable cells to inoculate a 50L fermenter. A frozen vial containing 10^7 cells viable cells could theoretically provide this cell number after 9 generations. However, because the initial viable cell number will generally be below 10^7 and because there is always some cell death the fermenter can be inoculated after 10-14 generations.

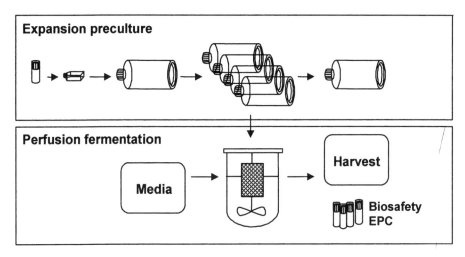

Figure 9.1. Target upstream process to generate monoclonal antibody as crude product in fermentation harvest

Standard criteria for the expansion preculture include a minimum seeding density for viable cells (target of 10^5/mL) that can run through three complete population doublings (reach 8 x10^5/mL) as part of the exponential growth phase. The mean viability during the expansion preculture should be above 90%. The mean doubling time for hybridoma and myeloma cells usually is in the range of 12 to 24 hours, for CHO cells more in the range of 24 to 36 hours. A mean population doubling time of 48 hours or longer is considered as non feasible because a standard expansion phase could then last for more than a month causing high clean room occupation costs while no product is generated in this period of expansion.

The stationary T-flasks and the roller bottles rotating on a bench are placed in an incubator at 36.5 ± 1°C. Usually the flasks are aerated with air containing 5% CO_2 as part of the transfer handling in a class 100 Biohazard LAF cabinet and placed in the incubator with closed lid. The aeration procedure causes some extra handling but eliminates the regulation of the humidity as parameter in the incubators.

Figure 9.2 shows the viable cell densities and viability of a standard expansion pre-culture for a mouse hybridoma during three consecutive expansions resulting in the inoculation of a 50L fermenter at day 9. A back-up culture is maintained for a few passages after inoculation of the fermenter for control on the condition of the cell suspension in rollers used as inoculum.

For some projects spinner flasks are used to generate larger volumes of cell suspensions but usually disposable materials are preferred at this scale instead of materials that require a validated cleaning process.

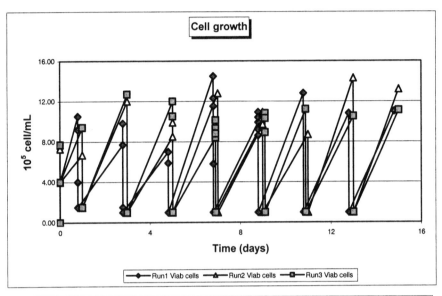

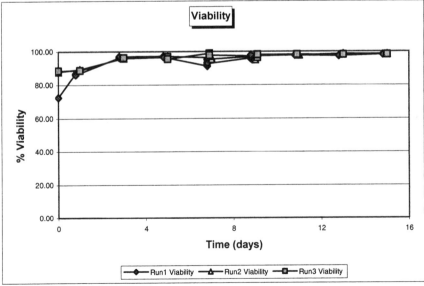

Figure 9.2. Viable cell density and viability during a standardized expansion preculture of hybridoma cells in serum-free culture medium

5.2 Upstream Target IgG process : 50L fermentation

The 5 to 10 L of cell suspension in roller bottles is collected in an inoculation bottle in a LAF hood and is connected to the 50L fermenter by connecting c-flex tubing from both systems with a sterile connection device (SCD). The target inoculation density of viable cells in the fermenter is 0.3 $x10^6$/mL and the starting working volume between 20 and 50 L. The fermenter is equipped with an internal spinfilter mounted on the stirrer axis for retention of the majority of the cells. Culture medium is added into the stirred cell suspension and the effluent is removed from the inside of the spinfilter. The media as well as the fermenter harvest containing crude product is connected and disconnected with the SCD.

The physical parameters such as temperature, DO, pH, and stirrer speed are maintained within preset ranges during the fermentation run. The flow rate of culture medium is increased with the increase in viable cell concentration to maintain a target refreshment of culture medium per cell during the growth phase (standard 0.3 nL/cell/day). When a target flow rate of one suspension volume per day is reached the medium flow rate is fixed and the suspension culture enters a stationary phase at a low growth rate. Dependent on the strength of the culture medium and the biomass removal rate a certain total cell concentration of 5 - 15 $x10^6$/mL is retained at 70-90% viability. A standard fermentation run length is 25 to 35 days, generating 1000-1500 L of fermenter harvest for a 50L working volume perfusion fermenter. For a cell line with a specific production rate of 10 to 20 pg/cell/day in the fermentation medium reaching a viable cell density of 10^6/mL this will yield 80 to 250 gram crude antibody product.

Figure 9.3 shows the viable cell density and the product concentration of IgG during three consecutive fermentation runs with spinfilter as cell retention device. Some differences in values can be observed but no major differences are found in the mean values (beyond the normal scatter for biological processes) for the specific perfusion rate and in the specific production rate (Figure 9.4), the parameters that will support a constant product quality provided that the physical parameters are constant and that the used cell line has good stability.

The fermenter harvest is stored at 2 - 8 °C, in the dark. The cells and cell debris are removed with dead-end filtration with filters in the range of 3.0 to 0.2 micrometer. The clarified harvest is concentrated by tangential flow filtration, using a 30 kD membrane for IgG and a 100 kD membrane for IgM. Dependent on the solubility of the antibody at higher concentrations the concentration factor is between 10 and 20.

For continuous perfusion fermentation at 250L or 500L scale the 50L working volume fermenter is used to inoculate the larger stirred tank reactors.

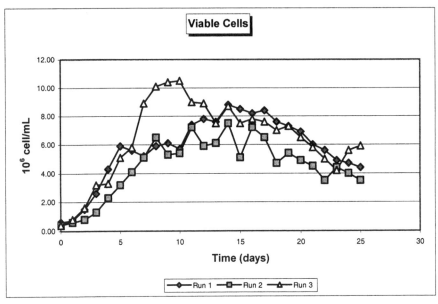
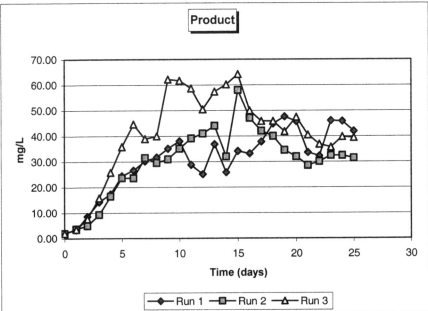

Figure 9.3. Viable cell density and antibody product concentration of hybridoma cells during three consecutive continuous perfusion fermentations

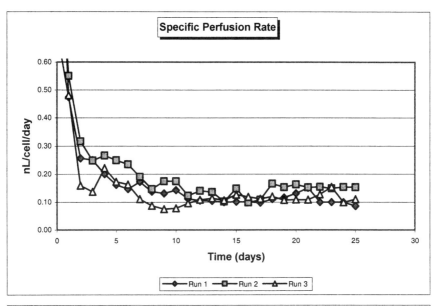

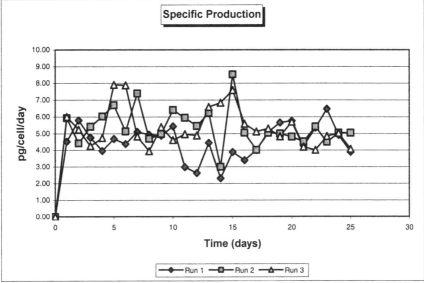

Figure 9.4. Specific perfusion rate and specific antibody production rate of hybridoma cells during three consecutive continuous perfusion fermentations

5.3 DSP process targets

A downstream process that is developed at a contract manufacturer is based on the experience of the customer with their product and based on the experience of the contract manufacturer with the development of IgG production processes. For the development of a purification process, targets for the product quality and for the process need to be defined. Close communications between the customer and the contract manufacturer on these targets should start as early as possible. Targets can be set on product parameters but also on process parameters like process yield and viral clearance. DSP targets are summarized in Table 9.1 and are discussed shortly below.

Antibody purity: The purity of the antibody is determined by the level of product-related impurities and by the level of impurities related to the process. Specifics of these impurities will be detailed below. In general, antibodies are purified to a high purity already early in the downstream process by specific affinity resins, like protein A-based resins. Therefore, the further downstream steps have to purify the antibody until the level of the impurities is below their target specification.

Potency: Therapeutic antibodies are selected to mediate certain biological activities in patients in such a manner that it is for the benefit of the patient. The potency, alternatively named the functional activity, of an antibody is the strength of the antibody to mediate this biological activity. An analytical assay that provides information on the potency of the product is necessary to demonstrate antibody stability throughout the production process, for example during process changes, process development and scale-up. For antibodies, assays such as ELISA and BiaCore demonstrating product binding to its target can be developed. More conclusive on the product potency is a biological assay (a bioassay) that shows that the product is active in a biological model that mimics the application of the product.

Product concentration: The concentration of the antibody in the final operation unit depends on the application where it is used for and on the stability of the antibody at higher concentrations.

Product-related impurities: The product-related impurities are either directly produced and secreted by the cells used for the production of the antibody or due to instability of the product after production and secretion. Product-related impurities that are directly produced by the cells, like aggregates or splicing variants need to be removed by the downstream process. Product-related impurities that are caused by the instability of the product are preferably minimized by employing process conditions that support the stability of the antibody. It is not always possible to find such process conditions and therefore the impurities have to be removed until acceptable levels by the downstream process.

Integrity of the carbohydrate moieties: The antibody molecules that are present in a final antibody preparation are not identical, but can be subdivided into discrete subsets of differently glycosylated molecules. This is not a specific characteristic of biopharmaceutical antibodies but is a general characteristic of all glycoproteins, including the natural counterparts of antibodies in the human blood. The carbohydrate chains of antibodies have a potential influence on the stability and functionality of antibodies and on the clearance of antibodies from the human body. Therefore, it is important to develop assays for the determination of the structure of the carbohydrates linked to the manufactured antibody. The structure of the carbohydrates that are linked to the manufactured antibody not only depend on the expression host but also on the production conditions.

Process related impurities: For the production of antibodies, materials like cell culture medium, resins, filters, and host cells are used. These materials or parts of these materials are potential impurities of the final preparation of the antibody. These impurities have potential effect on the safety of the antibody preparation and therefore need to be removed by the downstream process below their target limit. Among these impurities are the host cell proteins (HCPs) and DNA. HCPs and DNA are potential impurities because a part of the host cells lyses thereby releasing their content into the cell culture medium. In addition, HCPs are actively released into the cell culture medium because the cells secrete contaminating proteins upon propagation. Cell culture medium components that pose risks for the safety of the biopharmaceutical antibody need to be removed by the downstream process. Among these are the components derived from mammalian sources. In the past, these components were necessary for the propagation of the host cells. Current media are more and more free of serum and other components of mammalian source. Leachates of the filters and resins, like protein A ligand, have the risk that they cause adverse effects like immunogenic reactions and need to be minimized (The Biopharmaceutical Process Extrables Core Team, 2002). Finally, microbial contamination and endotoxin levels pose a potential risk for the safety of the product and therefore need to be controlled during manufacturing.

Process economic targets: The manufacturing costs of the antibody are determined for a large extent by the design of the production process. It is therefore important to keep control over the development of the downstream process by setting targets on the factors that determine the process economics. Important factors in the process economics are the raw material costs, the column life-time, the number of operation units and the process times, and the process yield.

Process robustness: Process robustness is the characteristic of the process that it is not effected by small changes to process parameters and that the process is relatively simple to operate. This robustness will result in a more reliable process, facilitating the process validation.

Holding times intermediates: Established holding times of intermediates increase the flexibility of the process, certainly when manufactured on a campaign basis. When a part of the process needs to be delayed, established holding times gives the manufacturer more flexibility without the product quality affected beyond established limits. This flexibility reduces the risk that a batch is rejected.

Viral clearance: Regulatory authorities provide guidelines to minimize any potential risks regarding viral safety. Next to the testing of the cell banks and the unpurified bulk for the presence of infectious viruses, the viral safety guidelines request that the downstream process is tested for its capacity to clear potential viruses (Sofer, 2003). The clearance of viruses by the downstream process happens by the inactivation of viruses, for example by a low pH treatment or a solvent/detergent treatment, and by the removal of viruses, for example by virus filtration and by affinity chromatography. The antibody DSP process needs to be designed in such a way that substantially more viruses are removed and/or inactivated than potentially present in the unpurified bulk. The capacity of a downstream process to clear viruses is demonstrated in a viral clearance study. For this, respective downstream unit operations in DSP are tested in a downscaled model for their capacity to clear (model) viruses that are spiked to the feed.

Table 9.1. The product and process targets to be set on an antibody downstream process

Product targets		Process targets	
Product purity		Holding time intermediates and final product	
Product potency		Total viral clearance	
Product concentration		Process robustness	
Product-related impurities			
Process related impurities:	Host cell DNA	Process economic targets:	Process yield
	Host cell proteins		Column life-time
	Impurities derived from cell culture components		Number of operation units
	Leachates		Raw material costs
	Endotoxin		
	Microbial contamination		

The characteristics of the product, the application of the product, the dosage, the dosage form, the site of application, and current FDA and international regulations determine where targets should be defined and the limits of these targets. Some targets can be set already early on in the development of a downstream process, other targets can only be set in later process development as knowledge of the product increases during process development and product manufacture. Moreover, some targets may be contradictory, like the process yield versus the product purity.

Not only the design of the downstream process is aimed by the above mentioned targets, also the development of the analytical assays is aimed by these product targets and their limits. The targets determine what kind of analytical tests are needed, the limits of the targets guides what limit of detection or quantification is needed for the respective analytical test. On the other hand, the current progress in the analytical assay technology for product characterization at a molecular level has a major impact on the requirements for testing of the product quality and the product consistency.

6. PROCESS VALIDATION

The standard validation work for the target upstream process producing crude antibody in fermenter harvest includes a Process Qualification study, a consistency study, a robustness study and specification setting runs, an Early, Mid, Late study, and stability studies for the cell line, the culture medium, and intermediate product. A robustness study will demonstrate the reproducibility at small scale of a selected process when run at set point, while testing worst case conditions for certain parameters. For the specification setting runs experimental design can be used as systematic approach to the validation of process control parameters, that is which combination of values for key process parameters will support the yield of antibody of constant product quality (Moran *et al.*, 2000). An Early, Mid, Late study has to demonstrate that product produced in an early phase of a fermentation run at scale is equivalent to product produced later during the run by comparing product quality from product purified by a down-scaled version of the DSP process.

The process validation work is not detailed in this chapter. In general for most larger validation studies that are scheduled before or associated to phase III production, limited process validation is performed as standardized development work or pre-validation study before phase I production.

7. PROCESS DEVELOPMENT

7.1 Development General

The process development for a biopharmaceutical product is a mixture of process development and pre-validation work that has to yield a feasible small-scale process that meets economic, time, and quality targets. Several quality targets are category "must have" because otherwise the approval of the product is at risk, potentially blocking all future revenues. If, however, the quality criteria are set much higher than necessary this can present a costly and time consuming exercise.

The investment made for a certain project in time and costs to develop an efficient and robust production process is dependent on:

1. application of the product (new versus second generation)
   If a product is the first in a certain application the time to market is the number 1 driver; if the product is a second-generation product there is more emphasis on cost of goods
2. amount of product required (dose per patient ; number of patients)
   The expected required scale for the market production of a biopharmaceutical antibody will influence the effort put in Development. A potential multi-kilogram blockbuster will justify more upfront Development than a single dose product for an orphan drug application.
3. product quality required for clinical performance
   Is it known what product quality (glycosylation or any other modification of protein) is required to support a desired clinical performance and are the assays to demonstrate the right quality available at a certain stage of process development.
4. process development during and after clinical phase I/II
   If it is accepted that a certain process is feasible for cGMP production because it is "only phase I" production what are then the potential consequences for further development with respect to the planning of validation studies and the demonstration of comparability or biochemical equivalence of the product.

A project plan is made indicating that a targeted approach for process development is followed defining feasibility criteria for standardized small-scale unit process steps or modules. The settings for the modules are based upon historical settings (previous antibody projects with comparable cells) and specific project requirements.

Actual additional R&D work is only started for modules that clearly do not meet the criteria. Process modifications will be tested to demonstrate feasibility of a revised process step. In addition the potential impact of the revised process has to be evaluated on other process steps and possible implications for the cGMP process.

7.2 Upstream process development activities

7.2.1 Adaptation

The adaptation program includes the transfer of mammalian cells from culture in serum-containing medium to growth in serum-free or MSF medium. The adaptation can also include the transfer from adherent to suspension culture and the shift from selective to non-selective culture medium.

The standard adaptation scheme starts with the culture of exponentially growing cells in 5% serum-containing medium in either T-flasks (150 cm^2, adherent cells) or roller bottles (suspension cells). The culture is split in a single-step transfer to a MSF medium, a gradual adaptation starting with the target MSF medium containing 2.5% serum and back up in the original medium. If the single step adaptation is successful for 3-5 passages a WCS of 20-30 vials is generated in MSF medium containing DMSO. When a successful test thaw procedure has been performed the gradual adaptation and the control culture are terminated.

If the single-step adaptation is not successful the gradual adaptation is continued via MSF medium containing target MSF medium. From 1% serum containing medium there should be sufficient exponential cell growth for the transfer to target MSF medium. If the criteria for sufficient exponential growth are not met this usually an indication that the target medium is not suitable for the successful culture of the cell line in MSF medium. Different formulations should be included to complete the adaptation program.

It is preferred to use a simple chemically defined target MSF medium for the adaptation of the standard mammalian suspension cell lines (hybridoma, myeloma, CHO, BHK). The advantages of adaptation to a basal MSF medium are : 1) regulatory accepted 2) low cost 3) some idea on basal nutrient requirements for cell growth 4) excellent freeze/thaw performance.

At present the time required to adapt cells to a target MSF culture medium on average is no longer than the time previously required to adapt cells to serum-free media.

7.2.2 Target Expansion preculture

The objective for the expansion preculture is to generate cell suspension from a frozen stock to inoculate a stirred bioreactor. With cells from the WCS it is tested whether an expansion preculture can be performed in a particular MSF medium that meets criteria for standard preculture, as listed in section 5.1. Another wording for the criteria for preculture would be that a 1:5 dilution is feasible after 3 days at minimum 90% viability

During the initial implementation of MSF media a lower performance with respect to growth rate and viability was accepted, provided that the reproducibility of the expansion pre-culture did qualify. Now the pre-culture in MSF media can meet the same criteria as for media containing components from mammalian source.

Besides the use of ASF/MSF media for the expansion preculture a change in the target process involves the replacement of the use of roller bottles or spinner flasks towards the culture in plastic bags. This is especially beneficial for if a sterile connection device (SCD) is already used during the fermentation process to connect and disconnect bags.

7.2.3 Target Fermentation process

In the target MSF medium a fermentation run at 4 L working volume is performed using standard settings for the type of suspension cell. The target seeding density is 0.3 $x10^6$/mL ; the viable cell concentration has to increase to a value above 5 $x10^6$/mL within 2 weeks. A stationary phase has to reached for at least two weeks at a medium flow rate of 1 volume per day, a mean viable cell density above 5 $x10^6$/mL and a mean viability above 75%. These setting usually result in harvest containing 25 - 250 mg/L antibody for cell lines with specific production rates in the range of 5 - 20 pg/cell/day.

7.2.4 Implementation of MSF Media in Fermentation

While serum-free but not protein-free media supported a robust performance of the majority of mammalian suspension cells, the implementation of chemically defined MSF media gave fast initial clogging of the spin-filter for a number of cell lines. Therefore a two-sided approach was taken for the additional R&D work on the continuous perfusion fermentation process. First the acoustic cell retention system was tested as external device instead of the internal spin-filter and secondly the MSF media and fermentation conditions were optimized to avoid the clogging of the filter.

The acoustic system was selected from various options for devices for the retention of mammalian suspension cells because it has no fixed complicated parts in the external loop that would cause difficult - if not impossible - cleaning validation and would give cells the opportunity to adhere to the retention system. The system has been used for continuous perfusion fermentations at 100 L scale for a multiple week run (to be published elsewhere).

The R&D work for the improvement of the spinfilter fermentation process was performed with a smaller pore-size filter to create worst-case conditions. After modification of the defined MSF medium and the mode of pH control the spinfilter performance in this simple culture medium were better with the small pore-size filter than with the larger pore-size filter in protein-containing fermentation medium. Additional beneficial effect is the faster growth phase because of the high initial cell retention (Figures 9.5, 9.6, and 9.7).

Though the shift to the use of MSF media initially caused longer time lines for projects and reduced process robustness the overall process performance in MSF is now yielding a mature and more efficient and controlled production process than in serum-free non-MSF media.

Contract manufacturing of biopharmaceutical grade antibodies 245

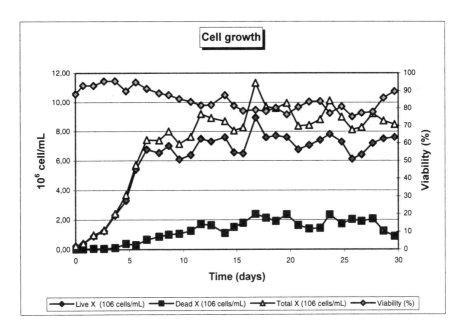

Figure 9.5. Cell densities and viability of myeloma cells in basal MSF medium during a continuous perfusion run with internal spin filter

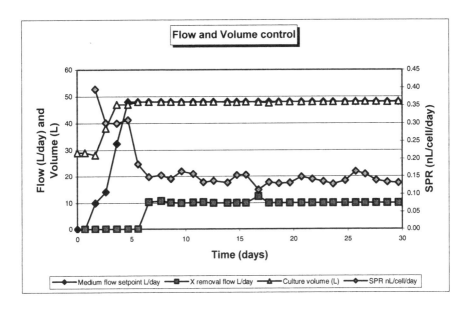

Figure 9.6. Culture medium, media flow rate, biomass removal flow and specific perfusion rate for myeloma cells in MSF medium during a perfusion run with spin filter

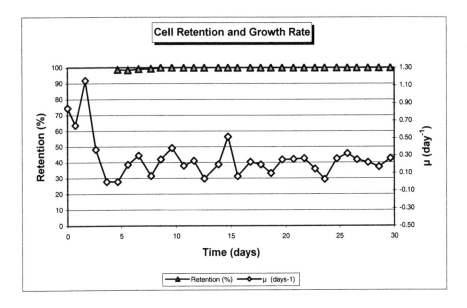

Figure 9.7. Cell retention and growth rate of myeloma cells in basal MSF medium during a continuous perfusion run with internal spin filter

8. CONCLUSIONS

An increase in the required capacity for the production of pharma-grade antibodies is expected. Pharmaceutical companies expand their in-house production capacity while new CMO's develop and existing CMO's are growing.

A CMO should provide a fast-track targeted approach towards a feasible production process according to cGMP guidelines that will yield product that will meet established criteria. Such a route has to work for the majority of antibody producing cell lines and antibody products. In addition a CMO has to offer R&D capacity that will provide feasible solutions for process activities that do not meet the initial pre-set criteria for a project.

For the coming years a continued focus on product quality is expected to establish a certain beneficial effect in the patient and avoid unwanted side effects, such as rapid clearance or an unwanted immunogenetic response (Adair and Ozanne, 2002). Such unwanted side effects can be related to the quality of the product (primary structure, glycosylation, other modifications) but also the presence of product-related and process-related impurities.

It is expected that the use of defined ASF/MSF media will facilitate the required process control to ensure the production of product of constant quality.

ACKNOWLEDGEMENT

The authors would like to thank Gerben Zijlstra for providing additional input for this chapter.

REFERENCES

Adair, F. Ozanne, D., 2002, The immunogenicity of therapeutic proteins. *BioPharm* **15 (2)**: 30-36.
Chisti, Y., 2000, Animal-cell damage in sparged bioreactors. *TibTech* **18**: 420-432.
Clayton, T., Jenkins, I., Steward, P., 1999, The improvement of aeration in 8000L animal cell culture vessels. In *Animal Cell Technology: Products from Cells, Cells as Products* (A. Bernard et al. eds.), Kluwer Academic Publ., p p.277-283.
Fahrner, R.L., Whitney, D.H., Vanderlaan, M. and Blank, G.S., 1999, Performance comparison of Protein A affinity-chromatography sorbents for purifying recombinant monoclonal antibodies. *Biotechnol. Appl. Biochem.* **30**: 121-128.
Gura, T., 2002, Magic bullets hit the target. *Nature* **417**: 584-586
Hahn, R., Schlegel, R. and Jungbauer, A., 2003, Comparision of protein A affinity sorbents. *Journal of Chromatography B* **790**: 35-51.
Hesse, F., Wagner, R., 2000, Developments and improvements in the manufacturing of human therapeutics with mammalian cell cultures. *TibTech* **18**: 173-180.
Iyer, H., Henderson, F., Cunningham, E., Webb, J., Hanson, J., Bork, C. and Conley, L., 2002, Considerations during development of a Protein A-based Antibody Purification Process. *BioPharm* **15 (1)**: 14-53.
Moran, E., McGowan, S.T., McGuire, J.M., Frankland, J.E., Oyebade, I.A., Waller, W., Archer, L.C., Morris, L.O., Pandya, J., Nathan, S.R., Smith, L., Cadette and M.L., Michalowski, J.T., 2000, A systematic approach to the validation of process control parameters for monoclonal antibody production in fed-batch culture of a murine myeloma. *Biotechnology &.Bioengeneering* **69**: 242-255.
van der Pol, L.A., Tramper, J., 1998, Shear sensitivity from a culture medium perspective. *TibTech* **16**: 323-328.
Rathore, A., and Velayudhan, A., 2003, Guidelines for Optimization and Scale-Up in preparative chromatography. *BioPharm* **16 (1)**: 34- 42.
Reichert, J.M., 2000, New biopharmaceuticals in the USA: trends in development and marketing approvals 1995-1999. *TibTech* **18**: 364-369.
Sofer, G., 2003, Virus Inactivation in the 1990s – Part 4, culture media, biotechnology products, and vaccines. *BioPharm* **16 (1)**:: 50-57.
The Biopharmaceutical Process Extractables Core Team, 2002, Evaluation of Extractables from Product-Contact Surfaces. *BioPharm* **15 (12)**: 22-34.
Walsh, G., 2000, Biopharmaceutical benchmarks. *Nature Biotechnology* **18**: 831-833
Warner, T.N., and Nochumson, S., 2003, Rethinking the economics of chromatography. *BioPharm* **16 (1)**: 58-60.

Chapter 10

THE PHARMACOKINETICS AND PHARMACODYNAMICS OF MONOCLONAL ANTIBODIES
Preclinical and clinical safety evaluations

David B. Haughey and Paula M. Jardieu
Prevalere Life Sciences, Inc., One Halsey Road, Whitesboro, N.Y.

1. INTRODUCTION

The genetic engineering of an immunoglobulin construct with the variable region of a mouse monoclonal antibody (mAb) and the constant region of a human immunoglobulin has resulted in the development and production of chimeric mouse/human mAbs with improved biologic activity, long residence times and reduced immunogenicity (Morrison *et al.*, 1984, Morrison, 1985). In an attempt to further reduce immunogenicity, recombinant DNA technology has been used to generate "humanized" mAbs with mouse sequences largely confined to the hypervariable regions.

Monoclonal antibodies have been targeted towards a diverse array of endogenous substrates, biologic receptors, malignant cell types, tumors, toxins, and drugs.

Antibodies do not undergo oxidative metabolism, they bind to cell surface receptors, and are then internalized, trafficked, and sorted within the cell for transcytosis, recycling, or lysosomal degradation (Fig. 10.1). In some cells, the entire membrane surface is internalized and replenished in approximately 30 minutes (Marsh and Helenius, 1980).

Monoclonal antibody clearance is a balance between the formation of mAb:antigen complex, binding to FcγR receptors that traffic IgG for lysosomal metabolism, and the protection from lysosomal degradation that occurs following binding of IgG to the FcRn receptor. It is thought that the

FcRn receptor recycles IgG from endosomes thus extending the plasma half-life of IgG and conserving antibody through a "salvage pathway".

Pharmacokinetic (PK) models have been extended to describe elements of physiologic processes such as receptor-mediated endocytosis, transcytosis, receptor salvage pathways, and neutralizing antibody formation that are unique to mAbs and other large molecules (Bauer et al., 1999, Mould et al., 1999).

PK models account for saturable uptake or binding to receptors to explain the disposition characteristics of mAbs and other macromolecules (Froehlich et al., 1995, Sharma et al., 2000, Mager and Jusko, 2002). Pharmacokinetic models are also used for dose selection in animal safety studies and to generate mAb exposure parameters (Baxter et al., 1995; Mordenti et al., 1999, Lin et al., 1999).

Immunogenic responses to therapeutic antibodies may have a pronounced effect on mAb disposition. A 5- to 100-fold increase in the clearance of an antitumor immunoconjugate resulted from the formation of neutralizing antibodies (NAB) after repeat administration in rats and dogs (Damle et al., 2000).

Pharmacodynamic (PD) models have been derived to provide a mechanistic approach to describe the effect versus time course of mAbs. PK/PD models offer a theoretical framework for understanding the mechanism of mAb action (Benincosa et al., 2000, Chow et al., 2002).

PK/PD modeling has been recommended by the FDA to identify possible toxicities in human safety studies, estimate the likelihood and severity of adverse mAb effects, determine the impact of immunogenic responses, and to identify a safe mAb starting dose and dose escalation schedules (Anon., 1997).

2. PHARMACOKINETICS

2.1 Absorption

Monoclonal antibodies are large proteins that range in molecular weight from approximately 150,000 to 970,000 daltons. Antibodies are subject to proteolytic degradation in the gastrointestinal tract and are not absorbed after oral administration.

Transcytosis of IgG across the fetal and neonatal small intestine and placenta is mediated via the neonatal Fc receptor (FcRn) to provide passive immunity transfer from mother to newborn.

The secretion and subsequent neonatal absorption of maternal antibodies from amniotic fluid and milk is reported in rodents. (Brambell, 1966) However, in humans, the passive transport of IgG from mother to fetus likely occurs via FcRn-mediated placental transfer (Ghetie and Ward, 2000).

In adults, the neonatal Fc receptor is present on the brush border of human small intestine, and is also expressed in the liver and mammary gland (Simister, 1989, Israel *et al.*, 1997, Berryman and Rodewald, 1995). The primary function of the human intestinal FcRn receptor in adults appears to be the maintenance of immunosurveillance and host defense at mucosal sites; and to maintain steady-state distribution of IgGs across the intestinal epithelial barrier of the small intestine. Binding to this receptor by immunoglobulin isotypes dramatically increases the immunoglobulin half-life (Table 10.1). Bidirectional transport of IgGs across polarized intestinal epithelial cells by FcRn-dependent transcytosis has been demonstrated using human cell lines (Dickinson *et al.*, 1999).

Monoclonal antibodies are slowly absorbed after subcutaneous (SC) or intramuscular (IM) injection. (Supersaxo *et al.*, 1990). Antibodies diffuse into the lymphatic fluid that drains the injection site, and are apparently absorbed into the circulation through junctional complexes that regulate the barrier function of the vascular wall in high endothelial venules (HEVs). HEVs contain intercellular complexes that are quite leaky, and are regulated by a novel protein family (JAM) that controls vascular permeability to lymphocytes and presumably macromolecules (Aurrand-Lions *et al.*, 2001).

Drug exposure in preclinical safety studies is assessed from area under the mAb plasma concentration versus time curve (AUC) which is directly related to the mAbs bioavailability. Exposure is also determined from the maximum mAb plasma concentration (C_{max}) which is a function of the rate and extent of absorption.

The bioavailability of an anti-respiratory syncytial virus mAb in rats was 83% after SC and 91% after IM injection, and was 82-100% in macaques following IM administration (Davis *et al.*, 1995). An anti-vascular endothelial growth factor mAb had a bioavailabilty of 69% in rats and 100% in mice and monkeys following SC administration (Lin *et al.*, 1999). A humanized mAb directed to human interlukin-5 had a bioavailability of 100% in monkeys (Zia-Amirhosseini *et al.*, 1999). However, after SC or IM doses the maximum plasma concentrations (C_{max}) of these mAbs were nearly 30-50% lower than an equivalent intravenous dose. The time of maximum plasma concentration (t_{max}) often exceeded 1 or 2 days (Davis *et al.*, 1995, Lin *et al.*, 1999, Zia-Amirhoseini *et al.*, 1999).

The prolonged absorption of mAbs following SC or IM injection must be considered in the design of safety studies. It is necessary to collect blood samples for PK evaluation over a sufficient time interval in order to obtain an accurate estimate of C_{max}.

Moreover, transplacental transfer of therapeutic monoclonal antibodies may have implications in the design of toxicology studies for the assessment of reproductive toxicology and teratogenicity.

2.2 Distribution

Upon IV administration mAbs initially distribute into a space that is equivalent to total plasma volume in most species (Eger *et al.*, 1987, Fox *et al.*, 1996, Lin *et al.*, 1999, and Davis *et al.*, 1995).

Antibodies exit the vascular space by diffusion through junctional complexes located within the endothelial cells of HEVs and other blood vessels. (Aurrand-Lions *et al.*, 2001).

Diffusion and specific transport mechanisms deliver mAbs across epithelial barriers to specific sites within the body (Baxter *et al.*, 1995). Saturable and non-saturable tissue binding and a bidirectional exchange of mAb between plasma and the extravascular compartment has been demonstrated (Eger *et al*, 1987, Zia-Amirhosseini *et al*, 1999, Davis *et al*, 1995).

Because mAbs distribute to plasma or to a lesser extent the more permeable interstitial fluid spaces of the liver, spleen, and lymph, the steady-state volume of distribution of many mAbs is less than extracellular fluid volume. (Egger *et al.*, 1987, Trang *et al.*, 1990, Tanswell *et al.*, 2001, Gobburu *et al.*, 1998).

The decline in plasma mAb concentrations is therefore multiexponential after intravenous administration. The initial decline in plasma concentration is a result of the movement of mAb from plasma to the extravascular space, and the result of tissue or cell binding of the antibody (Eger *et al*, 1987). A physiologic model approach has been proposed to account for the specific and non-specific tissue binding of antibodies (Baxter *et al.*, 1995).

The initial distribution half-life of a human monoclonal anti-respiratory syncytial virus was 6-7 hours in the rat, and 24 hours in the macaque after IV administration (Davis *et al*, 1995). The distribution half-life of a humanized anti-vascular endothelial growth factor mAb was approximately 1 hour in the mouse, 7 hours in the rat and ranged from 10 to 25 hours in the monkey (Lin *et al*, 1999). Safety studies to assess the mAb plasma/tissue ratio require a sufficient period of time (approximately 4-5 distribution half-lives) before distribution equilibrium is attained following an intravenous dose. It is only in the post-distributive phase that the fraction of drug in the plasma compartment is constant (Gibaldi, M. and Perrier, D., 1975).

2.3 Elimination

The cellular uptake, transport, and lysosomal degradation of an immunoglobulin occurs via receptor-mediated endocytosis. Phagocytes, granulocytes, monocytes, lymphocytes, and platelets express a family of IgG receptors with varying affinity for the IgG subclasses, and determine the rates of IgG clearance after the formation of immune complexes, (de Haas, M., 2001).

Moreover, immune complex-formation is not a pre-requisite for receptor mediated endocytosis. The binding of monomeric IgG to a high affinity receptor (FcγRI), in the absence of cross-linking is sufficient to recycle monomeric IgG and receptor. Cross-linking the occupied receptor results in lysosomal degradation of the immune complex whereas monomeric bound IgG and receptor undergo recycling (Harrison *et al.*, 1994).

Recycling of IgG is also mediated by the neonatal Fc receptor expressed by endothelial cells, hepatocytes, and intestinal epithelial cells (Dickinson *et al.*, 1999). The FcRn receptor performs a "scavenger function" to protect IgG from lysosomal degradation. IgGs that do not bind avidly to FcRns accumulate in lysosomes and have relatively short residence times (Ward *et al.*, 2003, Ober, *et al.*, 2001). Table 10.1 summarises the biologic half-life values estimated for endogenous human immunoglobulins.

Table 10.1. Biologic Half-life Values of Endogenous Human Immunoglobulins

Type/Isotype	Half-life, days	FcRn Binding
IgG1	23	+
IgG2	23	+
IgG3	8	+
IgG4	23	+
IgM	5	-
IgA1	6	-
IgA2	6	-
IgD	3	-
IgE	2.5	-

The disposition of antibodies used for therapeutic applications may also depend on the specific isotype of the mAb, host immunogenic responses, the amount of antigen or target receptor; the pleiotropic nature of the antibody preparation, and host receptor-mediated uptake/elimination. Many of these processes are species specific and care should be taken translating results between species.

A two-compartment PK model with linear or non-linear elimination kinetics is adequate to describe the time course of mAb exposure in animals and humans (Benincosa *et al.*, 2000, Gobburu *et al.*, 1998, Sharma *et al.*, 2000).

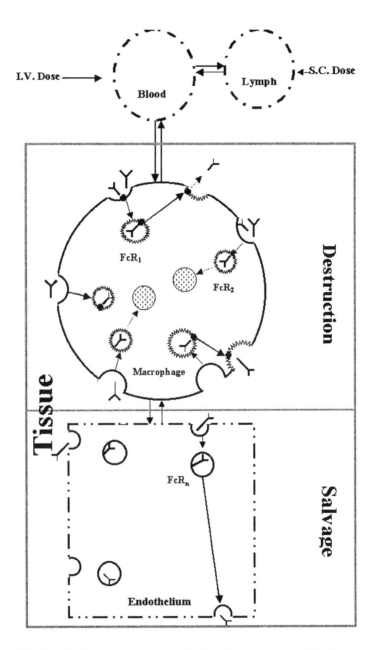

Figure 10.1. Simplified representation of mAb disposition and nonspecific clearance following intravenous and subcutaneous administration

Monoclonal antibodies bind with high affinity to receptors and target antigens. The molar ratio of receptor or target antigen to mAb is high compared to conventional low molecular weight drugs, and the disposition of some mAbs is sensitive to changes in the amount of antigen or receptor (Meijer et al., 2002).

The formation of neutralizing antibodies (NAB) directed against a therapeutic mAb may have a profound effect on the mAb's distribution and clearance. (Damle et al., 2000, Baert et al., 2003).

To illustrate the effects of NAB formation, data from the literature was used to develop a pharmacokinetic model. Model-based computer simulations were performed to describe the pharmacokinetics and immune response of a ^{131}I-chimeric mouse/human B72.3 (human γ4) monoclonal antibody directed against a colorectal tumor antigen (data extracted from Khazaeli et al., 1991).

Four patients received a single intravenous injection of 18mCi/m^2 of ^{131}I-ch-B72.3(γ4) that was followed by a second intravenous dose 8 weeks after the first dose (Khazaeli et al., 1991). A PK model was constructed that considered the distribution of antibody (AB) from the vascular space (p) into tissue (t) as a reversible first-order process and first order elimination of AB from plasma (k_{10}). After the second dose, the model was modified to account for the formation of neutralizing antibody (NAB) by a zero order process (R_{syn}/V_{NAB}).

The complexation of neutralizing antibody and ^{131}I-chimeric mouse/human B72.3 (NAB:AB) was described with a second order association rate constant (k_{on}) and first order dissociation rate constant (k_{off}). Elimination of NAB:AB and NAB were both assumed to occur by first order processes (k_{40} and k_{30}).

The model is a modification of a neutralizing antibody model reported previously to characterise the immunogenic responses to interferon-β in humans (Mager and Jusko, 2002). A schematic representation of the model is provided (Fig. 10.2)

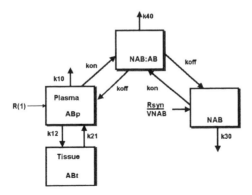

Figure 10.2. Proposed model used to simulate neutralizing antibody inactivation following repeat injection

After the first mAb dose, the disposition of B72.3 (human γ4) monoclonal antibody was described using a two-compartment model (Fig. 10.3). The central distribution volume of 0.0286 L/Kg indicates that the mAb initially distributed into a space less than plasma volume. A steady-state distribution volume of 0.085 L/Kg indicated that the mAb also distributed from the vascular space into a space less than extravascular fluid volume. Plasma clearance (CL_p) was approximately 0.282 mL/Kg/hr and distribution clearance (Cld) was 3.07 mL/Kg/hr. The terminal half-life was 163 hr, which is less than the half-life of endogenous IgG4 in humans (Morell *et al.*, 1970). In the post-distribution phase, the fraction of mAb in the plasma compartment was approximately 50% of the total amount of drug in the body.

After administration of the second dose of B72.3 (human γ4) monoclonal antibody at week 8 there was a marked alteration in its disposition. Administration of the second antibody dose stimulated a strong immune response to the B72.3 (human γ-4) monoclonal antibody. Prior to the second infusion of mAb, the plasma concentration of neutralizing antibody was approximately 947 pM/L. After the second mAb dose, the neutralizing antibosy (NAB) concentration increased to about 14900 pM/L and remained near this level for at least 6 weeks.

The "apparent" plasma mAb clearance after repeat infusion was increased to 5.52 mL/Kg/hr, the "apparent" Vc was increased to 0.128 L/Kg, and the "apparent" Vss was increased to 0.142 L/Kg.

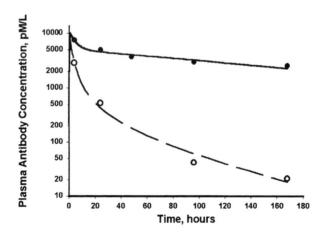

Figure 10.3. Observed and computer simulated plasma mAb concentrations following infusion of antibody on week 1 (closed circle, solid line) and week 8 (open circle, broken line)

The production of neutralizing antibody was considered a zero-order process for modeling purposes. The measured and computer simulated plasma concentrations of neutralizing antibody are displayed in Figure 10.4. Based on this simulation, it is obvious that maintaining exposure of the therapeutic mAb cannot be overcome by increasing the antibody dose. Likewise, it is unlikely that an adequate exposure ratio of mAb would be maintained in preclinical toxicology studies in the presence of NAB formation.

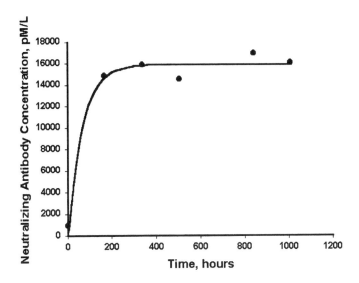

Figure 10.4. Observed (circles) and computer simulated (line) neutralizing antibody concentrations in plasma following repeat infusion of chimeric mouse/human B72.3 (human γ-4) antibody

The computer model was also used to simulate the time course of neutralizing antibody:B72.3 (human γ-4) mAb complex (Fig. 10.5).

There was an initial rapid increase in the predicted amount of immune complex formed, the amount of immune complex was predicted to reach a maximum at approximately 16 hours and then decline in parallel with plasma mAb concentrations.

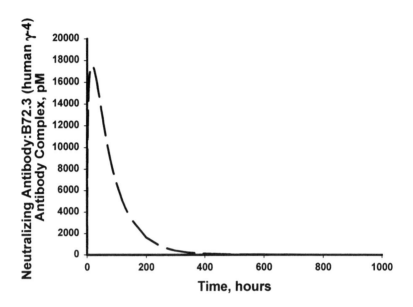

Figure 10.5. Computer simulation of the time course of neutralizing antibody:B72.3 (human γ-4) monoclonal antibody complex in a colorectal cancer patient following repeat mAb infusion.

Although chimerization can diminish anti-antibody responses, the foreign V region framework of some chimeric constructs is apparently sufficient to generate a strong anti-antibody response.

This concept was demonstrated in another study with a chimeric monoclonal IgG1 antibody directed against tumor necrosis factor that resulted in the formation of neutralizing antibodies in 61% of patients that received this mAb for the treatment of Crohn's disease. Moreover, patients with a high titre of NAB were 2.4 times more likely to have an infusion reaction. Patients that had an infusion reaction had a short duration of clinical response (38.5 days versus 65 days) compared to patients that did not have adverse reactions (Baert *et al.*, 2003).

2.4 Interspecies Scaling

Physiologic functions and anatomic parameters for small organic molecules frequently scale across species when expressed as a power function of body weight. (Adolph, 1949, Weiss *et al.*, 1977). Allometry and physiologic models have been applied to the interspecies scaling of small organic molecules but there are sparse published data on the interspecies scaling of mAbs (Mordenti, 1986, Bischoff *et al.*, 1971, Zaharko *et al.*, 1972).

Allometric scaling is particularly suited to the evaluation of preclinical data when the physical processes for drug disposition are linear and first order, such as biliary secretion, renal excretion, and pulmonary excretion. Allometry may have limited utility for compounds that are metabolised, exhibit non-linear or saturable disposition, and are subject to species specific or saturable binding (Mordenti *et al.*, 1991).

Monoclonal antibodies and other macromolecules exhibit linear and non-linear tissue uptake. The predominant clearance mechanism at concentrations exceeding ligand concentrations is Fcγ receptor-mediated. Monoclonal antibodies are not subject to significant renal excretion or hepatic oxidative metabolism.

In one study, allometric scaling was used to analyse the clearance and volume of distribution of five human proteins (recombinant CD4, CD4 immunoglobulin G, growth hormone, tissue-plasminogen activator, and relaxin) (Mordenti *et al.*, 1991). The CL, V_c, and V_{ss} for these 5 proteins was well described by an allometric relationship, and the animal data obtained in from 3 to 6 species was predictive of human data (Mordenti, *et al.*, 1991).

Allometric scaling involves the generation of pharmacokinetic parameters in several species using noncompartmental or compartmental methods. The pharmacokinetic parameters are then scaled to a function of body mass with a power function of the form $Y = a \bullet W^b$, Y represents the pharmacokinetic parameter of interest, W is the animal's body mass and b is an exponent. Using this approach, biologic time functions (*i.e.* half-life) typically have an exponent of 0.25, biologic rates have an exponent of about 0.75, and volumes tend to have an exponent of approximately 1.0 (Mordenti *et al.*, 1991).

Data was extracted from the literature to perform allometric scaling of an anti-respiratory syncytial virus human monoclonal IgG1 antibody in the rat, cynomolgus macaque, and infant baboon (Davis *et al.*, 1995). Linear transformation of the power function to an equation of the form $\log Y = \log a + b \bullet \log W$ was used to analyse the data by ANOVA regression analysis. The PK variables included CL, V_{ss}, and $t_{1/2}$, and approximate average body weights of each species were extrapolated from literature values in the rat (300 gm), adult macaque (5.9 Kg) and infant baboon (2.0 Kg). The log-log plots of CL, V_{ss}, and $t_{1/2}$ versus body weight are shown in Figure 10.6. The data was well described using the log transformations, and the r^2 values for CL, V_{ss} and $t_{1/2}$ versus body weight were 0.9790, 0.9979, and 0.8842, respectively. The exponent values were 0.751 for CL, 0.9868 for V_{ss}, and 0.2544 for $t_{1/2}$.

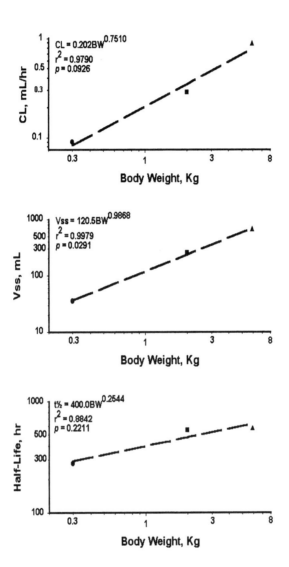

Figure 10.6. Allometric scaling of an anti-respiratory syncytial virus mAb in the Sprague-Dawley rat (circle), adult cynomolgus macaque (Macaca fasicularis, triangle), and infant baboon (Papio cyanocephalus, square).

These allometric exponents would be expected for small organic molecules and therapeutic proteins, that are eliminated by linear, first order processes without dose-dependent disposition or stimulation of an immune response (Mordenti *et al.*, 1991).

The allometric scaling results were used to predict the CL, V_{ss} and $t_{1/2}$ values in a 70 Kg human. The predicted values were compared to the PK parameters reported in the literature after intravenous administration of a single 1.25 mg/Kg dose (Everitt *et al.*, 1996).

In humans, the allometric scaling of V_{ss} was more reliable than the predictive value of the allometric model for CL and $t_{1/2}$. The observed mean $\pm$ SD and predicted values in a 70 Kg human were 8.54 $\pm$1.26 mL/hr versus 5.06 mL/hr for CL, 7280 $\pm$ 525 mL versus 7972 mL for V_{ss}, and 603 $\pm$ 115 hr versus 1179 hr, respectively.

Physiologic flow models provide an alternate approach to interspecies scaleup that is mechanism-based, and seeks to characterise the underlying anatomy, physiology and biochemistry of the drug disposition process.

A model is constructed that includes pertinent tissues and organs that eliminate or bind drug (Figure 10.7).

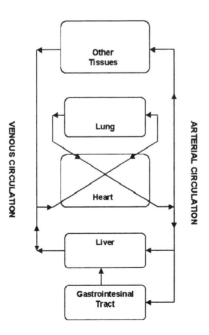

Figure 10.7. Schematic representation of a physiologic flow model.

These compartments are connected by an anatomically correct flow scheme to account for the arterial and venous transport, tissue and organ uptake, and/or elimination of drug in a single species.

The mathematical representation of the model is obtained by writing mass balance equations for the uptake and/or elimination of drug in each compartment and the differential equations are solved simultaneously by computer. Once the model is defined in a species, the physiologic parameters can be modified based on knowledge of human anatomy, physiology, and the drugs partitioning characteristics to predict the disposition characteristics in humans.

The physiologic approach is preferred for compounds that are highly lipid soluble, extensively metabolised, or when the distribution properties of the compound are important. The physiologic approach has some advantages in being able to characterise the disposition of compounds that exhibit non-linear distribution and elimination, or if there is only one relevant species to obtain animal data (Mordenti, 1986).

The extrapolation of results obtained in animals to predict the disposition characteristics of mAbs in humans should be performed with due caution. Antibodies are typically species specific, and the target antigens may not be expressed or may not be recognized to the same degree across species (Klingbeil and Hsu, 1999). For instance, the neonatal Fc receptor has different binding affinities for IgG in the mouse and human. Human FcRn binds to human, rabbit, and guinea pig IgG1 but not significantly to rat, bovine, sheep, or mouse IgG1. The mouse FcRn binds to each of the above species IgG1 (Ober *et al.*, 2001). Systematic studies with other human isotypes of IgG have not been reported.

Likewise, mouse FcγR receptors bind to human IgG1. Thus predictions of non-specific clearance rates for this antibody isotype in humans can often be made from mouse data.

Specific clearance data can only be obtained if the mAb binds target antigen across relevant species. For example, an anti-VEGF humanized mAb binds to primate but not rat or mouse vascular endothelial growth factor, therefore total clearance of anti-VEGF may not be accurately extrapolated from the mouse to humans (Ryan *et al.*, 1999).

The construct of transgenic animal models in which mice are genetically altered to express human target receptors may prove useful in establishing a pertinent species for the estimation of total clearance in mAb disposition studies (Davis *et al.*, 1996).

Coupled with exposure data from preclinical efficacy and toxicity models, sufficient information may be available from interspecies scaling to cautiously estimate a safe and efficacious dosing regimen in humans. Given the ease and reliability of simulating exposure using PK models, interspecies scaling from preclinical toxicology studies should be examined to provide an initial dose estimate for first-in-man studies.

3. PHARMACODYNAMICS

Knowledge of the relationship between drug concentration at the site of action and the drug's pharmacologic effects or side effects is essential to the design of safety and toxicity studies for drug development programs. The information is also used to identify effective and safe dosage regimens for first-in-man studies.

Pharmacokinetic (PK) /pharmacodynamic (PD) models seek to link the changes in drug concentration at the site of action and the intensity of observed response to describe the time course of effect (Levy, 1986, Derendorf and Meibohm, 1999). Pharmacodynamic models may include any desired or undesired effects that result from the drug or it's metabolites. The responses can be directly related to concentration of the drug or metabolite at the effect site without time-lag. The responses may be indirect, and not related to the concentration at the site of action, or by simply accounting for a distributional process (Gibaldi and Perrier, 1982, Derendorf and Meibohm, 1999). Indirect response modeling was first used by Nagashima *et al.*, to describe the kinetics of prothrombin complex activity synthesis and degradation to define the anticoagulant action of warfarin (Nagashima *et al.*, 1969).

If the observed effects are directly related to the concentration of drug at the site of action, and the effect site and plasma drug concentrations are in rapid equilibrium, under steady-state conditions the sigmoid E_{max} model is an empirical function that can be used to describe the plasma drug concentration-effect relationship: $E = E_{max} \cdot C^n / (EC_{50}^n + C^n)$. E_{max} is the maximum effect, EC_{50} is the concentration of the drug that produces half-maximum effect, and n is a constant used to impart adequate shape to the effect versus concentration curve.

Many drugs, however, act indirectly by altering the rate of production or loss of response from a baseline value. Some drugs inhibit one or more factors controlling the rate of input or dissipation of drug response, others may stimulate these factors (Dayneka *et al.*, 1993). For such drugs, the drug effects have been shown to depend on both the rate of production (k_{in}) and rate of loss (k_{out}) of the response factor as well as the time course of drug concentrations (Dayneka *et al.*, 1993).

Indirect response models describe the pharmacodynamics of many biotechnology derived products that modulate the production or dissipation of blood cells, endogenous compounds, hormones, or other substances

(Sharma *et al.*, 2000, Zia-Amirhosseini, 1999, Gobburu *et al.*, 1999, Gobburu *et al.*, 1998).

The kinetic characteristics of a drug, including the biophase kinetics, the response turnover rate, potency, and intrinsic activity may be discerned in the absence of measured drug concentrations from response versus time data, (Gabrielsson *et al.*, 2000). The use of kinetic forcing functions in pharmacodynamic modeling for the purpose of characterising drug response data may have some utility in early preclinical studies that are conducted before sensitive analytical procedures can be developed (Gabrielsson *et al.*, 2000).

3.1 Pharmacodynamic Markers

Pharmacodynamic models provide information about the mechanism of action of a drug and dose-response relationship. The responses may be a direct or indirect measure of efficacy, safety or toxicity. A pertinent response variable has clinical relevance to the drug's efficacy or toxicity. To be useful response variables used in preclinical animal studies must provide information that can extrapolate to humans.

For example, many mAbs exhibit interspecies differences in affinity and specificity. Although humans and other primates express the CD4 antigen on T cells, the administration of an anti-CD4 mAb depleted circulating T cells at high doses in monkeys, but did not cause T cell depletion in the chimpanzee. The differences in T cell depletion between monkey and chimpanzee were shown to result from species differences in the expression of CD4 antigen (Fishwild *et al.*, 1999).

Response variables have been categorised as biologic markers (biomarkers), surrogate end-points, or clinical end-points (Derendorf *et al.*, 2000). Biomarkers are a measure of laboratory, biochemical or physiologic response not related to the therapeutic or toxic effects of a drug in a specific disease or process. Biomarkers are generally not acceptable end-point for evaluating effectiveness or safety, but they can provide insight regarding the mechanism of action. An example of this, are the studies aimed at suppression of eosinophil growth factor (IL-5) as a treatment for asthma. The PK/PD relationship for an anti-IL-5 antibody was developed to predict the level of suppression of eosinophils following anti-IL-5 treatment (Foster *et al.*, 2002). While the PK/PD model was useful for predicting eosinophil suppression among patients, the model had no correlate with clinical benefit (Leckie *et al.*, 2000).

A surrogate end-point is a specific effect that may substitute for a clinical end-point and can be used to reliably predict clinical effectiveness or safety (Derendorf and Meibohm, 1999). Surrogate end-points are typically physiologic (*i.e.* blood pressure) or laboratory measurements (*i.e.* serum cholesterol), or biochemical indices (*i.e.* prostate specific antigen).

In order for a surrogate end-point to be used to support efficacy or safety it must be validated, and also demonstrate relevance, reliability, and accuracy (Derendorf *et al.*, 2000, Colburn, 1997). It is essential to establish a strong link between the surrogate end-point measure and the clinical effectiveness or safety of the drug product. In the case of anti-CD4 treatment, saturating the CD4 receptor on T cells with a mAb to CD4 is a determinant of clinical response. Surprisingly, clinical response does not correlate well with CD4 cell depletion. This speaks to the need to validate and show the clinical relevance of the surrogate (Mason *et al.*, 2002).

Clinical end-points provide a direct measure of patient response such as survival, symptom remission rate, cure rate, onset of adverse effects or any other clinical outcome measure. These end-points may be categorical, a response rate, or survival curve, and may be difficult to accurately quantify and integrate into PK/PD models.

Regulatory guidelines for the pharmacodynamic modeling of prospective drug candidates have been established for the pharmaceutical industry describing the use of dose- or concentration-response data in the drug development and registration process (Anonomous, 1994).

3.2   PK/PD Modeling

PK and PD models are by necessity an oversimplification of the complex physiologic processes and molecular reactions that they seek to characterise. An integrated PK/PD model is constructed to understand the underlying mechanisms of drug action and to arrive at a mechanism-based approach to predicting drug action so that extrapolations to other species or clinical situations is possible.

There are excellent reviews in the literature that provide a comprehensive and conceptual approach to PK/PD modeling (Derendorf and Meibohm, 1999, Derendorf *et al.*, 2000).

The concentration of a drug or an active metabolite in plasma may or may not represent the concentration at the site of action. There may exist a temporal dissociation between the time course of measured plasma concentrations and the observed physiologic responses. Integrated PK/PD models are therefore linked (directly or indirectly) to jointly account for the time course of drug concentrations and pharmacologic effects (Derendorf and Meibohm, 1999, Derendorf *et al.*, 2000).

The link between a PK and PD model has been further characterised by Derendorf *et al.* as hard or soft. The soft link PK/PD models are typically "effect compartment" models that are descriptive in nature. They have been used to account for the hysteresis in concentration versus effect relationship that arises when the site of drug action is kinetically distinct from the site of PK sampling (Holford and Sheiner, 1982, Sheiner et al., 1979).

Hard link models are mechanism-based and use laboratory-derived parameters such as receptor binding measurements, minimum inhibitory concentration values, and receptor density values, in addition to PK information to predict the time course of drug effect (Xu et al., 1995).

PK/PD models are further identified by the time-dependent nature of their PD-parameters. Time invariant models infer an effect intensity that is secondary to the drug concentrations and the PD parameters are stationary (Derendorf and Meibohm, 1999). Most PK/PD models exhibit time-invariant characteristics.

The pharmacodynamic parameters of time-variant models are not stationary. Therefore, the effect intensity at any given drug concentration at the site of action may not be constant. A decrease in effect intensity may arise due to tolerance (clockwise hysteresis of the effect versus concentration curve) that occurs after multiple dosing. A mechanism based PK/PD model was used to describe the hemodynamic tolerance to nitroglycerin (Bauer and Fung, 1994).

Sensitization (counterclockwise hysteresis of the effect versus concentration curve) is an increase in drug intensity at the same drug concentration.

Racine-Poon et al. constructed a time-invariant, hard-link, direct response PK/PD model to describe the time-course of free IgE serum concentrations in patients with seasonal allergic rhinitis that received biweekly doses of an anti-immunoglobulin E chimeric monoclonal antibody (Racine-Poon, 1997).

The PK component was a two-compartment model, consistent with that used to characterise the kinetics of IgG antibodies in humans. The predicted population mean (SE) PK parameters of the anti-IgE antibody were $\alpha = 0.365$ (0.116) d^{-1}, $\beta = 0.046$ (0.014) d^{-1}, $V_c = 3.45$ L, and $k_{21} = 0.161(0.061)$ d^{-1} for an 80kg patient with baseline IgE levels of 250 IU/mL. A modified (inhibitory) E_{max} model was used to describe the serum concentrations of IgE:

$$IgE = IgE_0 \bullet (1 - (C^{\eta}/(C^{\eta} + IC_{50}^{\eta})))."$$

IgE_0 represents the baseline serum IgE concentration and C represents the plasma mAb concentration. IC_{50} is the concentration of mAb necessary to produce a 50% reduction in serum free IgE concentration. The variable η is a parameter used to define the shape of the IgE response curve. The baseline IgE$_0$ value was 250 IU/mL, the IC$_{50}$ value was 179 ng/mL and η was 0.516 (Racine-Poon, 1997).

We used the PK/PD model of Racine-Poon *et al.* to simulate the expected time course of anti-IgE mAb after multiple 60 mg IV doses in an 80 Kg patient with baseline IgE$_0$ levels of 250 U/mL and 1000 U/mL (Figure 10.8).

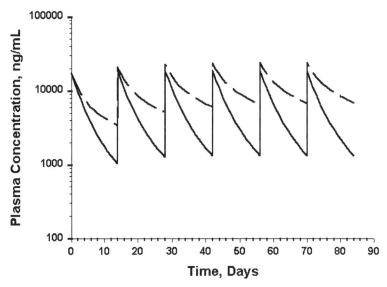

Figure 10.8. Model predicted time course of anti-IgE mAb serum concentrations following 60 mg doses of anti-IgE mAb in an 80 Kg patient (IgE$_0$ = 250 IU/mL, broken line; IgE$_0$ = 1000 IU/mL, solid line)

The predicted serum anti-IgE mAb concentrations after the third dose and for all subsequent doses were above the level needed to achieve a clinical response (~ 5200 ng/mL) for a patient with baseline IgE$_0$ levels of 250 U/mL. In comparison, the model predicted serum concentrations of mAb in an 80 Kg patient with baseline IgE$_0$ levels of 1000 U/mL are subtherapeutic for approximately 9 days during each 14-day dosing interval.

The model simulated values for percent reduction of free serum IgE concentrations are provided in Figure 10.9.

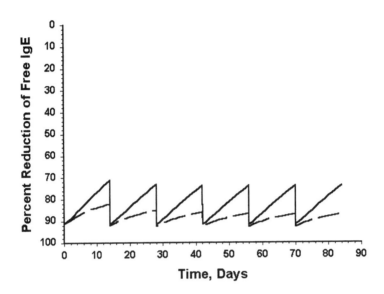

Figure 10.9. Model predicted reduction in serum IgE levels in an 80 Kg patient following multiple 60 mg doses of anti-IgE mab (broken line, IgE_0 = 250 IU/mL; solid line, IgE_0 = 1000 IU/mL)

An immediate reduction (>90%) of free IgE is predicted following each dose and a sustained reduction in serum IgE beyond the clinically relevant threshold value of 85% was predicted when the baseline IgE serum concentration was 250 IU/mL. At a baseline IgE_0 level of 1000 U/mL, the there was an initial rapid reduction in free serum IgE but subtherapeutic responses (<85% reduction in free serum IgE) were predicted for much of the dosing interval.

The outcome of this analysis revealed that dosing by body weight alone would not result in efficacious levels of the anti-IgE antibody for all patients. Not until the PD marker (baseline IgE level) is included in the model, could the model be used to predict the therapeutic dose needed to achieve a clinically significant reduction in serum IgE. This approach demonstrates the utility of PK/PD modeling to enhance the probability of clinical success in the drug development process.

4. CONCLUSIONS

PK/PD models jointly account for the time course of mAb plasma concentrations and the direct and indirect effects of mAbs. In contrast to low molecular weight drugs, mAbs are eliminated via receptor-mediated endocytosis and lysosomal degradation. The low clearance and long biologic half-life values of mAbs may in part arise from FcRn receptor-mediated recycling. The disposition kinetics of most mAbs is described by linear and stationary first-order elimination. Nonlinear disposition may occur from the saturation of receptor-mediated clearance or capacity-limited mAb transport. Heterolgous antibody proteins are immunogenic, and can evoke the formation of NABs after repeat administration. The formation of NABs can enhance the clearance of mAbs and diminish their effectiveness. PK studies can be useful for the early identification of an immune response, and thus help to identify a problematic antibody construct at an early stage of drug development. Species differences in mAb disposition and pharmacodynamics can arise from the variations in target antigen and antigen affinity between species, and differences in Fc receptor subtype affinity for IgG subclasses among species.

A PK/PD approach can clearly lend value to the drug development process and provide useful insight into the mechanisms of mAb action and for the prediction of safe and efficacious dosage regimens. In the current health care environment, companies are under pressure to provide treatments that add value for cost. Given the high risk and high cost of mAb development, it is imperative to identify early in this process the clinical candidates that have the best chance of success. A thorough understanding of mAbs through PK/PD modeling and simulation represents such an opportunity. The application of these models can be beneficial throughout preclinical and clinical drug development programs resulting in the early identification of optimal dosing and potential shortening of drug development time.

REFERENCES

Adolph, E.F., 1949, Quantitative relations in the physiological constitutions of mammals. *Science*, **109**:579-585

Anonomous, 1994, Dose-response information to support drug registration. *Federal Register* **59**:55972-55976

Anonomous, 1997, Points to consider in the manufacture and testing of monoclonal antibody Products for human use. *FDA Center for* Biologics *Evaluation and Research Document*, 94D-0259, Rockville, MD

Aurrand-Lions, M., Johnson-Leger, C., Wong, C., Du Pasquier, L., and Imhof, B.A., 2001, Heterogeneity of endothelial junctions is reflected by differential expression and specific subcellular localization of three JAM family members. *Blood*, **98**:3699-3707

Baert, F., Noman, M., Vermeire, S., Van Assche, G.V., D'Haens, G., Carbonez, A., and Rutgeerts, P., 2003, Influence of immunogenicity on the long-term efficacy of infliximab in Crohn's disease. *N. Eng. J. Med.*, **348**:601-608

Berryman, M. and Rodewald, R., 1995, Beta-2-microglobulin co-distributes with the heavy chain of the intestinal IgG-Fc receptor throughout the transepithelial transport pathway of the neonatal rat. *J. Cell Sci.*, **108**:2347-2360

Bauer, R.J., Dedrick, R.L., White, M.L., Murray, M.J., and Garovoy, M.R., 1999, Population pharmacokinetics and pharmacodynamics of the anti-CD11a antibody hull24 in human subjects with psoriasis. *J. Pharmacokinet. Biopharm.*, **27**:397-420

Bauer, J.A. and Fung, H.L., 1994, Pharmacodynamic models of nitroglycerin-induced hemodynamic tolerance in experimental heart failure. *Pharm. Res.* **11**:816-823

Baxter, L.T., Zhu H., Mackensen, D.G., Butler, W.F., and Jain, R.K., 1995, Biodistribution of monoclonal antibodies: sacle-up from mouse to human using a physiologically based pharmacokinetic model. *Cancer Res.*, **55**:4611-4622

Benincosa, L.J., Chow, F-S., Tobia, L.P., Kwok, D.C., Davis, C.B., and Jusko, W.J., 2000, Pharmacokinetics and pharmacodynamics of a humanized monoclonal antibody to factor IX in cynomolgus monkeys. *J. Pharmacol. Exp. Ther.*, **292**:810-816

Bischoff, K.B., Dedrick, R.L., Zaharko, D.S., and Longstreth, J.A., 1971, Methotrexate pharmacokinetics. *J. Pharm. Sci.*, **60**:1128-1133

Brambell, F.W., 1966, The transmission of immunity from mother to young and the catabolism of immunoglobulins. *Lancet*, **2**:1087-93

Chow, F-S., Benincosa, L.J., Sheth, S.B., Wilson, D., Davis, C.B., Minthorn, E.A. and Jusko, W.J., 2002, Pharmacokinetic and pharmacodynamic modeling of humanized anti-factor IX antibody (SB 249417) in humans. *J. Pharmacol. Ther.*, **71**:235-245

Colburn, W.A., 1997, Selecting and validating biologic markers for drug development. *J. Clin. Pharmacol.*, **37**:355-362

Damle, B., Tay, L., Comereski, C., Warner, W., and Kaul, S., 2000, Influence of immunogenicity on the pharmacokinetics of BMS-191352, a *Pseudomonas* exotoxin immunoconjugate, in rats and dogs. *J. Pharm. Pharmacol.*, **52**:671-678

Davis, C.B., Hepburn, T.W., Urbanski, J.J., Kwok, D.C., Hart, T.K., Herzyk, D.J., Demuth, S.G., Leland, M., and Rhodes, G.R., 1995, Preclinical pharmacokinetic evaluation of the respiratory syncytial virus-specific reshaped human monoclonal antibody RSHZ19. *Drug Metab. Dispo.*, **23**:1028-1036

Davis, C.B., Garver, E.M., Kwok, D.C., and Urbanski, J.J., 1996, Disposition of metabolically radiolabeled CE9.1-a macaque-human chimeric anti-human CD4 monoclonal antibody- in transgenic mice bearing human CD4. *Drug Metab. Dispo.*, **24**:1032-1037

Dayneka, N., Garg, V., and Jusko, V., 1993, Comparison of four basic models of indirect pharmacodynamic responses. *J. Pharmacokinet. Biopharm.*, **21**:457-478

DeHaas, M., 2001, IgG-Fc receptors and the clinical relevance of their polymorphisms. *Wien. Klin. Wochenschr*, **113**:825-31

Dedrick, R.L. and Bischoff, K.B., 1980, Species similarities in pharmacokinetics. *Fed. Proc.*, **39**:54-59

Derendorf, H. and Meibohm, B., 1999, Modeling of pharmacokinetic/pharmacodynamic (PK/PD) relationships: concepts and perspectives. *Pharm. Res.*, **16**:176-185

Derendorf H., Lesko, L.J., Chaikin, P., Colburn, W.A., Lee, P., Miller, R., Powell, R., Rhodes, G., Stanski, D., Venitz, J., 2000, Pharmacokinetic/pharmacodynamic modeling in drug research and development. *J. Clin. Pharmacol.*, **40**:1399-1418

Dickinson, B.L., Badizadegan, K., Wu, Z., Ahouse, J.C., Zhu, X., Simister, N.E., Blumberg, R.S., and Lencer, W.I., 1999, Bidirectional FcRn-dependent IgG transport in a polarized human intestinal epithelial cell line. *J. Clin. Invest.*, **104**:903-911

Eger, R.R., Covell, D.G., Carrasquillo, J.A., Abrams, P.G., Foon, K.A., Reynolds, J.C., Schroff, R.W., Morgan, A.C., Larson, S.M., and Weinstein, J.N., 1987, Kinetic model for the biodistribution of an ^{111}In-labeled monoclonal antibody in humans. *Cancer Res.*, **47**:3328-3336

Everitt, D.E., Davis, C.B., Thompson, K., DiCicco, R., Ilson, B., Demuth, S.G., Herzyk, D.J., and Jorkasky, D.K., 1996, The pharmacokinetics, antigenicity, and fusion-inhibition activity of RSHZ19, a humanized monoclonal antibody to respiratory syncytial virus, in healthy volunteers. *J. Infect. Dis.*, **174**:463-469

Fishwild, D.M., Hudson, D.V., Deshpande U., Kung, A.H., 1999, Differential effects of administration of a human anti-CD4 monoclonal antibody, HMG6, in nonhuman primates. *Clin. Immunol.* **92**:138-152

Foster, P.S., Hogan, S.P., Yang, M., Mattes, J., Young, I.G., Matthaei, K.I., Kumar, R.K., Mahalingam, S., and Webb, D.C., 2002, Interleukin-5 and eosinophils as therapeutic agents for asthma. *Trends. Mol. Sci.*, **8**:162-167

Fox, J.A., Hotaling, T.E., Struble, C., Ruppel, J., Bates, D.J., and Schoenhoff, M.B., 1996, Tissue distribution and comples formation with IgE of and anti-IgE antibody after intravenous administration in cynomolgus monkeys. *J. Pharmacol. Exp. Ther.*, **279**:1000-1008

Froelich, J., Schoenhoff, M., Tremblay, T., Ruppel, B.A., and Jardieu, P., 1995, Initial human study with a humanized recombinant anti-IgE monoclonal antibody: safety, tolerance and pharmacokinetic (PK)/Dynamic profile. *Clin. Pharmacol. Ther.*, **67**:162

Gabrielsson, J., Jusko, W.J., and Alari, L., 2000, Modeling of dose-response-time data: four examples of estimating the turnover parameters and generating kinetic functions from response profiles. *Biopharm. Drug Dispos.*, **21**:41-52

Ghetie, V. and Ward, E.S., 2000, Multiple roles for the major histocompatability complex class I-related receptor FcRn. *Ann. Rev. Immunol.*, **18**:739-766

Gibaldi, M. and Perrier, D., 1975, Pharmacokinetics. In *Drugs and the Pharmaceutical Sciences* (J. Swarbrick, ed.), Marcel Dekker, New York, pp. 55-59

Gibaldi, M. and Perrier, D., 1982, Pharmacokinetics. In *Drugs and the Pharmaceutical Sciences* (J. Swarbrick, ed.), Marcel Dekker, New York, pp. 221

Gobburu, J.V.S., Tenhoor, C., Rogge, M.C., Frazier, D.E., Thomas, D., Benjamin, C., Hess, D.M., and Jusko, W.J., 1998, Pharmacokinetics/dynamics of 5c8, a monoclonal antibody to CD154 (CD40 ligand) suppression of an immune response in monkeys. *J. Pharmacol. Exp. Ther.*, **286**:925-930

Gobburu, J.V.S., Agerso, H., Jusko, W.J., and Ynddal, L., 1999, Pharmacokinetic-pharmacodynamic modeling of ipamorelin, a growth hormone releasing peptide, in human volunteers., *Pharm. Res.*, **16**:1412-1416

Harrison, P.T., Davis, W., Norman, J.C., Hockaday, A.R., and Allen, J.M., 1994, Binding of monomeric immunoglobulin G triggers FcγRI-mediated endocytosis. *J. Biol. Chem.*, **269**:24396-24402

Holford, N.H.G. and Sheiner, L.B., 1982, Kinetics of pharmacological response. *Pharmacol. Ther.* **16**:143-166

Israel, E.J., Taylor, S., Wu, Z., Mizoguchi, E., Blumberg, R.S., Bhan, A., and Simister, N.E., 1997, Expression of the neonatal Fc receptor, FcRn, on human intestinal epithelial cells. *Immunology*, **92**:69-74

Khazaeli, M.B., Saleh, M.N., Liu, T.P., Meredith, R.F., Wheeler, R.H., Baker, T.S., King, D., Secher, D., Allen, L., Rogers, K., Colcher, D., Schlom, J., Shochat, D., and LoBuglio, A.F., 1991, Pharmacokinetics and immune response of ^{131}I-chimeric mouse/human B72.3 (human γ4) monoclonal antibody in humans. *Cancer Res.*, **51**:5461-5466

Klingbeil, C. and Hsu, D., 1999, Pharmacology and safety assessment of humanized monoclonal antibodies for therapeutic use. *Toxicol. Path.*, **27**:1-3

Leckie, M.J., ten Brinke, A., Khan, J., Diamant, Z., O'Connor, B.J., Walls, C.M., Mathur, A.K., Cowley, H.C., Chung, K.F., Djukanovic, R., Hansel, T.T., Holgate, T., Sterk, P.J. and Barnes, P.J. *Lancet,* **356**:2144-2148

Levy, G., 1986, Kinetics of drug action: an overview. *J. Allergy Clin. Immunol.,* **78**:754-761

Lin, Y.S., Nguyen, C., Mendoza, J-L., Escandon, E., Fei, D., Meng, Y.G., and Modi, N.B., 1999, Preclinical pharmacokinetics, interspecies scaling, and tissue distribution of a humanized monoclonal antibody against vascular endothelial growth factor. *J. Pharmacol. Exp. Ther.,* **288**: 371-378

Mager, D.E. and Jusko, W.J., 2002, Receptor-mediated Pharmacokinetic/pharmacodynamic model of interferon-β 1a in humans. *Pharm. Res.,* **19**:1537-1543

Marsh, M. and Helenius, A., 1980, Adsorptive endocytosis of Semliki Forest virus. *J. Mol. Biol.,* **142**:439-454

Mason, U., Aldrich, J., Breedveld, F., Davis, C.B., Elliott, M., Jackson, M., Jorgensen, C., Keystone, E., Levy, R., Tesser, J., Totoritis, M., Truneh, A., Weisman, M., Wiesenhutter, C., Yocum, D., and Zhu, J., 2002, CD4 coating, but not CD4 depletion, is a predictor of efficacy with primatized monoclonal anti-CD4 treatment of active rheumatoid arthritis. *J. Rheumatol.,* **29**:220-229

Meijer, R.T., Koopmans, R.P., Ten Berg, I.J.M., and Schellekens, P.T.A, 2002, Pharmacokinetics of murine anti-human CD3 antibodies in man are determined by the disappearance of target antigen. *J. Pharmacol. Exp. Ther.,* **300**:346-353

Mordenti, J., 1986, Man versus beast:pharmacokinetic scaling in mammals. *J. Pharm. Sci.,* **75**:1028-1040

Mordenti, J., Thomsen, K., Licko, V., Chen, H., Meng, Y.G., and Ferrara, N., 1999, Efficacy and concentration-responseof murine anti-VEGF monoclonal antibody in tumour-bearing mice and extrapolation to humans. *Toxicol. Pathol.,* **27**:14-21.

Mordenti, J., Chen, S.A., Moore, J.A., Ferraiolo, B.L., and Green, J.D., 1991, Interspecies scaling of clearance and volume of distribution data for five therapeutic proteins. *Pharm. Res.,* **8**:1351-1359

Morell, A., Terry, W.D., and Waldmann, T.A., 1970, Metabolic properties og IgG subclasses in man. *J. Clin. Investig.,* **49**:673-680

Morrison, S.L., Johnson, M.J., Herzenberg, L.A., and Oi, V.T., 1984, Chimeric human antibody molecules: mouse antigen-binding domains with human constant region domains. *Proc. Natl. Acad. Sci.* **81**:6851-6855

Morrison, S.L., 1985, Transfectomas provide novel chimeric antibodies. *Science.* **229**:1202-1207

Mould, D.R., Davis, C.B., Minthorn, E.A., Kwok, D.C., Elliott M.J., Luggen, M.E., and Totoritis, M.C., 1999, A population pharmacokinetic-pharmacodynamic analysis of single doses of clenoliximab in patients with rheumatoid arthritis. *Clin. Pharmacol. Ther.,* **66**:246-257

Nagashima, R., O'Reilly, R.A., Levy, G., 1969, Kinetics of pharmacologic effects in man: the anticoagulant action of warfarin. *Clin. Pharmacol. Ther.,* **10**:22-35

Ober, R.J., Radu, C.G., Ghetie, V., and Ward, E.S., 2001, Differences in promiscuity for antibody-FcRn interactions across-species: implications for therapeutic antibodies. *Int. Immunol.,* **13**:1551-1559

Ryan, A.M., Eppler, D.B., Hagler, K.E., Bruner, R.H., Thomford, P.G., Hall, R.L., Shopp, G.M., O'Neill, C.A., 1999, Preclinical safety evaluation of rhuMAbVEGF, an antiangiogenic humanized monoclonal antibody. *Toxicol. Pathol.,* **27**:78-86

Sharma, A., Davis, C.B., Tobia, L.A., Kwok, D.C., Tucci, M.G., Gore, E.R., Herzyk, D.A., and Hart, T.K., 2000, Comparative pharmacodynamics of keliximab and clenoliximab in transgenic mice bearing human CD4. *J. Pharmacol. Exp. Ther.,* **293**:33-41

Sheiner, L.B., Stanski, D.R., Vozeh, R.D., Miller, R.D., Ham, J., 1979,Simultaneous modeling of pharmacokinetics and pharmacodynamics: application to d-tubocurarine. *Clin. Pharmacol. Ther.*, **25**:358-371

Simister, N.E., 1989, An Fc receptor structurally related to MHC class I antigens. *Nature*, **337**:184-187

Supersaxo, A., Hein, W., and Steffen, H., 1990, Effect of molecular weight on the lymphatic absorption of water-soluble compounds following subcutaneous administration. *Pharm. Res.*, **7**:167-169

Tanswell, P., Garin-Chesa, P., Rettig, W.J., Welt, S., Divgi, C.R., Casper, E.S., Finn, R.D., Larson, S.M., Old, L.J., and Scott, A.M., 2001, Population pharmacokinetics of antifibroblast activation protein monoclonal antibody in cancer patients. *Br. J. Clin. Pharmacol.*, **51**:177-180

Trang, J.M., LoBuglio,A.F., Wheeler, R.H., Harvey, E.B., Sun, L., Ghrayeb, J., and Khazaeli, M.B., 1990, Pharmacokinetics of a mouse/human chimeric monoclonal antibody (C-17-1A) in metastatic adenocarcinoma patients. *Pharm. Res.*, **7**:587-592

Ward, E.S., Zhou, J., Ghetie, V., and Ober, R.J., 2003, Evidence to support the cellular mechanism involved in serum IgG homeostatis in humans. *Int. Immunol.*, **15**:187-195

Weiss, M., Sziegoleit, W., and Forster, W., 1977, Dependence of pharmacokinetic parameters on body weight. *Int. J. Clin. Pharmacol.*, **15**:572-575

Xu, Z.X., Sun, Y.N., DuBois, D.C., Almon, R.R., and Jusko, W.J. Third-generation model for corticosteroid pharmacodynamics: Roles of glucocorticoid receptor mRNA and tyrosine aminotransferase mRNA in rat liver. *J. Pharmacokinet. Biopharm.*, **23**:163-181

Zaharko, D.S., Dedrick, R.L., and Oliverio, V.T., 1972, Prediction of the distribution of methotrexate in the sting rays Dasyatidae sabrina and sayi by use of a model developed in mice. *Comp. Biochem. Physiol A.*, **42**:183-194

Zia-Amirhosseini, P., Minthorn, E., Benincosa, L.J., Hart, T.K., Hottenstein, C.S., Tobia, L.A.P, and Davis, C.B., 1999, Pharmacokinetics and pharmacodynamics of SB-2404653, a humanized monoclonal antibody directed to human interleukin-5, in monkeys. *J. Pharmacol. Exp. Ther.*, **291**:1060-1067.

Chapter 11

REGULATORY AND LEGAL REQUIREMENTS FOR THE MANUFACTURE OF ANTIBODIES

Lincoln Tsang
Of Counsel, Arnold & Porter, Tower 42, 25 Old Broad Street, London EC2N 1HQ,, England

1. INTRODUCTION

Monoclonal antibodies are antibodies which have a defined single amino sequence, specificity and affinity. They can be obtained from immortalised hybridoma or B lymphocytes or by recombinant DNA technology. The development of these techniques has paved the way for the design and production of specific monoclonal antibodies with the requisite antigenic determinants for the treatment and diagnosis of a range of clinical indications.

Hybridoma technology, first described in 1975 by Kohler and Milstein, used for the production of monoclonal antibodies heralded a new era in research and clinical development of antibodies. However, most of the monoclonal antibodies developed and subsequently authorised in the late 80s and early 90s were used as diagnostic agents to establish and monitor the progress and conditions of diseases ranging from cancer to infectious diseases.

Thanks to a better understanding of disease aetiology at molecular level (see below), newer types of monoclonal antibodies have been developed for therapeutic purposes. Some of these have been developed to target specific receptors for oncological indications, for example, Her-2 and CD-52 respectively for the treatment of metastatic breast cancer and chronic lymphocytic leukaemia. The list of therapeutic antibodies against cancer and chronic inflammatory diseases such as rheumatoid arthritis and Crohn's Disease is growing.

Innovative engineering techniques have enabled structural designs to improve *in vivo* pharmacokinetics, expand immune repertoires and permit screening against refractory targets (see Review by Hudson and Souriau 2003). New molecular strategies have also produced molecules with greater affinity and stability. Most of the recently developed antibodies are humanised or fully human in order to minimise or to overcome the problem of human anti-murine antibody (HAMA) associated with the mouse derived or chimeric antibody that is not a desirable clinical feature, particularly for products intended for long-term use.

Life sciences industry is tightly regulated. Navigating an ever-changing regulatory landscape is becoming an increasingly complex and essentially unavoidable task for industry. This chapter, therefore, reviews and highlights principally the related regulatory and legal issues in the European Union for biological products with particular emphasis on antibodies such as monoclonal antibodies. In addition, references are drawn to the United States regulatory requirements, where appropriate.

2. REGULATORY REQUIREMENTS

Under the single market provision of the Treaty of Rome, the first European Directive- harmonising the national laws governing the regulation of medicinal products- was passed in 1965 under Council Directive 65/65/EEC, which has progressively been amended, and most recently consolidated into Directive 2001/83.

This Directive defines the characteristics that constitute a *"medicinal product"*, and the legal requirements and obligations for granting a marketing authorisation. European Directive 87/22/EEC, which has now been repealed by Directive 93/41 and is the predecessor of the European Centralised Procedure established by Regulation 2309/93, defined a new category of medicinal products manufactured by a biotechnological process. This includes the use of hybridoma technology for the production of monoclonal antibodies. The first monoclonal antibody authorised in Europe under the procedure as set out in Directive 87/22, the Concertation Procedure, is Orthoclone (OKT3). The monoclonal antibody targets the surface antigen CD3 for the prevention of allograft transplant rejection. The mode of manufacture is *in vivo* by harvesting the monoclonal antibody from murine ascitic fluids. The emergence of recombinant technologies has revolutionised the selection, humanisation and production of antibodies and has gradually phased out the use of hybridoma technology and *in vivo* techniques for producing antibodies. Council Directive 86/609/EEC sets out the objective of animal welfare and minimising animal use in the manufacture. Although this is not a consideration for the purpose of granting a marketing authorisation, the European Centre for the Validation of Alternative Methods (ECVAM) has issued a report containing recommendations to phase out the use of *in vivo* method in the manufacturing process. The CPMP guideline, referred to in the following paragraph, also recommends *"In vitro production is the preferred method of production...If in vivo production is chosen, it must be justified by the manufacturer."* This recommendation appears to take into account the possibility that there are circumstances under which a monoclonal antibody cannot be manufactured by an *in vitro* method. This is interpreted in such a way to mean that the choice of mode of manufacture would be a matter for the applicant company to justify, including consideration to quality safeguards as recommended in the guidance note.

2.1 CONVENTIONAL MONOCLONAL ANTIBODIES

Irrespective of the method of manufacture, the grant of a marketing authorisation of any therapeutic or diagnostic monoclonal antibody is based on satisfying three objectively defined criteria of safety, quality and efficacy in the interest of public health protection. The European regulatory guidance entitled *"Production and Quality Control of Monoclonal Antibodies"* (the Monoclonal Antibody Guideline) was developed by the Committee for Proprietary Medicinal Products (CPMP) in 1994 and has been into operation since 1995. This guideline should be read in conjunction with other regulatory guidelines progressively developed and implemented by the CPMP and by the International Conference on Harmonisation (ICH)

The preamble of *"The Rules Governing Medicinal Products in the European Union. Volume III"* states that guidelines are not legally binding and *"has been prepared in order to maintain an element of flexibility and not to place undue legislative restraints on scientific progress. It is recognised that in some case, as a result of scientific developments, an alternative approach may be appropriate."* By virtue of their reference in the Annex to Directive 2001/83, its importance should not be under-estimated in that it sets out the regulatory standards that authorities would anticipate in any marketing authorisation applications.

The Monoclonal Antibody guideline mentioned above describes the technical requirements and scientific principles, necessary to ensure the quality and safety of this class of medicinal products produced by both *in vitro* and *in vivo* methods. It addresses issues pertaining to the method of production and types of monoclonal antibodies. From a safety perspective, it is emphasised *"important considerations for the clinical use of monoclonal antibodies include the possible unintentional immunological cross-reactivity of the antibody with human tissue antigens other than those desired, and the possible presence of viruses in the products*". It is with these specific considerations in mind, the guideline elaborates further on these safety issues in the body of the document. Although some of the regulatory recommendations may not be directly applicable to antibodies produced by means of a more modern technique, the underlying principles may nevertheless be generally applicable. The guideline emphasises three complementary regulatory principles that underpin the safety, quality and efficacy of biological products, namely

- Safe sourcing and characterisation of the starting materials
- Validation and control of the manufacturing process
- Defining the biological and physico-chemical characteristics of the product

Safe sourcing and characterisation of the starting materials include the control of all biological materials that are used at all stages of the manufacturing process. These include the source cells used for producing the antibodies and reagents used for cultivation. In addition to their qualification for microbiological purity (i.e. free from contamination with mycoplasma, fungi and bacteria), reagents of biological origin should be tested for relevant viruses likely to be present). For example, bovine sera used in tissue culture, reference, should be made to the recently adopted CPMP Note for Guidance on Bovine Serum Albumin. The amendment of the Annex I to Directives 2001/82/EC and 2001/83/EC by virtue of Directives 1999/104/EC and 1999/83/EC has rendered compliance with the Note for Guidance on "*minimising transmitting animal transmissible spongiform encephalopathy agents via human and veterinary medicinal products*" a mandatory requirement. The amending Directives enacted in 1999 require that ruminant materials or materials derived from animals susceptible to infection by animal spongiform encephalopathy agents comply with the requirements as set out in the latest version of the Committee for Proprietary Medicinal Products and Committee for Veterinary Medicinal Products (CVMP) guidance.

For other processing reagents, the Monoclonal Antibody guideline specifically states that it is undesirable to use agents, which are known to provoke sensitivity reactions (such as beta-lactam antibiotics) in certain individuals. Moreover, the use of antibiotics in cell culture is not desirable as this may be seen to be a means to circumvent compliance with good manufacturing practice in so far as microbiological safety is concerned.

The guidance also recommends adequate characterisation of the producing cell line. A two-tiered banking system, consisting of a master cell bank and a working cell bank, is recommended to ensure continuity in the supply of a well-defined, consistent starting material.

Cell-lines may include immortalised transformed cells, such as B-lymphocytes, and those used for producing recombinant monoclonal antibodies. In the case of the use of an immortalised cell-line, the method of immortalisation will determine the requirements for the level and nature of characterisation. For example, the use of Epstein-Barr virus in the immortalisation method will necessitate validation studies to be conducted to determine the overall capacity of the process to remove residual viral DNA. The results form part of the overall risk assessment because of their potential to induce oncogenesis.

For monoclonal antibodies produced by means of a recombinant technique, reference is made to section 5 of the guideline as well as the Guideline on Quality of biotechnological products: analysis of the expression construct in cells used for production of r-DNA- derived protein products already adopted by the International Conference on Harmonisation (ICH). To summarise, there is a need to provide a description of the origin, isolation and cloning strategy of the gene inserts, for example, heavy and light chains, complementarity determining regions (CDRs). The stability of the host/vector genetic and phenotypic characteristics should be demonstrated up to, and beyond the population doubling levels or generation numbers expected during full-scale production. The following aspects should be addressed in the genetic stability studies:

- Gene copy number in relation to productivity of the culture
- Characterisation of the monoclonal antibody at both polypeptide and nucleic acid levels
- The level and consistency of expression of both the heavy and light chain

With respect to the characterisation and control of the monoclonal antibody, reference is made to section 7 of the Monoclonal Antibody guideline and those principles already developed by the ICH, namely:

- Guideline on Specification: Test Procedures and Acceptance Criteria for Biotechnological /Biological Products (ICH Q6B)
- Preclinical Safety Evaluation of Biotechnology-Derived Pharmaceuticals (ICH S6)

These guidelines have been in operation for sometime following their adoption by the European Committee for Proprietary Medicinal Products

(CPMP) and incorporated into the United States Federal Register. See 62 Fed Reg 61515 (November 18, 1997); 64 Fed Reg. 44928 (August 18, 1999). The Q6B and S6 guidelines also form the regulatory basis of the Common Technical Document for global submissions in the USA, the European Union and Japan (ICH M4).

2.2 GENETICALLY ENGINEERED ANTIBODIES IN GENE TRANSFER

Besides cloning and genetic modification of antibodies for improving the pharmacokinetic and pharmacodynamic properties, antibody engineering using innovative structural designs has also opened up an immense opportunity for its application to gene transfer by directing the expression of specific antibody fragments in target cells for therapeutic interventions (Pelegrin *et al* 1998). An attempt had been made by using virally mediated delivery of a gene encoding a single chain immunologlobulin (sFv) which is directed against a specific oncogene, erbB-2, for its potential to treat ovarian and extraovarian cancer patients (Alvarez and Curiel 1997).

In the European Union, a gene transfer product can be regulated as a medicinal product under the harmonised Community rules if it meets the legal definition of a medicinal product pursuant to Article 1 of Directive 2001/83. The European Commission, has formulated a legal definition in the revision of Annex I to Directive for a *"gene therapy medicinal product"*, which is:

"For the purposes of this Annex, gene therapy product shall mean a product obtained through a set of manufacturing processes aimed at the transfer, to be performed either in vivo or ex vivo, of a prophylactic, diagnostic or therapeutic gene (i.e. a piece of nucleic acid), to human / animal cells and its subsequent expression in vivo. The gene transfer involves an expression system contained in a delivery system known as vector, which can be of viral, as well as non-viral origin. The vector can also be included in a human or animal cell"

The CPMP Note for Guidance, for gene transfer for medicinal products defines gene transfer as the deliberate introduction of genetic material into cells for diagnostic, prophylactic or therapeutic purposes. In this sense, it covers gene transfer products for cell tracking; prophylactics such as DNA vaccines; and therapeutic products such as cancer vaccines. Gene transfer of an intracellular antibody to be expressed *in situ* for therapeutic intervention will again fall within the regulatory definition of a gene transfer medicinal product.

In the United States, the Food and Drug Administration (FDA) approves biological products by review of biologics licence applications (BLAs) pursuant to Section 351 of the Public Health Service (PHS) Act, 42 U.S.C. 262(a). For purposes other than approval, biological products are regulated under the Federal Drug and Cosmetic Act.

The FDA utilises PHS provisions to enable it to regulate gene therapy. The statutory criteria for assessment for products licensed through BLA are purity, safety and potency. The FDA interprets these terms to require (with rare exceptions) clinical evidence of safety and effectiveness as well as appropriate non-clinical investigations. Because of the increasingly rapid innovative development in this area, Center for Biologics Evaluation and Research (CBER) of the FDA has used guidance document such as a Points to Consider for cell and gene therapies and Federal Register Notice (58 Fed Reg 53,248 of October 14, 1993) issued respectively in 1991 and 1993 to regulate gene therapy products. Gene Therapy is defined as *"a medical intervention based on modification of the genetic material of living cells"*. The 1993 Federal Register Notice introduced the possibility of less stringent regulatory oversight for biologics, depending on the use of a given product. Reagents used in the preparation of gene transfer are considered to be components of the final product although by design they are not intended to be part of the product. Nevertheless, the Agency's view is that such materials might affect the *"safety, purity or potency"* of the finished product.

Notwithstanding the legal position, gene transfer medicinal products belong to a sub-set of the recombinant DNA derived products and biological products. As such, the regulatory principles underpinning the safety, quality and efficacy of gene transfer products principally follow those already applied to conventional biological products. However, it should be recognised that the active ingredient in the finished product consists of genetic material (see review by Tsang *et al* 2001).

2.3 TRANSGENICS

The use of transgenics technology, including transgenic plants and animals, has offered an alternative manufacturing strategy for the production of monoclonal antibodies. The US FDA and the CPMP guidelines on transgenic animals were developed in the early and mid 1990s whereas the guidelines for transgenic plants were only developed as recently as 2002.

In relation to the use of transgenic animals as the host for producing monoclonal antibodies, both the FDA and the CPMP recommend the following:

- microbiological status, including the risk of transmission of zoonoses, of the production animals
- housing and animal care
- characterisation of the expression system
- creation of the transgenic animal and maintenance of the gene expression from generation to generation
- quality control of the active substance and validation of the downstream processing

In relation to antibodies derived from transgenic plants, the guidance issued by the FDA and CPMP addresses aspects that are pertinent to ensuring the quality, safety and efficacy of proteins derived from transgenic plants. Both documents emphasise the importance of characterising the gene construct particularly in the establishment of the Fo generation of the transformant in terms of:

- the copy number
- the loci of insertion
- sequence arrangements including point mutations, deletions and insertions
- expression properties and levels, including post-translational modifications
- the likely effects of inserted sequences on the expression of flanking endogenous genes
- effects of the transformation and of the transgene-expressed protein on the biology of the transgenic plant compared with the untransformed host
- fate of the marker sequence in the context of environmental risk assessment

Similar to products derived from other recombinant DNA technology platforms, the guidelines recommend the necessity for a properly conducted study to address genetic stability. In the draft CPMP guidance, it states:

"The design of the genetic stability studies should follow a global strategy which takes into account relevant parameters characterising the expression construct and the plant, with genotypic and phenotypic markers being monitored at different levels from the expression construct up to, or beyond, the limit of normal production conditions."

The FDA guidance similarly recommends an investigation into the stability of the transgenic plant derived through stable transformation.

In addition, both the FDA and CPMP, have made a specific reference to the applicable rules governing environmental risks associated with the use of

Regulatory and legal requirements for the manufacture of antibodies   283

transgenic plants. The CPMP guidance considers that a purified transgene-expressed protein, is not expected to fall within the scope of the European Deliberate Release Directive 2001/18/EC. This appears to be consistent with the scope of the legislation in that a purified derivative is not considered to be a biological entity capable of replication or transmitting genetic material within the meaning of the Directive. That said, the transgenic plants cultivated in the open field may, nevertheless, fall within the scope of the legislation.

The US guidance makes a specific reference to the applicable rules promulgated by various Federal agencies, including

- the Animal and Plant Health Inspection Service (APHS) of the US Department of Agriculture (USDA)
- Biotechnology Regulatory Service Division of the USDA/APHIS

According to 7 CFR 340.4, growing plants in an enclosed environment such as a greenhouse does not require a permit from USDA/APHIS/BRS. However, this exemption does not apply to importation or interstate movement of bioengineered pharmaceutical plants. The guidance also cross-refers to requirements made under the National Environmental Policy Act in relation to environmental assessment (see 21CFR part 25). Considerations should also be given to the potential environmental impact of all aspects of the manufacturing process, including but not limited to transport of seeds and plants, planting, growing, harvesting, processing.

2.4   GOOD MANUFACTURING PRACTICE

Under the European law, the Commission Directive 91/356/EEC lays down the principles and guidelines of good manufacturing practice.

Chapter II of the Directive sets out the principles and guidelines of good manufacturing, relating to:

- the establishment and implementation of an effective pharmaceutical quality assurance system;
- the need for appropriately qualified personnel to achieve the quality assurance objective;
- an appropriately constructed, designed and qualified manufacturing facilities to avoid in general any adverse effect on the quality of the product;
- proper documentation;
- a validated production process including its in-process control;
- quality control;

Article 3 provides:

"For the interpretation of these principles and guidelines of good manufacturing practice, the manufacturers and the agents of the competent authorities shall refer to the detailed guidelines referred to in Article 19a of Directive 75/319/EEC. [now Article 47 of Directive 2001/83/EC]*"*

The European Commission has issued further regulatory guidance in Volume IV of the *Rules governing medicinal products in the European Union* to supplement the general legal principles as set out in the Directive. Annex 2 and Annex 13 concern respectively the manufacture of biological medicinal products and investigational medicinal products, and are relevant to the manufacture of monoclonal antibodies.

Annex 2 emphasises the difference between a chemically synthesised product and a biological product in terms of the level of control. It states the following in the preamble:

"Unlike conventional medicinal products, which are reproduced using chemical and physical techniques capable of a high degree of consistency, the production of biological medicinal products involves biological processes and materials, such as cultivation of cells or extraction of material from living organisms. These biological processes may display inherent variability, so that the range and nature of by-products are variable. Moreover, the materials used in these cultivation processes provide good substrates for growth of microbial contaminants.
Control of biological medicinal products usually involves biological analytical techniques which have a greater variability than physico-chemical determination. In-process controls therefore take on a greater importance in the manufacture of biological medicinal products."

Annex 13 is being revised to take account of the regulatory requirements necessary for the implementation of the Clinical Trials Directive 2001/20, in which Article 13(3)(a) provides:

"in the case of investigational medicinal products manufactured in the Member State concerned, that each batch of medicinal products has been manufactured and checked in compliance with the requirements of Commission Directive 91/356/EEC..."

In the United States, as mentioned previously, biological products are regulated by the Public Heath Service Act. In 42 USC 262(j), it states that Federal Food, Drug, and Cosmetic Act applies to a biological product except that biological products shall not be required to obtain approval of a new drug application. USC 262(2)(B) provides:

"The Secretary shall approve a biologics licence application on the basis of demonstration that...
(II) the facility in which the biological product is manufactured, processed, packed or held meets standards designed to assure that the biological product continues to be safe, pure and potent..."

Section 501(a)(2)(B) of the Federal Food, Drug, and Cosmetic Act (21 USC 351(a)(2)(B)) provides:

"if it is a drug and the methods used in, or the facilities or controls used for, its manufacture, processing, packing, or holding do not conform to or are not operated or administered in conformity with current good manufacturing practice to assure that such drug meets the requirements of this chapter as to safety and has the identity and strength, and meets the quality and purity characteristics, which it purports or is represented to possess..."

The rules applicable to current good manufacturing practice are set out in Title 21 Part 210 of the Code of Federal Regulations (21 CFR 210). Section 210.2(a) states, amongst other things, that the regulations pertaining to drugs and those pertaining to biological products *"shall be considered to supplement, not supersede, each other"*. The combined effect of these provisions seems to suggest that GMP is mandatory for both biological products and drugs to ensure their safety and purity.

2.5 MUTUAL RECOGNITION AGREEMENTS

There has been in the recent years a renewed interest in international co-operation in the areas of standards, conformity assessment, and the elimination of technical barriers to trade by encouraging international trading partners to adopt standards and regulatory approaches based on, or compatible with international and European practice. For example, the ICH in the pharmaceutical sector has been an important platform in the harmonisation of technical requirements, resulting in the development of a number of international guidelines. These include the Guidance on Good Manufacturing Practice for Active Pharmaceutical Ingredients (Q7A), which has been in operation since 2001. Q7A applies to chemically synthesised active ingredients but the principles will equally apply to biotechnology-derived active substances. The objectives of Q7A were to minimise variations in interpretation among industry and regulatory agencies in the three jurisdictions, the USA, the European Union and Japan as well as those countries and regions, which recognise ICH guidelines. Most importantly, this guidance defines the reworking and re-processing and the role of agents and brokers. Where agents or brokers are used, the origin of the material needs to be established, hence the requirement for certificates of analysis. Blending of the passed and failed batches of an active ingredient is not acceptable. Furthermore, there must be clearly defined responsibilities for the QA/QC units and for manufacturing.

The European Commission has indicated its endeavour to promote international trade between the Community and third countries. For regulated products, this is achieved through the conclusion of Mutual Recognition Agreements (MRAs) on the basis of Article 133 of the Treaty. MRAs are agreements on the mutual recognition of conformity assessment of regulated products. Through an MRA, each importing party is given the authority to test and certify products against the regulatory requirements of the other party, in its own territory and prior to export. In cases where testing is conducted by a third party, each importing party agrees by the terms of an MRA, to recognise the tests and results obtained thereof.

At the time of writing this chapter, an MRA had been signed between the European Union and Switzerland in relation to conformity assessment. An MRA has also been signed between the European Union and Australia. The MRA between the EU and the USA is subjected to a satisfactory assessment of equivalence. Equivalence is defined in Article 1 of the Sectoral Annex to the US-EC MRA for Pharmaceutical Good Manufacturing Practices. It states:

"'Equivalence' of the regulatory systems means that the systems are sufficiently comparable to assure that the process of inspection and the ensuing inspection reports will provide adequate information to determine whether respective statutory and regulatory requirements of the authorities have been fulfilled. "Equivalence" does not require that the respective regulatory systems have identical procedures."

Equivalence is assessed against the criteria as set out in the Appendix 4 of the MRA. Article 6(3) provides that the assessment for equivalence will include the following:

- information exchange (including inspection reports)
- joint training

- joint inspection for the purpose of assessing regulatory systems and the capabilities of the authorities

3. CONCLUSIONS

This chapter is intended to provide an overview of the European framework for the regulation of monoclonal antibodies, including the technical and legal requirements for marketing authorisation. Research and Development of pharmaceuticals is a global business. ICH regulatory guidelines, which set out the standards for safety, quality and efficacy, have greatly facilitated international product development and movement of pharmaceuticals across national boundaries. The on-going discussions for mutual recognition agreement between the US and the EU will further streamline the GMP approval of two major economic regions.

REFERENCES

Alvarez R D, Curiel DT (1997) Human Gene Therapy 8:229-242

Committee for Proprietary Medicinal Products Guideline "Production and Quality Control of Monoclonal Antibodies" Eudra/B/94/014

Committee for Proprietary Medicinal Products Guideline "Use of Transgenic Animals in the Manufacture of Biological Medicinal Products for Human Use" Eudra/B/93/17

Committee for Proprietary Medicinal Products Note for Guidance on Plasma-Derived Medicinal Products (CPMP/BWP/269/95)

Committee for Proprietary Medicinal Products Not for Guidance on Quality of biotechnological products: analysis of the expression construct in cells used for production of r-DNA-derived protein products (CPMP/ICH/139/95)

Committee for Proprietary Medicinal Products (CPMP) Note for Guidance on Preclinical Safety Evaluation of Biotechnology-derived Pharmaceuticals (ICH S6 CPMP/ICH/302/95)

Committee for Proprietary Medicinal Products (CPMP) Note for Guidance on Specifications: Test Procedures and Acceptance Criteria for Biotechnological/Biological Products (ICH Q6B CPMP/ICH/365/96)

Committee for Proprietary Medicinal Products Note for Guidance on the Quality, Preclinical and Clinical Aspects of Gene Transfer Medicinal Products (CPMP/BWP/3088/99)

Committee for Proprietary Medicinal Products Note for Guidance on Development Pharmaceutics Annex: Development Pharmaceutics for Biotechnological and Biological Products (CPMP/BWP/328/99)

Committee for Proprietary Medicinal Products Points to Consider on Quality Aspects of Medicinal Products Containing Active Substances Produced by Stable Transgene Expression in Higher Plants (CPMP/BWP/764/02)

Committee for Proprietary Medicinal Products Note for Guidance on Minimising the Risk of Transmitting Animal Spongiform Encephalopathy Agents via Human and Veterinary Medicinal Products (EMEA/410/01/2)

Committee for Proprietary Medicinal Products Note for Guidance on the use of Bovine Serum in the manufacture of Human Biological Medicinal Products (CCPMP/BWP1793/02)

Commission Directive 2003/63/EC OJ L159/46
Commission Directive 91/356/EEC OJ L193/30
Council Regulation (EEC) 2309/93 OJ L214/1
Directive 2001/83/EC of the European Parliament and of the Council OJ L311/67
European Commission: The Rules Governing Medicinal Products in the European Union Volume IV: Good Manufacturing Practice for Medicinal Practice
Food and Drug Administration Points to Consider in Human Somatic Cell Therapy and Gene Therapy (1991)
Food and Drug Administration Points to Consider in the Manufacture and Testing of Therapeutic Products for Human Use Derived from Transgenic Animals (1993)
Food and Drug Administration Guidance for Industry: Drugs, Biologics and Medical Devices Derived from Bioengineered Plants for Use in Humans and Animals (2002)
Hudson PJ, Souriau C (2003) *Nature Medicine* **9**(1):129-134
Kohler G and Milstein C (1975) *Nature* **256**:495-497
Pelegrin M, Marin M, Noel D, Peichaczyk M (1998) *Human Gene Therapy* **9**:2165-2175
Tsang L, Knudsen LH, Theilade MD (2001) *Regulatory Affairs Journal* **13**(4):275-278

Index

Abciximab (ReoPro), 41, 42, 55
Abrin, 39
Absorption pharmacokinetics, 250–252
Acetate production, E. coli fermentation, 52
Acetylethyleneimine (AEI), 213
Acoustic cell retention system, 244, 245, 246
Additives, 77, 127
    capture of antibodies, 104
    fermentation, 53, 90
    quality control testing, 171
Adenoviruses, 202, 223
ADEPT (antibody directed enzymatic prodrug therapy), 40–41
Administration route, pharmacokinetics, 251–252
Adsorption
    chromatography, 230; *see also* Binding affinity; specific methods
    fragments, 58, 60–61
Adverse reactions, anti-antibody response, 258
Affinity, antibody, 275
    fragment design, 30, 35; *see also* Avidity, fragment
    interspecies differences, 140, 264
Affinity capture, 60, 79; *see also* Protein A capture chromatography
Affinity chromatography, 106–107, 128, 134; *see also* Protein A chromatography
    antibody construction, 15
    cost, 12
    fragment purification, 57, 58–59
    IMAC, 106–107
    methods, *see* Chromatography, methods
    virus removal/inactivation, 203, 204
Affinity macroligand (AML), 159, 160

Affinity precipitation techniques, 158–160
Agarose matrices, chromatography, 150
Agarose media, 89, 95
Aggregated antibody
    fragments, 30, 47, 88
    quality control, 170, 171, 175–176, 180
Aggregates, protein impurities
    ion exchange resin reuse, 121
    process steps, 127; *see also* Contaminants and impurities, process
Aglycosylated IgG, 46–47
Agribacterium tumefaciens, 55
Albumin, 135, 138, 139, 213
Alcohol precipitation, virus removal/inactivation, 203, 207
Allometric scaling, 259, 261
Amino acid analysis, product characterisation, 178, 179
Amino acid modifications, 47, 48
Amino acid sequence, 275
Ammonium sulfate precipitation, 92, 151
Analytical methods, 177–184; *see also* Quality control
Animal care, regulatory and legal requirements, 276, 282
Animal products, 104
    regulatory and legal requirements, 278
    removal of, Protein A chromatography, 112, 113
Animal proteins, 135
Animals
    immunoglobulin binding, comparison of, 140
    transgenic, 7, 56
Animal source-free (ASF) medium
    cell culture systems, 54
    contract manufacturing, 227

product considerations, 228
    upstream processes, 244
Anion exchange chromatography, 91, 127, 150
    manufacturing strategies
        customising, 16, 19
        generic processes, 14
    polishing, 93
    scale-up
        flowchart, 103
        polishing, 105
Anion exchange membrane, 93
Anti-antibodies, chromatography ligands, 145
Anti-antibody response
    HAMA, 1, 2, 276
    pharmacodynamics/pharmacokinetics, 253–258, 266–268
Antibiotic-free plasmid maintenance, 51
Antibiotics
    fermentation, 53
    regulatory and legal requirements, 278
Antibody binding, *see* Binding capacity; specific chromatographic methods
Antibody capture, *see* Capture methods
Antibody characterisation, quality control, 177–184
Antibody-dependent cellular cytotoxicity (ADCC), 54
    anti-D antibodies, 190–196
    fragment design, 35, 36
Antibody directed enzymatic prodrug therapy (ADEPT), 40–41
Anti-CD20, 39
Anti-CD33, 40
Antifoam additives, 53
Antigen-antibody complex
    pharmacokinetics, 249, 253, 254–255
Antigen binding
    fragment design, 29, 31
        glycoproteins and, 41
        pharmacokinetics, 32, 33, 34, 35, 40
    IgG1 structure, 26
    pharmacokinetics, 249, 252, 253, 254–255, 262
Antigens, chromatography ligands, 134, 138
Anti-Rh (D) antibodies, 190–196
    carbohydrates and effector function of recombinant antibodies, 194–196
    modulation of effector functions,
192–193, 194
    screening, ADCC assay, 190–192
Anti-TNFα antibody, 41
ApA (Artificial Protein A), 142–144
Approval of product, 76
Area under curve (AUC), 251
Artificial IgG-binding proteins (pA(AB)[1-6]), 141
Artificial Protein A (ApA), 142–144
Ascites, 135, 151, 152
Assays
    quality control
        antibody characteristics, 177–184
        impurity control, 170–177
    virus removal/inactivation studies, 216, 221, 218–219
Automation, manufacturing strategies, 20
Avidity, fragment, 29, 31, 32, 34, 35
    increasing, 28
    radionuclide attachment, 39

Bacterial products, contaminant removal, 141
Bacterial protein ligands, 58, 97
Bacterial systems, *see* Escherichia coli systems; Microbial systems
Bacterial toxins, 39, 104
Batch culture, 229
Batch fed systems, 54
B cells, 275, 279
Bed height, 128
    chromatography scale-up, 110, 111
    modification of, 87–88
Bench scale production, scale-up, 9–11, 106–107
Beta propiolactone, 209, 214
Bexxar (^{131}I-tositumomab), 39
BHK cells, 4–5, 243
Bind and elute mode, customising manufacturing, 17
Binding, antigen, *see* Antigen binding
Binding, nonspecific, 34, 89–90
Binding capacity
    chromatography, 103, 128; *see also* specific chromatography methods
        capture of antibodies, 104
        ion exchange resins, 114, 116–117, 118
        mechanism, 117–118
        scale-up, 104, 109–110
    manufacturing strategies, customising, 17
Binding strengths, Protein A and G, 140, 141

Index

Bioanalytical methods, *see* Assays;
  Quality control
Bioavailability, pharmacokinetics, 251
Bioburden, quality control testing, 170,
  171
Biological product regulations, 284–285
Biomarkers, pharmacodynamics, 264
Biomass levels, fermentation, 52
Biomass removal, 244, 245
Bioreactors, 228–239
Biotin, 38, 59
Bispecific antibodies
  fragment design, 30, 32, 33, 36–37
    effector function
      engineering, 35–36
    pharmacokinetics, 43
    radionuclide attachment, 38
  hydrophobic interaction
    chromatography, 153–154
Blocking antibodies, 40–41, 62
Blood products
  high-performance monolith affinity
    (HPMA) chromatography, 155
  virus removal/inactivation, 207,
    209, 214, 222
  virus safety issues, 199
Blood tumors, fragment design, 34
  radionuclide attachment, 39
  toxin attachment, 40
Blot techniques, 133
Bluetongue virus, 215, 223
Body weight
  interspecies scaling, 258–259
  pharmacodynamics, 268
Bovine components, 135
  industry trends, contract production
    considerations, 228
  removal of, Protein A
    chromatography, 112, 113
Bovine serum albumin, 5
Bovine viruses, 202, 215, 223
Breakdown products, 77
Broad-spectrum pulsed light treatment,
  209, 211
Bromoethylamine, 213
Buffer exchange, 14
Buffers
  chromatography, *see also* Elution;
    specific methods
      elution strategies, 149
      scale-up, 109
  virus removal/inactivation, 205–
    206, 223

Cache valley virus (CVV), 202
Calicheamicin, 40
Caliciviruses, 223
Caprylate, 209, 213
Capsid proteins, 213
Capture methods, 127, 128, 136
  downstream processing, 103, 104–
    105
  fragment production, 62–63
  optimising, 82–87; *see also*
    Purification and recovery,
    optimising
  Protein A chromatography, 81–90
    bed height modification, 87–
      88
    elution conditions, 88
    intermediate washing, 89–90
    ligand leaching, 90
    media lifetime
      (chromatography), 89
    optimising, 82–87
    virus removal, 90
Carbohydrates, 133, 136; *see also*
  Glycosylation
    anti-Rh (D) antibodies, and effector
      function, 194–196
    contract manufacturing, process
      targets, 239
    IgG1, 26
    quality control, product
      characterisation, 178, 180–181
    toxin attachment, 40
Carbon source, fermentation, 52
Cation exchange chromatography, 79, 92,
  127, 128
    binding mechanisms, 117
    fragment purification, 60
    manufacturing strategies,
      customising, 17, 19
    quality control, product
      characterisation, 179, 180
    scale-up
      flowchart, 103
      intermediate purification,
        105
      resin screening, 118–121
CD3 cells, 36, 41
CD4 cells, 41, 42
CD20 antibodies, 39
CD33 antibody, 40
CD52 receptors, 275
CDR, *see* Complementarity-determining
  regions
Cell banking system, 11
Cell binding pharmacokinetics, 252, 253
Cell culture, 134
  anti-Rh (D) antibodies in different

cell lines, 189–196
continuous annular chromatography, 154–155
contract manufacturing
    industry trends, 228
    upstream expansion, 232–234
    upstream processes, 242–243
contract manufacturing, targeted approach of DSM Biologics, 231; see also Manufacturing process, contract
expended (fluidised) bed chromatography, 157
expression system comparisons, 7
fragment production, 45, 54–55
fragment purification, 58, 61
impurities in antibody preparations, 135
industry trends, contract production considerations, 228
manufacturing strategies, 4–5, 7
regulatory and legal requirements, 278, 278–279
virus safety issues, 202
Cell debris, see Contaminants and impurities, process
Cell density
    contract manufacturing
        fifty liter fermentation, 235, 236
        upstream expansion preculture, 232–234
    fermentation, 51, 52, 53
Cell membranes, virus removal/inactivation, 213
Cell protein contaminants, see Contaminants and impurities, process
Cell retention device, 235
Cellular contaminants and impurities, see Contaminants and impurities, process
Cellular uptake and trafficking, 34, 35
    fragment design, 41, 42
    pharmacokinetics, 42, 249, 253, 254
Cellulose matrices, chromatography, 150
Center for Biologics Evaluation and Research (CBER), 281
Centrifugation, 12, 78
cGMP, see Good Manufacturing Practices
Chaperones, 48, 49, 53
Charge density, ion-exchange matrices, 151
Chase molecules, 38

Chelating Sepharose® fast flow, 107
Chelators, 38, 152
Chemical cross linking of fragments, 29, 34, 37
Chemical inactivation of viruses, 90, 209, 211–212
Chemically defined media, 228, 244, 245, 246
Chemically synthesized product, 284
Chemical resistance, affinity chromatography matrix properties, 147
Chimeric antibodies, 1, 2
    anti-antibody response, 258
    fragment design
        blocking antibodies, 41
        pharmacokinetics, 43
    pharmacokinetics/pharmacodynamics, 249
    proteolytic digestion, 55
CHO cells, 134, 169
    anti-Rh (D) antibody effector function, 192
    cell culture systems, 54, 55
    contract manufacturing, 243
    DNA content, 172
    impurities in antibody preparations, 135
    industry trends, contract production considerations, 228
    manufacturing strategies, 8
    quality control testing, 173, 174
    recombinant cell lines, 4–5
    virus removal/inactivation studies, 222, 223
    virus sources, 215
Chromatography, 127
    antibody construction, 15
    cleanability of resin, 104
    contract manufacturing
        product quality, 239
        purification of IgG, 229–230
    fragments
        adsorption chemistry, 58
        affinity ligands, 58–59
        modes of operation and process integration, 60–61
        non-affinity ligands, 59–60
    manufacturing strategies, 11
        cost, 12
        customising, 17, 19
        generic processes, 13, 14
        innovations, 20
    scale-up
        flowchart, 103
        miscellaneous methods, 106–107

Index   293

stability and reuse of media, 113–114
virus removal/inactivation, 203, 205–206, 208, 213–214, 223
Chromatography, methods
    affinity chromatography elution, 149–150
    affinity chromatography ligands, 137–147
        anti-antibodies, 145
        antigens, 138
        Fc receptors, 138–141
        histidin, 145
        lectins, 147
        metals, 145–146
        Protein A mimetic, 141–145
        thiophilic interactions, 146–147
    affinity chromatography stationary phases, 147–148
    affinity precipitation technique, 158–160
    antibody characteristics, 136
    applications, 133
    continuous annular chromatography, 154–155
    expended (fluidised) bed chromatography, 157–158
    high-performance monolith affinity (HPMA) chromatography, 155–156
    hydrophobic interaction chromatography, 152–153
    hydroxyapatite (pseudo-affinity) chromatography, 151–152
    ion exchange chromatography, 150–151
    sources of antibodies and impurities, 135
    stages of process, 136
Chromatography, optimising, 77, 79
    post-affinity process steps, 91–93
        contaminant removal, 91
        ion exchange, 91–92
        other chromatographic methods, 92–93
    Protein A capture chromatography
        bed height modification, 87–88
        elution conditions, 88
        intermediate washing, 89–90
        ligand leaching, 90
        media lifetime (chromatography), 89
        optimising, 82–87
        virus removal, 90

Chromatography supports/matrices/stationary phases, *see* Matrices/stationary phases/supports
Chromosome integration, 46
Circoviruses, 202
Clarification, 78, 79, 136
    manufacturing strategies, 14
    optimising purification and capture process, 80
Cleaning, chromatography column, 89, 104, 205
    contract manufacturing, 240
    production scale, 127
    Protein A, 113–114
Cleaning, filter, 244
Clearance, antibody, *see* Half-life and clearance rates of antibodies
Clearance (clarification) procedures, *see* Clarification
Cleaved antibody, *see* Proteolysis
Clinical end-points, pharmacodynamics, 265
Clinical and therapeutic applications, fragments, 29, 34–41
Clinical trials, 76
    fragment production, 62
    virus removal/inactivation, 215
Clinical Trials Directive, 284
Cloning (animal) methods, 56
CM-HyperD™, 20, 151
Cohn fractionation, 94, 207
Column cleaning, *see* Reuse of chromatography columns
Column elution, *see* Elution
Column packing, large scale, 125–127
Combinatorial libraries, Protein A mimetic ligands, 141
Commercial products
    cation exchange resins, 118, 119
    production scale columns, 126
    Protein A chromatography resins, 110–111, 112
Committee for Proprietary Medicinal Products (CPMP), 277, 278, 281–283
Committee for Proprietary Veterinary Products (CPVP), 278
Compartment models, 265–266
Competitive elution, 149–150
Complementarity-determining regions (CDR), 29; *see also* Humanised antibody
    IgG1 structure, 26
    manufacturing strategies, 1, 2
Complement-dependent cytotoxicity,

fragment design, 35, 36
Compression, column material, 76
Computer simulations/modeling
 manufacturing costs, 12, 13
 pharmacokinetics, 255, 256, 257
 Protein A mimetic ligands, 141
Concentration, product, 178, 179, 238
Concentration-effect relationship, pharmacodynamics, 263
Concentration process, antibody purification
 fragments, 57
 generic processes, 14
Conductivity, CEC feed, 92
Conjugates, fragment, 29
 pharmacokinetics, 43
 purification considerations, 57
Consistency of product, 11
Constant region
 antibody construction, 15
 fragment design, 31, 32
 fragment production, 28
 IgG1 structure, 26
 purification, 58
Construct stability, 50, 51, 52
Contaminants and impurities, process, 77, 78, 105, 108, 127
 chromatography matrix, 134, 135
  ion exchange resin reuse, 121, 123
  removal of, 141
  Protein A, *see* Protein A ligand, leached/residual antibodies, 88
 contract manufacturing, 239, 240
  process targets, 238, 239, 240
  product quality, 239
 manufacturing strategies
  customising, 16–17
  downstream processing principles, 8–9
  generic processes, 14
 optimising purification and capture process, 91
 polishing, 93
 post affinity purification steps, 91
 quality control, 170–177; *see also* Quality control
  contract manufacturing, 239
  DNA, host cell, 171–172
  proteins, 173–174
  testing, 171, 173–174
 scale-up, 112, 113
 viruses, *see* Virus safety issues/virus clearance studies

Continuous annular chromatography, 154–155
Continuous culture systems, 54
Continuous perfusion fermentation at high medium flow rate, 229, 235
Contract manufacturing, *see* Manufacturing process, contract
Controls, process
 glycosylation, 180–181
 manufacturing strategies, 11
 regulatory and legal requirements, 278
Controls, virus removal, 216, 217, 219
Convective Interaction Media (CIM™) disks, 155
Cooling, fermentation, 51
Copper leaching, 107
Copy number, gene
 cell culture systems, 54
 fragment production, 50
 recombinant cell lines, 5
 regulatory and legal requirements, 279, 282
Costs, 4, 76
 cell culture systems, 54
 contract manufacturing considerations, 239, 240
 fragment production, 45, 46
 fragment purification, 61
 manufacturing strategies, 12–13
  customising, 19
  expression system comparisons, 7
  generic processes, 14
  scale-up from bench/laboratory production, 10
 purification processes, 58, 60, 79, 230
  affinity purification, 58, 60
  fragments, 61
  Protein A chromatography, 110
  scale-up considerations, 103
 virus removal/inactivation, 209
Creutzfeld-Jacob Disease, 228
Cross-linking, 29
 fragments, 34
  bispecific antibodies, 37
  blocking antibodies, 41
  pharmacokinetics, 43–44
 matrices, 60–61
 pharmacokinetics, 43–44, 253
 T cells, 41
Crystallization methods, 94
Culture medium, *see* Medium
Cyanogen bromide, 59, 148

Cysteine groups, 29, 32, 40
Cytokines, 41
Cytoplasmic expression, fragment production in E. coli, 48–49
Cytotoxicity, 54, 134
    anti-D antibodies, 190–196
    bispecific antibodies, 36
    fragment design, 35, 36
    virus removal/inactivation studies, 216, 217

Dead-end filtration, 235
DEAE chromatography matrices, 150–151
DEAE Sephadex columns, virus removal/inactivation, 213–214
Degradation, *see also* Proteolysis
    contaminants, process, *see* Contaminants and impurities, process
    pharmacokinetics/pharmacodynamics, 249, 253
    quality control testing, 170, 171
Deletions, regulatory and legal requirements, 282
Delivery systems, manufacturing strategies, 12
Density, cell, *see* Cell density
Density of ligands, chromatography matrix properties, 147
Derivatization, 44; *see also* Polyethylene glycol/PEGylation
Design of fragments, format, 27–29, 30–33
Design of process, *see* Process design
Detergents, virus removal/inactivation, 203, 204, 207–208
Development phase, contract manufacturing, 231, 232
Dewatering, 57
Dextrans, 43
Diabody, 29, 30
    bispecific antibodies, 36
    pharmacokinetics, 43
Diafiltration, 58, 95
Diagnosis, 133
Dialysis fermentation, 51
Diethylaminoethyl (DEAE)-type chromatography supports, 150–151
Diffusion pharmacokinetics, 252
Dihydrofolate reductase, 54
Dilution, fragment purification, 58
Dimeric antibody fragments
    design, 31, 32
    production, 28

Diphtheria toxin, 39
Dissociation, VH and VL domains, 27
Distribution pharmacokinetics, 252, 255
Distribution half-life, *see* Half-life and clearance rates of antibodies
Disulfide bonds, 177
    fragment design, 29
        bispecific antibodies, 37
        pharmacokinetics, 43–44
        stabilisation, 27, 28
    fragment production
        cell culture systems, 55
        E. coli systems, 46, 48–49
    manufacturing strategies, 4
    quality control
        cleavage of, 180
        product characterisation, 178
Disulfide isomerase, 53
Divalent antibodies, 30, 36, 38
    $F(ab')_2$ production, 28–29
    cell culture systems, 55
    pharmacokinetics, 43
    yeast production systems, 53–54
DNA removal, *see* Contaminants and impurities, process
DNA viruses, 90, 212, 213, 215, 222, 223
Documentation
    contract manufacturing, 231
    regulatory and legal requirements, 283
Doped sol-gel glass, 148
DOTA, 38
Dot blot hybridisation, 171, 172
Downscaling, virus removal/inactivation, 209
Downstream processing
    design, 102–103, *see also* Purification and recovery
    manufacturing strategies, 8–15
        cost, 12–13
        generic processes, 13–14
        purity, potency, and identity, 11–12
        R&D laboratory versus industrial processes, 9–11
    optimising, *see* Purification and recovery, optimising
    regulatory and legal requirements, 282
DPTA, 38
Dry heat, virus removal/inactivation, 203
Dual antigen specificity, *see* Divalent antibodies
Dyes, virus removal/inactivation, 209, 212
Dynamic capacity, 18, 83

Economic targets, contract manufacturing, 239
Economies of scale, 10
Economics, see Costs
Effect compartment models, 265–266
Effect-concentration curve, 266
Effector function engineering, 35
Efficacy, product, 4, 263
Efficiency
    manufacturing strategies, 10, 18
    process, 76
Egg yolk, 135
Electrophoresis
    HPMC product, 155–156
    quality control testing, 171, 173, 178, 182–184
Elimination, pharmacokinetics, 253–258
ELISA, 90, 112, 133, 171, 173, 174, 178
Elution
    affinity chromatography, 149–150
    fragment purification, 58, 59
    manufacturing strategies, customising, 15, 17
    optimising purification and capture process, 88
    Protein A chromatography, 83
    step-wise, 138
    virus removal/inactivation, 203, 208
Emerging methodologies, 76
Endocytosis, 253
Endoglycosidase H, 195
Endosomes, 42
Endotoxins, 77
    chromatography, nonspecific binding, 90
    contract manufacturing, 240
    ion exchange resins, 114
    polishing, 93
    post affinity purification steps, 91
    quality control testing, 170, 171
    scale-up, 104
End-points, surrogate, 264–265
Enhanced ultrafiltration (EUF), 94–95
Enteroviruses, 202
Enveloped viruses, 213
Environmental risk, 282–283
Enzymes, 40
    fragment design, 29
    fragment production
        E. coli systems, cytoplasmic expression, 48–49
        E. coli systems, periplasmic expression, 47
    reagents, viruses in, 202
Epithelial barriers, 252

Equipment, 10, 76, 108
Escherichia coli systems, 135
    fragment production, 26, 45, 46–53, 46–53
        bispecific antibody design, 36
        cytoplasmic expression, 48–49
        fermentation, 51–53
        general considerations, 46–47
        periplasmic expression, 47–48
        plasmid biology, 50–51
        purification, 57, 58, 61
    manufacturing, targeted approach of DSM Biologics, 231; see also Manufacturing process, contract manufacturing strategies, 6
Ethanol fractionation, 207
Ethyleneimine, 213
Eudragit S-100, 159
European Centre for the Validation of Alternative Methods (ECVAM), 277
European Commission, 280
European Committee for Proprietary Medicinal Products (CPMP), 279
European Deliberate Release Directives, 283
European Directive, 276–277
Expanded bed adsorption (EBA), 79
    chromatography, 230
    fragment purification, 61
    manufacturing strategies, customising, 18
    optimising purification and capture process, 96
    Protein A chromatography, 112
    scale-up, 113
Expansion preculture, 232–234, 243–244
Expended (fluidised) bed chromatography, 60, 61, 157–158, 230
Expression levels, 75
    recombinant cell lines, 5
    regulatory and legal requirements, 279, 282
Expression of recombinant proteins
    fermentation, 52
    fragment production, 62
Extracellular proteins, 135
Extraction, 136
Extravascular compartment pharmacokinetics, 252

Index

Fab fragments/region
    blocking antibodies, 41
    crystallization, 94
    design, 29, 41
    production, 62
        cell culture systems, 55
        E. coli plasmid biology, 50
        E. coli systems, cytoplasmic expression, 49
        E. coli systems, periplasmic expression, 47–48
        yeast production systems, 53
    IgG1 structure, 26
    microbial expression systems, 6
    purification, 58, 94
Fab´ fragments/region
    design, 34
        PEGylation, 44–45
        pharmacokinetics, 43–44
    production
        cell culture systems, 55
        E. coli systems, cytoplasmic expression, 49
        fermentation, 53
    purification, 58, 60
F(ab´)$_2$
    cell culture systems, 55
    design, 33
        blocking antibodies, 42
        full length, 32
        PEGylation, 44–45
        pharmacokinetics, 43–44
    production, 28–29, 55
Fab-ScFv fragment design, 33
Facilities, 76
    regulatory and legal requirements, 283
    scale-up considerations, 10, 108
FastMabs A®, 20, 144–145
Fc domains, 29, 140
    anti-Rh (D) antibody effector function, 195
    cell culture systems, 55
    chromatography ligands, 138–141
    fragment design
        blocking antibodies, 41
        effector function engineering, 35
        pharmacokinetics, 42
    IgG1 structure, 26
    interspecies scaling, 262
    ligands for affinity purification, 138
    neonatal, 251
    pharmacokinetics, 249–250, 253
    purification, 58, 137

Fcα receptor
    anti-Rh (D) antibody effector function, 190–191, 193, 194, 195, 196
    fragment design
        bispecific antibodies, 36
        blocking antibodies, 41, 42
        effector function engineering, 35
        pharmacokinetics, 42
    neonatal, 29
    pharmacokinetics/pharmacodynamics, 249, 253
Fed-batch culture, 229
    cell culture systems, 54
    fermentation, 51, 53
Feedstock conditioning, 57, 58, 79
Fermentation
    contract manufacturing
        fifty liter fermentation, 235–237
        industry trends, 229
        upstream processes, 244
    direct application to chromatography column, 230
    fragments
        production, 51–53
        purification, 61
    purification of product, *see* Purification and recovery
Fetal antibodies
    anti-Rh (D) antibodies, 189–196
    pharmacokinetics, 250–251
FF Sepharose A, 82
Fiberglass supports, chromatography, 148
FIDA (fluorescence-intensity-distribution analysis), 175, 176
Fill and draw, 229
Filtration, 78
    contract manufacturing
        fifty liter fermentation, 235
        product quality, 239
        upstream processes, 244, 245, 246
    manufacturing strategies
        customising, 19
        generic processes, 14
    purification processes, optimising, 79–80, 81–82
    scale-up
        capture of antibodies, 104
        flowchart, 103
    virus removal/inactivation, 90, 199, 203, 206–207
Finished product
    manufacturing steps, 103, 127

manufacturing strategies, 10, 11, 12
  quality control, 184–185
First-order pharmacokinetics, 255
Fixed bed adsorption, fragment purification, 60
FkpA, 48
FLAG tag, 59
Flanking genes, regulatory and legal requirements, 282
Flaviviruses, 215, 222
Flow dispersion properties, 94
Flow filtration, 78, 79
Flow rate, chromatography, 81, 83, 84, 230
  ion exchange resins, 114, 115
  scale-up, 109, 110
    flowchart, 103
    Protein A chromatography, 111
  virus removal/inactivation studies, 223
Fluidised (expended) bed adsorption, 157–158
  fragment purification, 60, 61
  chromatography, 230
Fluorescence-intensity-distribution analysis (FIDA), 175, 176
Foldases, 49
Folding, fragments, 46, 47, 48, 49
Foot and mouth diease virus, 213
Formats, fragments, 27–29, 30–33, 29, 34–41
  bispecific antibodies, 36–37
  blocking antibodies, 40–41
  effector function engineering, 35
  fragments, *see also* Fragment production
  pharmacokinetics, 43
  radionuclide attachment, 37–39
  tissue targeting and penetration, 34–35
  toxin attachment, 39–40
Formulation
  manufacturing steps, 103, 127
  manufacturing strategies, 10, 11, 12
  quality control, 184–185
Fouling, 79
Fractionation, generic processes, 13
Fractogel® EMD Chelate, 107
Fractogel® EMD TA, 106
Fractogel® products, 106, 107, 115, 116–117, 118, 119, 120, 124
  cleaning and stability, 122
  production scale columns, 126

Fragment production, 25–63
  crystallization, 94
  degradation and cleavage products, 88, 170
  format, 27–29, 30–33
  format function and therapeutic applications, 29, 34–41
    bispecific antibodies, 36–37
    blocking antibodies, 40–41
    effector function engineering, 35
    radionuclide attachment, 37–39
    tissue targeting and penetration, 34–35
    toxin attachment, 39–40
  future prospects, 62–63
  pharmacokinetics, 42–45
    comparisons of fragments with whole IgG, 43–44
    half-life modulation by PEGylation, 44–45
  production, 45–56
    cell culture, 54–55
    E. coli, 46–53
    transgenic technology, 55–56
    yeasts, 53–54
  purification strategies, 137
  recovery and purification, 56–62
    adsorption chemistry, 58
    affinity ligands, 58–59
    modes of operation and process integration, 60–61
    non-affinity ligands, 59–60
    primary recovery, 57–58
  structure of IgG, 26
Framework regions, fragment purification, 58
Freeze-thaw performance, 243
Frozen cells, 243
Fusion products
  bispecific antibodies, 36
  production, 28
  yeast production systems, 53–54
Future prospects
  fragments, 62–63
  manufacturing process design, 20–21
  optimising purification and capture process, 97
Fv domain
  cell culture systems, 55
  fragments
    design, 29
    E. coli systems, periplasmic

Index

expression, 47–48
production, 28

Gastrointestinal tract, Fc receptors, 250
Gel electrophoresis, 155–156, 171, 173, 178, 182–184
Gel filtration chromatography, 151
   fragment purification, 60
   virus removal/inactivation, 204
Gelonin, 39
Gene copy number, 279
Generic processes
   contract manufacturing, 242–243
   manufacturing strategies, 13–14, 15–17
   optimising purification and capture process, 78–79
Gene therapy medicinal product, definition, 280
Genetic engineering
   pharmacokinetics/pharmacodynamics, 249
   regulatory and legal requirements, 280–281
Genetic stability
   fermentation, 52
   regulatory and legal requirements, 282
Gentuzumab (Mylotarg, ozogamixin, 40
Glass beads, expended (fluidised) bed chromatography, 157–158
Glass supports, 148
Glutamine synthetase, 54
Glutaredoxin, 48–49
Glutathiones, 49
Glycolytic pathway, 52
Glycoproteins
   chromatography ligands, 138
   receptor binding, 41
Glycosylation, 133, 136, 177
   anti-Rh (D) antibody effector function, 192–193, 194–196
   contract manufacturing process targets, 239
   expression system comparisons, 7
   fragments
      E. coli systems, 46–47
      effector function engineering, 35
   heat treatment and, 205
   IgG1 sites, 26
   manufacturing strategies, 4, 7
   microbial expression systems, 6
   quality control, 178, 180–182
   toxin attachment, 40
   transgenic systems, 55, 56
   yeast production systems, 54
Good Laboratory Practice standards, virus removal/inactivation studies, 216
Good Manufacturing Practices (GMP)
   contract manufacturing, 227, 229, 232
   fermentation processes, 52, 229
   regulatory and legal requirements, 278, 283–285
Group C and G streptococcal antigens, 58, *see* protein G
Growth rate, 229
   contract manufacturing, 244, 245, 246
   fermentation, 52
   manufacturing strategies, 4

Half-life, biological, 253
Half-life and clearance rate of antibodies
   fragments, 31, 32, 34, 35, 54, 62
      bispecific antibodies, 36
      blocking antibodies, 42
      neonatal Fc receptors and, 43
      PEGylation, 44–45
      pharmacokinetics, 42, 43–44
      radionuclide attachment, 39
   pharmacokinetics, 252, 253, 249, 255
Haloacetaldehydes, 209, 213–214
Hard link PK/PD models, 266
Hardware requirements, 76
Harvesting
   customising, 19
   generic processes, 14
Heat generation, fermentation, 51
Heat treatment, virus removal/inactivation, 203, 204, 205, 210
Heavy chains
   antibody construction, 15
   crystallization, 94
   fragments
      bispecific antibodies, 36
      E. coli plasmid biology, 50
      VH/CH1 interface, 47–48
   IgG1 structure, 26
   immunoglobulin G subclasses, 177
   regulatory and legal requirements, 279
Height equivalent to a theoretical plate (HETP), 125
HEK293, 228
Hematopoietic malignancies, 34, 39, 40

Hepatitis B virus, 207, 212, 214
Hepatitis C virus, 199, 207, 213, 222
Hepatitis E virus, 223
Her-2, 275
Herpesviruses, 215, 222
Heterodimerisation, 36
Heterohybridoma, anti-Rh (D) antibody effector function, 192
High charge density ion exchange chromatography, 20
High-performance liquid chromatography (HPLC), 153
   hydrophobic interaction, 153
   quality control testing, 171, 175
      product characterisation, 178, 180
      product isoforms and purity, 179–180
High-performance matrices, 20
High-performance monolith affinity (HPMA) chromatography, 155–156
High pH anion exchange chromatography with pulsed amperometric detector (HPAEC-PAD), 181–182
High pressure virus removal/inactivation, 209
High Temperature Short Time (HTST) microwave treatment, 210
Hinge region
   crystallization, 94
   fragments, 32
      bispecific antibodies, 37
      divalent fragments, 28–29
      pharmacokinetics, 43
   IgG1, 26
   proteolytic digestion, 55
Histidine chromatography ligands, 145
Histidine tagged scFv, 59
HIV, safety issues, 199, 207, 212, 214, 222
Holding times of intermediates, contract manufacturing, 240
Holistic approach to process design, 18–20
Homodimerization, fragment design, 32
Host cell contaminants, *see* Contaminants and impurities, process
HPAEC-PAD, 181–182
HPLC, *see* High-performance liquid chromatography
HPMA chromatography, 155–156
HTST microwave treatment, 210
Human antibodies
   anti-Rh (D) antibodies, 190–196
   industry trends, contract production considerations, 228
   manufacturing strategies, 1, 2
Human anti-murine antibody (HAMA) reaction, 1, 2, 276
Human cell lines, 228
Human components, medium, 135, 228
Humanized antibody (CDR-grafted), 29
   cell culture systems, 55
   contract manufacturing, industry trends, 228
   fragments, 62
      E. coli systems, periplasmic expression, 47, 48
      purification, 58
   manufacturing strategies, 1, 2
   pharmacokinetics, 252
   pharmacokinetics/pharmacodynamics, 249, 252
   regulatory and legal requirements, 279
Human T-cell lymphotrophic viruses, 212, 222
Human use standards, 169–185; *see also* Quality control
Human viruses, 199, 202, 207, 210, 212, 214, 222, 223
Hybrid hybridomas, 153
Hybridisation assays, quality control testing, 171, 172, 173, 174
Hybridomas, 134, 135, 153, 169, 275
   contract manufacturing
      fifty liter fermentation, 235–237
      industry trends, 228
      upstream expansion, 232–234
      upstream processes, 242–243
   HAMA reaction, 276
   virus removal/inactivation studies, 223
Hydrazone, 40
Hydrophobic charge induction chromatography, 21, 97, 107, 230
Hydrophobic interaction chromatography, 92–93, 107, 151
   fragment purification, 60
   methods, 152–153
   scale-up flowchart, 103
   virus removal/inactivation, 203
Hydrophobicity, antibody, 136
Hydroxyapatite (pseudo-affinity) chromatography, 79, 92, 107, 151–152
HyperD, 20, 151
Hypericin, 209, 213

Index

Hypersensitivity reaction
    infusion reaction, anti-antibody response, 258
    HAMA, 1, 2, 276
Hypervariable region, 177, 249
Hysteresis, pharmacodynamics, 266

Ibritumomab tiuxetan (Zevalin), 39
Identity, product
    manufacturing strategies, 11–12
    quality control, 178–179
IMAC (immobilized metal affinity chromatography), 79
Imaging studies, fragment design for, 39
Imines, virus removal/inactivation, 209
Immobilised metal-ion affinity chromatography (IMAC), 58
Immobilised protein A, fragment purification, 58
Immune complex pharmacokinetics, 253
Immune effector cells, fragment design, 35
Immunoadsorbents, 138
Immunogenicity, 276
    fragment design, 30, 31, 32, 33
        streptividin, 39
        toxin attachment, 40
    fragment production, 62
    HAMA, 1, 2, 276
    pharmacokinetics/pharmacodynamics, 249, 250
Immunoglobulin classes (IgA, IgE, etc), 177, 253
    chromatography, 230
        hydroxyapatite (pseudo-affinity) chromatography, 153
        relative binding strengths of Protein A and G, 140, 141
    IgY, 135, 140, 141
    quality control, product isoforms, 177, 178
Immunoglobulin G
    fragments
        bispecific, 36–37
        blocking antibodies, 41
        E. coli plasmid biology, 50
        pharmacokinetics, 42
        proteolytic digestion, 55
    pharmacokinetics, 249–250
    structure, 177
Immunoglobulin G, whole molecule
    crystallization, 94
    yeast production systems, 53
Immunoglobulin G[2a], chromatography binding mechanisms, 117
Immunoglobulin G receptor pharmacokinetics, 253
Immunoglobulin G subclasses, 177
    fragment design, 43
    hydrophobic interaction chromatography, 153
    pharmacokinetics, 43, 253
    relative binding strengths of Protein A and G, 140, 141
Immunoligand assays, 171, 173, 174
Impurities, *see* Contaminants and impurities, process
Inclusion bodies, 48, 52
Indirect response models, 263–264
Indirect (secondary) affinity precipitation, 159–160
Inducers, fragment production, 50, 52, 53
Industrial production, *see* Manufacturing strategies
Inflammatory diseases, 41–42, 62, 275
Infliximab (Remicade), 41
Infusion reaction, 258
Inheritance of plasmids, 51
Initial capture, 78, 79–80
In-line dilution, 58
Inoculum, fifty liter fermentation, 235
Insect cells, 7
Insertion loci, regulatory and legal requirements, 282
Inspections, 286, 287
Insulin, 171
Integration site
    cell culture systems, 54
    recombinant cell lines, 4–5
Inteins, 59
Intensification of process, 18
Interference effects, virus removal/inactivation studies, 216, 217
Interleukin-1, 41
Interleukin-2, 157–158
Intermediate purification, 105, 136
Intermediates, holding times of, 240
Intermediate washing, 89–90
Internalization of antibody
    fragment design, 34, 35
    pharmacokinetics/pharmacodynamics, 249
International Conference on Harmonization, 231, 277, 279
Interspecies differences
    binding affinities, 140, 264
    pharmacodynamics, 264
Interspecies scaling, pharmacokinetics, 258–263

Intestinal Fc receptors, 251
Intracellular proteins, 135
Intracellular trafficking, *see* Cellular uptake and trafficking
Intracellular viruses, 213
Intramuscular administration, 251–252
Intravenous administration, 252
Iodinated antibody fragments, 34, 39
Iodoacetaldehyde, 214
Iodobenzoic acid, 59
Ion exchange chromatography, 134
    fragment purification, 60
    methods, 150–151
    optimising purification and capture process, 91–92
    scale-up, 114–117
        capacity for mAbs, 116–117
        capture of antibodies, 104
        cation exchange resin screening, 118–121
        flowchart, 103
        stability and reuse of media, 121–123
    virus removal/inactivation, 203, 204
Ion exchange HPLC, 178
Ionic strength
    chromatography, *see* specific chromatography methods
    fermentation conditions, 61
    scale-up, capture of antibodies, 104
Irradiation
    tumor cells, *see* Radiolabeled antibodies
    virus removal/inactivation, 202, 209, 210–211
Isoelectric focusing, 178, 180
Isoelectric point (pI), 15, 136
Isoforms, 77
    immunoglobulin G, *see* Immunoglobulin G subclasses
    quality control, 178, 179–180
Isotypes
    immunoglobulin (IgA, IgE, etc), *see* Immunoglobulin classes
    interspecies scaling, 262

Kappa light chain, 153, 177
Kidney metabolism, 38, 39
Kinetics of activity, *see* Pharmacokinetics and pharmacodynamics
Kinetics of virus inactivation, 220

LAL testing, 171
Lambda light chain, 177

Large-scale processes, *see* Manufacturing process, contract
    manufacturing strategies, 9–11
    purification of product, optimising, *see* Purification and recovery, optimising
    scale-up, *see* Scale-up
Leachates, 77, 107
    contract manufacturing, 239, 240
    optimising purification and capture process, 90
    Protein A, *see* Protein A ligand, leached/residual
    quality control, 171, 174–175
    scale-up, capture of antibodies, 104
Lectin ligands, 147
Legal definitions, 280
Legal requirements, *see* Regulatory and legal requirements
Legislation, US, 284–285
Leucine zippers, 28, 29, 31
Libraries, Protein A mimetic ligands, 141
Life time, column, 240
Ligands, chromatography
    anti-antibodies, 145
    antigens, 138
    Fc receptors, 138–141
    histidin, 145
    leachates, *see* Leachates
    lectins, 147
    metals, 145–146
    Protein A mimetic, 141–145
    thiophilic interactions, 146–147
Light chains
    affinity purification, 58
    antibody construction, 15
    fragment design, bispecific antibodies, 36
    hydrophobic interaction chromatography, 153
    immunoglobulin G, 26, 177
    regulatory and legal requirements, 279
Light treatment, virus removal/inactivation, 209, 211
Linkers, fragment design, 30
    cross-linking, *see* Cross-linking
    pharmacokinetics, 43
Lipids, 133, 135
Lipoproteins, 121, 135
Liver metabolism
    fragment design, 39
    pharmacokinetics, 251, 252
Load controls, virus removal/inactivation studies, 216, 217
Loading conditions, 92

Index

Lymphatics, antibody distribution, 251, 252
Lymphocytes, 36, 41, 42, 253
Lyophilisation
    quality control considerations, 185
    virus removal/inactivation, 203
Lysosomal metabolism, 249, 253

α2-Macroglobulin, 135, 139
Macrophages, 41
Macroprep® HS, 118, 119, 123
Maedi visna virus, 222
MALDI-TOF, 178
Maleimide reagents, 29, 34, 44
Mammalian antibodies, relative binding strengths of Protein A and G, 140
Mammalian cell systems, *see also* Cell culture; Hybridomas
    contract manufacturing, 231, 242–243; *see also* Manufacturing process, contract
    fragment production, 45, 61
    manufacturing strategies, 4–5, 6, 7
Mammalian products, 104
Mammalian source-free (MSF) medium, 227
    industry trends, 228
    upstream processes, 242–243, 244, 245, 246
Mammary gland Fc receptors, 251
Manufacturing process
    purification of product, optimising, *see* Purification and recovery, optimising
    regulatory and legal requirements, *see* Regulatory and legal requirements
    virus introduction during, 202
    virus removal/inactivation studies, 221, 223
Manufacturing process, contract, 227–247
    advantages and disadvantages of target process, 231
    phases in process, 231
    process development, 241–246
        general, 241–242
        upstream, 242–245, 246
    process validation, 241
    target process, 232–241
        downstream, 238–241
        upstream, 50L fermentation, 235–237
        upstream, expansion procedure, 232–234
    trends in production process, 228–231
    bioreactors, 228–239
    cells, 228
    culture medium, 228
    purification of IgG, 229–230
    regulatory issues, 2
Manufacturing strategies, 1–21
    applications of concepts, 15–20
        adaptation of generic processes, 15–17
        holistic approach to process design, 18–20
        optimisation, 18, 19
    downstream processing, 8–15
        cost, 12–13
        generic processes, 13–14
        purity, potency, and identity, 11–12
        R&D laboratory versus industrial processes, 9–11
    evolution of mAb therapeutics, 2
    future of process design, 20–21
    number of products in development, 2–3
    upstream processing, 4–8
        mammalian cell systems, 4–5, 7
        microbial expression systems, 1, 7
        other sources, 6, 7, 8
Markers
    cell culture systems, 54
    E. coli plasmid biology, 51
    pharmacodynamics, 254–265
    recombinant cell lines, 5
    regulatory and legal requirements, 282
Mass spectrometry, 178, 180
Master Validation Plan, contract manufacturing, 232
Maternal-fetal transfer of antibodies, 133, 250–251
Matrices/stationary phases/supports
    affinity chromatography, 147–149
    affinity precipitation technique, 159–160
    contract manufacturing product quality, 239
    fragment purification, 57, 60–61
    impurities in, 134
    ion-exchange chromatography, 150–151
    manufacturing strategies
        customising, 17
        innovations, 20
        matrix lifetime, 11

pore size, 109, 148
Protein A chromatography, 110, 111
resin screening, 128
Maximal concentration (C[max]), 252
Media lifetime (chromatography), 89
Medium, 77
fragment purification, 57, 61
impurities in antibody preparations, 135
industry trends, contract production considerations, 228
manufacturing strategies
contract, 227, 242–243, 244, 245, 246
expression system comparisons, 7
product contaminants, *see* Additives and impurities, process
recombinant cell lines, 5
regulatory and legal requirements, 278
Medium additives, 77, 90, 171
Membranes, 21, 79
chromatography, 230
crosslinkers, virucides, 213
polishing, 93
scale-up flowchart, 103
Metal affinity chromatography, 145–146
Metal leachates, 107
Methionines, N-terminal, 48, 49
Methionine sulphoxime (MSX), 5
Methotrexate (MTX), 5, 54, 138
Methylene blue, 212
Microbial systems, 75
comparisons of systems, 7
fragments, 46–54
bacteria/E. coli, 46–53; *see also* Escherichia coli systems
bispecific antibodies, 36
production, 45
yeasts, 53–54
manufacturing strategies, 1, 7
product contaminants, 199; *see also* Contaminants and impurities, processing
Microbiological testing, quality control, 171
Microfiltration, scale-up, 104
Microwave treatment, virus removal/inactivation, 209, 210
Millistack HC+ system, 81
Minibodies
design, 31, 32
production, 28

Mixed mode adsorbents, 144–145
Modeling
computer, *see* Computer simulations/modeling
pharmacokinetics/pharmacodynamics, 265–268
Mode of action, fragment design, 29
Molecular weight, antibody, 136
fragment PEGylation, 45
product characterisation, 178, 179
Monoclonal antibodies
anti-Rh (D), 189–196
manufacturing strategies, *see* Manufacturing strategies
pharmacokinetics, *see* Pharmacokinetics and pharmacodynamics
regulatory and legal requirements, 277–280
virus safety issues, 202, 215
virus safety issues, *see also* Virus safety issues/virus clearance studies
Monocytes, 253
Monomeric binding, fragment design, 32
Mono Q anion exchanger, 151
Mucosal defense, 251
Multi-chain proteins, fragment production, 50
Multimeric fragments, 34
Multiple dosing, pharmacodynamics, 255, 256, 266
Multiple specificity, fragment design, 30, 33, 37
Multiple toxin attachment, 40
Multivalent antibody fragments, 28, 29, 62
Murine antibodies
binding strengths, comparative, 140, 262
chimeras, *see* Chimeric antibodies
HAMA reaction, 1, 2, 276
pharmacokinetics/pharmacodynamics, 249, 262
Murine hybridomas, *see* Hybridomas
Murine leukemia virus, 204
Murine myeloma cells, 4–5, 8, 54, 55, 153; *see also* Myeloma cells
Murine viruses, removal/inactivation, 202, 215, 222
Muromomab (OKT3), 276
Mutations, 282
Mutual recognition agreements, regulatory and legal requirements, 285–287
Myeloma cells, 4–5, 8, *see also*

Hybridomas
   cell culture systems, 54, 55
   contract manufacturing, 244, 245, 246
   hydrophobic interaction chromatography, 153
   recombinant cell lines, 4–5
Mylotarg (gentuzumab ozogamicin), 40

Nanofiltration, virus removal/inactivation, 203, 204, 206–207
Natural killer cells, 190, 191
Negative flow through mode, 17
Neoantigen formation, 210
Neonates, 133
   anti-Rh (D) antibodies, 189–196
   Fc receptors, 29, 42, 43, 253
   pharmacokinetics, 250–251
Neutralizing antibody model, 250, 255–258
NIPP (nucleation-induced protein polymerisation), 175, 176
NK cells, 190, 191
Non-affinity ligands, fragments, 59–60
Nonspecific binding, 89–90
   chromatography, 90
   fragment design, 34
Normal flow filtration, 78
NS0 cells, 4, 5
   cell culture systems, 54, 55
   manufacturing strategies, 8
NS1 cells, hydrophobic interaction chromatography, 153
N-terminal methionines, 48, 49
Nucleation-induced protein polymerisation (NIPP), 175, 176
Nucleic acids, viruses, 213, 215, 222, 222
Null glycosylation, 55

OKT3 (Orthoclone), 276
Oncology/tumor biology, 134, 275
   fragment design, 29, 30, 31, 34
      radionuclide attachment, 37–39
      toxin attachment, 39
   fragment production, 62
   tumor antigens, 134, 138
Optimization
   capture and purification, *see* Purification and recovery, optimising
   chromatography, *see* Chromatography, optimising
   manufacturing strategies, 15–18, 19
Orthoclone (OKT3), 276
Overexpression, yeast production systems, 53
Ovine-derived materials, virus removal, 222
Oxidised forms, quality control testing, 171
Oxygen requirements, fermentation, 51, 52
Ozogamicin (Mylotarg, gentuzumab), 40

pA(AB)$_4$-Sepharose, 141
Packed bed chromatography, 21
Packing density, production scale columns, 126–127
PAM (Protein A Mimetic, TG19318), 142
Papain, 55
Papova viruses, 223
Parallel phases, contract manufacturing, 232
Paramyxoviruses, 202, 215, 222
Particle size
   ion exchange media, 114
   Protein A media, 109
Partitioning process, virus removal, 203, 205, 207
Parvoviruses, 203–204, 210, 211, 215, 223
Passive immunity
   neonates, 133
   pharmacokinetics, 250–251
Pasteurization, virus removal/inactivation, 203, 205, 213
Pathogen contaminants, 77
PCR
   quality control testing, 171, 172
   virus removal, 90, 201, 205
PEGylation, *see* Polyethylene glycol/PEGylation
Peptide H, 142
Peptide linker
   fragment design, 30, 31, 33
   scFv production, 27, 28
Peptide mapping, 171, 178, 180
Peptostreptococcus magnus, 58
PER.C6, 228
Perfusion fermentation, 233
Perfusion production systems, 54
Perfusion rate, 236, 237, 244, 245
Periplasmic expression, fragments, 47–48
   fermentation, 53
   purification, 57
pH, 128
   affinity precipitation technique,

159
    antibody capture scale-up, 104
    antibody construction, 15
    chromatography binding and
        elution, 92
            affinity purification, 58
            ion exchange resin binding,
                117
            manufacturing strategies,
                customising, 16, 17
            protein A stability, 230
            scale-up, 109
    finished product, 185
    fragment design, pharmacokinetics,
        42
    product stability, 136
    virus removal/inactivation, 90, 203,
        204, 206, 208, 213, 223
Phage display technology, 15, 59, 97, 134
Phage proteins, 135
Phagocytosis, 35, 253
Pharmacokinetics and
pharmacodynamics, 249–269
    fragments, 29, 34, 42–45
        comparisons of fragments
            with whole IgG, 43–44
        half-life modulation by
            PEGylation, 44–45
        production, 62
        radionuclide attachment, 38,
            39
    pharmacodynamics, 263–268
        markers, 254–265
        modeling, 265–268
    pharmacokinetics, 250–263
        absorption, 250–252
        distribution, 252
        elimination, 253–258
        interspecies scaling, 258–
            263
        models, 250
Phased clinical trials
    evolution of mAb therapeutics, 2
    virus removal/inactivation, 215
Phenothiazine dyes, 209, 212
Phenyl-Sepharose, 151
Photoreactive chemical agents, virus
    removal/inactivation, 209, 211–
    212, 213
Physical inactivation methods, virus, 209
Physical inducers, plasmids, 50
Physiological flow models, interspecies
    scaling, 261–262
Pichia pastoris, 53–54
Picornaviruses, 203–204, 208, 211, 223
Pilot scale production, 76

Pinocytosis, 42
Pipeline products, 2, 3
Placental transfer, pharmacokinetics,
    250–251
Plants, transgenic, 55
    expression system comparisons, 7
    fragment production, 45
    regulatory and legal requirements,
        283
Plasma pharmacokinetics, 251, 252; *see
    also* Half-life and clearance rates of
    antibodies
Plasma and serum products, 5, 112, 113
    contract production considerations,
        228
    impurities, 135
    virus removal/inactivation, 202,
        207, 208, 222
Plasmid DNA
    chromatography, 230
    contract manufacturing, targeted
        approach of DSM Biologics, 231;
        see also Manufacturing process,
        contract
    fragment production, 46, 50–51
Point mutations, 282
Pokeweed anti-viral protein (PAP), 39
Polishing
    chromatography, 136, 151
    generic processes, 14
    large-scale production, 91
    scale-up, 103, 105–106
Polyclonal anti-D antibodies, 189–190,
    191, 192
Polycyclic quinone, 213
Polyelectrolyte complex (PEC), affinity
    precipitation technique, 159–160
Polyethylene glycol/PEGylation, 6
    fragments, 44–45
        pharmacokinetics, 43
        production, 62
    virus removal/inactivation, 203,
        207
Polyethylene terephthalate, 211
Polymeric matrices, affinity precipitation
    technique, 159–160
Polystyrene, virus removal/inactivation,
    211
Porcine viruses, 202, 215, 222
Pore size, chromatography matrices
    affinity chromatography matrix
        properties, 148
    Protein A media, 109
Pore size, filter
    contract manufacturing, 244, 245,
        246

virus removal/inactivation, 203, 207
Post-translational modification, *see also* Disulfide bonds; Glycosylation
  anti-Rh (D) antibody effector function, 192–193
  fragment design
    pharmacokinetics, 43
    production, 45
  manufacturing strategies, 4
    expression system comparisons, 7
    microbial expression systems, 6
  regulatory and legal requirements, 282
Potency, product
  contract manufacturing, 238, 240
  manufacturing strategies, 11–12
  quality control, 184
  regulatory and legal requirements, 281
Pox viruses, 222
Precipitation
  antibody, 92, 151
  primary effect affinity, 158–159
  secondary (indirect) affinity, 159–160
  virus removal/inactivation, 203, 207
Preclinical trials
  evolution of mAb therapeutics, 2
  quality control testing, 170
Preconditioning, feedstock, 79, 81
Preculture, upstream expansion, 232–234
Pressure treatment, virus removal/inactivation, 209
Primary capture, fragment purification, 57
Primary effect affinity precipitation, 158–159
Process controls, *see* Controls, process
Process design, 76
  downstream, 102–103
  future prospects, 20–21
  holistic approach, 18–20
  manufacturing strategies, *see* Manufacturing strategies
  purification and capture
    optimising, *see* Purification and recovery, optimising
    scale-up from bench/laboratory production, 106–107
  quality control testing, 170
Process development plan, contract manufacturing, 232

Process features, contract manufacturing, *see* Manufacturing process, contract
Processing, intracellular, 249
Process integration, fragments, 60–61
Process steps, virus removal/inactivation, 203, 221, 223
Process validation studies, scale-up, 104
Pro-drugs, ADEPT, 40–41
Product accumulation, fermentation, 52, 53
Production systems, *see* Manufacturing process
  contract, *see* Manufacturing process, contract
  fragments, 45–56; *see also* Fragment production
    cell culture, 54–55
    E. coli, 46–53
    transgenic technology, 55–56
    yeasts, 53–54
  purification, *see* Purification and recovery, optimising
Productivity
  manufacturing strategies, 4
  Protein A chromatography, 82–87
Product properties
  contract manufacturing process targets, 238
  quality control, *see* Quality control
Product yield, *see* Yield, product
Promoters
  E. coli plasmid biology, 50
  fermentation, 52
Pronuclear injection, 56
Propiolactone, beta, 214
PROSEP A HC, 82, 82–83, 85, 86, 87
PROSEP A ULTRA, 85, 86, 87
Prosep® Protein A chromatography matrices, 110, 111
Protease removal, 127
Protein A (ligand), 138
  cell culture systems, 55
  fragment design, 42
  fragment purification, 58, 59, 60
  high-performance monolith affinity (HPMA) chromatography, 156
  leached/residual, 14, 89, 90, 127, 141
    product contaminants, 239
    quality control, 171, 174–175
    stability and reuse of media, 113–114
  manufacturing strategies, generic

processes, 13
thermoresponsive affinity macroligands, 160
virus removal/inactivation, 208
Protein A capture chromatography
  bed height modification, 87–88
  elution conditions, 88
  intermediate washing, 89–90
  ligand leaching, 90
  media lifetime (chromatography), 89
  optimising, 82–87
  virus removal, 90
Protein A chromatography, 79, 81–90, 127, 128
  antibody construction, 15
  commercial media, 110–111
  contract manufacturing, industry trends, 229–230
  ligands for affinity purification, 138, 139–140
  manufacturing strategies
    customising, 19
    generic processes, 13, 14
  media lifetime (chromatography), 89
  relative binding strengths of Protein A and G, 140
  scale-up, 108–112
    capture of antibodies, 104
    flowchart, 103
    stability and reuse, 113–114
  stability and reuse of media, 113–114
Protein A mimetic ligands, 20, 141–145
Protein binding capacity, 103, 128; *see also* Binding capacity
Protein concentration
  quality control, 178, 179, 238
  virus removal/inactivation studies, 223
Protein denaturation, virus removal/inactivation, 205, 210
Protein-free medium, 5, 228
Protein G, 60, 139–140
  fragment purification, 58
  high-performance monolith affinity (HPMA) chromatography, 156
Protein impurities, *see* Contaminants and impurities, process
Protein L, 58, 97
  high-performance monolith affinity (HPMA) chromatography, 156
  ligands for affinity purification, 139
Protein load, 128

Protein trafficking, *see* Cellular uptake and trafficking
Proteolysis, 77
  cell culture systems, 55
  fragment purification, 58
  gastrointestinal, 250–251
  quality control, 180
  quality control testing, 170
Pseudo-affinity (hydroxyapatite) chromatography, 79, 92, 107, 151–152
Pseudomonas exotoxin, 39
Psoralens, 209, 212
Public acceptance
  fragment production, 62
  transgenic systems, 56
Purification and recovery
  chromatographic methods, 133–161; *see also* Chromatography, methods
  contract manufacturing, 238–241
  fragments, 56–62; *see also* Fragment production
    adsorption chemistry, 58
    affinity ligands, 58–59
    design, 30, 32, 33
    modes of operation and process integration, 60–61
    non-affinity ligands, 59–60
    primary recovery, 57–58
    production, 62–63
  industry trends, contract production considerations, 229–230
  manufacturing strategies, 11, 13–14
  scale-up
    antibody capture, 104–105
    cation exchange resin screening, 118–121
    column packing, large scale, 125–127
    downstream process design, 102–103
    intermediate purification, 105
    ion-exchange chromatography, 114–116
    ion exchanger capacity for mAbs, 116–117
    newer models of antibody binding mechanism, 117–118
    other methods, 106–107
    polishing, 105–106
    process steps and purpose, 127, 128, 127

Index

Protein A chromatography, 108–112
size exclusion chromatography, 123–125
stability and reuse of ion exchange media, 121–123
stability and reuse of Protein A media, 113–114
virus removal/inactivation, 205
Purification and recovery, optimising, 75–98
  capture chromatography, Protein A, 81–90
    bed height modification, 87–88
    elution conditions, 88
    intermediate washing, 89–90
    ligand leaching, 90
    media lifetime (chromatography), 89
    optimising, 82–87
    virus removal, 90
  demand for product, 75–76
  methods, other, 94–97
    crystallization, 94
    enhanced ultrafiltration (EUF), 94–95
    expanded bed adsorption, 96
    future prospects, 97
  polishing, 83–94
  post-affinity process steps, 91–93
    contaminant removal, 91
    ion exchange, 91–92
    other chromatographic methods, 92–93
  processes, 77–80
    clarification process compression, 80
    generic processing, 78–79
    goals and challenges, 77–78
    initial capture, 79–80
Purity, product, 79
  contract manufacturing, 238, 240
  manufacturing strategies, 9, 11–12
  quality control, 179–180
  regulatory and legal requirements, 281
Pyrogens, 141

Q-membrane, 103
Q-One Biotech, 206, 208
Q-Sepharose® FF, 151
Q-Sepharose® HP, 123
Quality control, 4, 169–185
  bioanalytical methods for antibody characterisation, 177–184
    glycosylation, 180–182
    HPLC methods, isoforms and purity, 179–180
    identity, 178–179
    peptide mapping, 180
    potency, 184
    protein concentration, 179
    SDS-PAGE electrophoresis, 182–184
  bioanalytical methods for impurity control, 170–177
    aggregated antibody, 175–176
    DNA, host cell, 171–172
    protein A, residual, 174–175
    proteins, host cell, 173–174
  contract manufacturing, 240, 242
  fermentation, 52
  filled and finished product, 184–185
  manufacturing strategies, 11
  regulatory and legal requirements, 282, 283
  regulatory guidelines, 169
  testing, stages of, 167–170
  virus removal/inactivation, 210
Quantitative PCR
  quality control testing, 171, 172
  virus safety, 201, 205

Racine-Poon PK/PD model, 267–268
Radiation, virus removal/inactivation, 209
Radiolabeled antibodies, 76, 133, 134
  fragment design, 29, 34, 36, 37–39
Raw materials, *see* Source materials
Reagent contamination, 77
Receptor binding, 254–255
Receptor-mediated endocytosis, 253
Recombinant Fab′2, 29
Recombinant products, 275
  manufacturing strategies, 4–5
  pharmacokinetics/pharmacodynamics, 249
  Protein A ligand, 109, 110
  virus safety issues, 202, 215, 223
Recovery, fragments, *see* Purification and recovery
Recycling of antibody, 249, 253, 254
Reducing environment, E. coli cytoplasm, 48–49
Reference batches of antibody, 11
Reliability, 76; *see also* Quality control
Regulatory and legal requirements, 76, 79, 97, 275–287

conventional mAbs, 277–280
European Directive, 276–277
expression system comparisons, 7
fragment production, 45, 62
genetically engineered products in gene transfer, 280–281
good manufacturing practices, 283–285
industry trends, contract production considerations, 231
manufacturing strategies, 7, 9, 10–11
mutual recognition agreements, 285–287
quality control, 169–185; *see also* Quality control
pharmacodynamic modeling for, 265
transgenic systems, 56, 281–283
virus safety issues, 200, 201, 215, 221, 223–224
Remicade (infliximab), 41
Renal filtration, 38, 39
ReoPro (abciximab), 41, 42, 55
Reovirus Type 3, 215, 223
Repeated batch culture, 229
Repeated doses, 255, 256, 266
Repressor titration, 51
Research and Development, *see also* Scale-up
comparison with industrial processes, 9–11
contract manufacturing, 232, 242
Residence time, chromatography column, 83, 84, 110, 111, 128
Residence time, fermenter, 229
Resins, *see* Matrices/stationary phases/supports
Resolution, manufacturing strategy innovations, 20
Response factor, pharmacodynamics, 263
Response variables, pharmacodynamics, 264
Retroviruses, removal/inactivation, 202, 204, 207, 211, 215, 222
Reuse of chromatography columns, 103
cleaning, 104, 122
Protein A leaching, *see* Protein A ligand, leached/residual
virus removal/inactivation, 205, 206
Reverse phase chromatography, 203
Rhabdoviruses, 222
Rh factor, anti-Rh (D) antibodies, 189–196
Riboflavin, virus removal/inactivation, 209, 212–213
Ricin, 39
Risks
contract manufacturing, 231
fragment production, 62
RNA viruses, 213, 215, 222, 223
Robustness, 76
contract manufacturing, 239, 240
manufacturing strategies, customising, 19
Route of administration, 251–252
Runaway plasmid replication, 51

Saccharomyces cerevisiae, 53, 54
Safety, 4
fragment production, 62
pharmacodynamics, 263–268
quality control, 180; *see also* Quality control
regulatory and legal requirements, 281
viral, *see* Virus safety issues/virus clearance studies
Salting out, 134, 151
Sanitisation, virus removal/inactivation, 203, 208
Saporin, 39
ScAb fragment design, 31
Scale of production, 76
fragment production, 45
manufacturing strategies, 9–11
purification and recovery, *see* Purification and recovery, optimising
virus removal/inactivation, 209
Scale-up
contract manufacturing, target process, 232–241
downstream, 238–241
upstream, 50L fermentation, 235–237
upstream, expansion procedure, 232–234
manufacturing strategies
from bench to industrial scale, 9–11
cost, 12–13
customising, 19
generic process modification, 13–17
optimisation and simplification, 15–18, 19
quality, 11–12
purification process, 101–129
antibody capture, 104–105

Index

cation exchange resin screening, 118–121
column packing, large scale, 125–127
downstream process design, 102–103
intermediate purification, 105
ion-exchange chromatography, 114–116
ion exchanger capacity for mAbs, 116–117
newer models of antibody binding mechanism, 117–118
optimising, *see* Purification and recovery, optimising
other methods, 106–107
polishing, 105–106
process steps and purpose, 127, 128
Protein A chromatography, 108–112
size exclusion chromatography, 123–125
stability and reuse of ion exchange media, 121–123
stability and reuse of Protein A media, 113–114
quality control testing, 170
Scaling, interspecies, 258–263
ScFvFc fusion antibody, 53
ScFv format, 29
cell culture systems, 55
design, 29, 30, 31, 33
bispecific antibodies, 37
dimers, 28, 31
trimers, 32
formats, 27–28
production, 57
E. coli plasmid biology, 50
E. coli systems, cytoplasmic expression, 49
E. coli systems, periplasmic expression, 47–48
yeast systems, 53
regulatory and legal requirements, 280
ScFv-IL2, cell culture systems, 55
ScFv-zipper, 31
Screening, resin, 128
SDS-PAGE electrophoresis, 155–156, 171, 173, 178, 182–184
Secondary filtration, 81
Secondary (indirect) affinity precipitation, 159–160

Second dose, pharmacokinetics, 255, 256,
Security of production, fragment production, 62
Sedimentation, 78
Selection markers, *see* Markers
Selectivity, manufacturing innovations, 20, 21
Sensitivity of virus assay, 221
Sensitization, pharmacodynamics, 266
Sepharose® products, 118, 119, 138, 141
Sequence arrangements, regulatory and legal requirements, 282
Sequencing, product characterisation, 178
Serum additives, 77; *see also* Contaminants and impurities, process
Serum antibodies
clearance rates, *see* Half-life and clearance rates of antibodies
high-performance monolith affinity (HPMA) chromatography, 155–156
Serum-free media
cell culture systems, 54
contract manufacturing upstream processes, 242–243
high-performance monolith affinity (HPMA) chromatography, 156
industry trends, contract production considerations, 228
Serum products, *see* Plasma and serum products
Shear forces, fragment purification, 57
Short batch, 229
Simulated moving bed chromatography, 97
Sindbis virus, 222
Single-chain Fv, *see* ScFv format
Site-specific recombination, 54
Size exclusion chromatography, 127
manufacturing, generic processes, 14
quality control testing, 171, 175, 179
scale-up, 123–125
flowchart, 103
polishing, 105–106
Size of construct, fragment design, 34
PEGylation, 45
pharmacokinetics, 43
Skp, 48
Sodium hydroxide, virus inactivation, 206, 208
Soft link PK/PD models, 265–266
Sol-gel glass supports, 148
Solubility, antibody, 136

antibody construction, 15
E. coli systems, periplasmic
expression, 47
Solvents, virus inactivation, 203, 204,
207–208
Sorting, intracellular, 249
Source materials
raw materials for manufacture, 9,
76
regulatory and legal requirements,
278
virus safety issues, 200
Species specificity, 262, 264
Specificity, antibody, 264, 275
Speed, manufacturing strategies, 18, 19
Spin filter
fifty liter fermentation, 235
upstream processes, 244, 245, 246
Spleen, 252
Spongiform encephalopathies, 278
SP Sepharose® products, 118, 119
Stabilisers, finished product, 184
Stability of antibody, 136
fragment design, 30
fragment stabilisation, 27–28
quality control testing, 170
scale-up from bench/laboratory
production, 10
Stability of construct, E. coli plasmid
biology, 50, 51, 52
Stability of Protein A columns, 89; *see
also* Protein A ligand,
leached/residual
Staphylococcus aureus Protein A, *see*
Protein A ligand
Stationary cells, 229
Stationary phases, *see* Matrices/stationary
phases/supports
Steady-state conditions,
pharmacodynamics, 263
Step-wise elution, 138
Sterilizing filter, 81
Stirred tank reactor, 228–229, 235
Storage stability of product, 170
Streamline® rProtein A column, 110, 112
Strep-tag, 59
Streptavidin, 38
Structure, 177
fragments, 26
immunoglobulins, 137
Subcutaneous administration, 251–252
Sulfhydryl groups, *see also* Disulfide
bonds; Thiol and sulfhydryl groups
Superdex-20, 151
Supports, cell culture, 229
Supports, chromatography, *see*
Matrices/stationary phases/supports
Surfactants, 77
Surrogate end-points, pharmacodynamics,
264–265
SV40 virus, 199, 223
Synthetic ligands, 59

Tangential flow filtration, 78
Target approach, manufacturing, *see*
Manufacturing process, contract
Targeted delivery
fragment design, 29, 30, 31, 34–35,
36, 37–39
pharmacokinetics, *see*
Pharmacokinetics and
pharmacodynamics
tumor cells, 134
Targeting, 134
T cells, 36, 41, 42
Temperature
gene induction, E. coli plasmid
biology, 50
heat generation by fermentation, 51
Protein A chromatography scale-
up, 109
scale-up, capture of antibodies, 104
thermoresponsive affinity
macroligands, 160
virus removal/inactivation, 205,
210, 223
Temperature stability, 30, 31, 136
Tetrabody fragment design, 37
Tetradomas, 153
Tetramaleimide reagents, 29
Tetrameric IgG-binding proteins
(pA(AB)[1-6]) of Protein A, 141
TFM (tris-maleimide), 29, 34
TG19318, 142
Therapeutic applications, fragments, 29,
34–41
Thermoresponsive affinity macroligands,
160
Thiol agents, 59
Thiol and sulfhydryl groups, 59; *see also*
Disulfide bonds
fragment cross linking, 29
product characterisation, 178
Thiophilic chromatography, 106, 146–
147, 230
Threshold® System, 172
Throughput, 76, 78
chromatography flow rate, 81
downstream processing principles,
8
Protein A chromatography, 82–87

purification of product, *see* Purification and recovery, optimising
Time course of neutralizing antibody, 257, 258
Time to market, 76
Tissue culture infective dose assay, 218
Tissue distribution
    fragment production, 62
    pharmacokinetics, 252; *see also* Pharmacokinetics and pharmacodynamics
Tissue targeting, *see* Targeted delivery
Titrations, virus removal, 218–219
TNFα, 41, 62
Togaviruses, 222
Tolerance, pharmacodynamics, 266
Tositumomab-I^{131} (Bexxar), 39
Total Organic Carbon technique, 123
Toxicity
    fragment design, 34, 35, 41
    pharmacodynamics, 263–268
Toxicology, virus removal, 209, 210, 212
Toxins, 76, 77
    capture of antibodies, 104
    fragment design and production, 29, 39–40, 62
Toyopearl® products, 118, 119
Trafficking, intracellular, *see* Cellular uptake and trafficking
Training, regulatory and legal requirements, 286
Transcriptional activation, cell culture systems, 54
Transcytosis, 249
Transfection, 5, 46
Transferrin, 135, 138, 171
Transgenic technology, 75, 134
    expression system comparisons, 7
    fragment design and production, 45, 55–56, 62
    industry trends, contract production considerations, 228
    interspecies scaling, 262
    regulatory and legal requirements, 281–283
Transplantation biology, 276
Transport pharmacokinetics, 252
Treaty of Rome, 276
Tresylates, 44
Triabody, fragment design, 30, 37
Trimaleimide reagents, 29, 34
Trispecific antibodies, fragment design, 33
Trivalent Fab´ fragment design, 34
Trypsin, porcine, 202

Tumor antigens, 134, 138
Tumor targeting, *see* Oncology/tumor biology
Two-compartment model, 253, 266–268

Ultrafiltration, 77, 128
    enhanced (EUF), 94–95
    manufacturing strategies
        customising, 19
        generic processes, 14
Ultraviolet light
    absorbance assays, product characterisation, 178, 179
    virus removal/inactivation, 211, 214
United States standards
    quality control, 169–185; *see also* Quality control
    regulatory and legal requirements, 280, 281–283
Upstream processes
    contract manufacturing, target process, 232–234
        fifty liter fermentation, 235–237
    manufacturing strategies, 4–8
        mammalian cell systems, 4–5, 7
        microbial expression systems, 1, 7
        other sources, 6, 7, 8
Uptake and processing of antibody
    fragment design, 34
        pharmacokinetics, 42
        toxin attachment, 41
    pharmacokinetics, 249, 253

Validation, process
    contract manufacturing, 232, 241
    manufacturing strategies, 11
    regulatory and legal requirements, 278, 282
    scale-up, capture of antibodies, 104
Variable domains
    affinity purification, 58
    antibody construction, 15
    formats, 27
    IgG1 structure, 26
    purification strategies, 137
    VH/CH1 interface, 47–48
    VL-VH bispecific fragments, 36
Vector, recombinant cell lines, 4–5
Virus antibodies, pharmacokinetics, 251
Virus removal/inactivation, 77, 108, 127,

135
  cell culture systems, 54
  manufacturing strategies
    expression system
      comparisons, 7
    generic processes, 14
  Protein A column media, 113–114
  purification and capture process
    optimisation, 90, 93
  regulatory and legal requirements,
    278
  scale-up flowchart, 102, 103
Virus safety/virus clearance studies, 199–
  224
  approaches to control, 200
  cell culture systems, 54
  contract manufacturing, 240
  design, 201–214
    methods in development,
      208–214
    process steps, 203–204
    removal and inactivation,
      205–208
  mAb study, virus choice for, 214–
    215
  performance, 216–224
    calculation of virus
      clearance, 219–220
    interpretation and limitations
      of, 220–224
    preliminary studies, 216–
      217
    spiked process runs, 218–
      219
    virus models for, 222–223
  regulatory guidelines, 201
  viruses and products, 199
  viruses of concern, 202, 222–223

Viscous feed stocks, 29
Vitamin B2 (riboflavin), 212–213
Volume of harvest product, 78
Volume reduction, 104

Washing, intermediate, 89–90
Weight, pharmacodynamics, 268
Western blots, 173, 174

Yeast systems
  fragment design, 45
  fragment production, 53–54
  manufacturing strategies, 7
Yield, product, 76
  contract manufacturing, 240
    fifty liter fermentation, 234,
      236
  fragmentation and aggregation and,
    88
  fragments, 30, 31, 32, 33
    bispecific antibodies, 36–37
    E. coli plasmid biology, 50,
      51
  manufacturing strategies
    customising, 18
    downstream processing
      principles, 8
  yeast production systems, 53

Zero-order pharmacokinetics, 257
Zevalin (ibritumomab tiuxetan), 39
Zipper, leucine 28, 29, 31